A to Z Health Guide

A to Z Health Guide

For TIME Weekly
Managing Editor: James Kelly
Deputy Managing Editor: Stephen Koepp
Sciences Editor: Philip Elmer-DeWitt
Senior Writers: Christine Gorman, Jeffrey Kluger, Michael D. Lemonick
Contributors: Dan Cray; Frederic Golden; Sanjay Gupta, M.D.
Senior Reporters: Alice Park, David Bjerklie
Reporter: Sora Song
Graphics Director: Jackson Dykman
Graphics: Ed Gabel, Joe Lertola (Associate Graphics Directors); Lon Tweeten, Kathleen Adams (Reporter)
Additional Writing: John Cloud, Richard Corliss, Richarad Lacayo; J. Madeleine Nash, Joel Stein; Claudia Wallis

For Time Inc. Home Entertainment
Editor: Kelly Knauer
Associate Editor: Alice Park
Design: Ellen Fanning
Picture Editor: Patricia Cadley
Writer/Researcher: Matthew McCann Fenton
Copy Editor: Bruce Christopher Carr
Research Assistant: Rudi Papiri

Special Thanks:
Bozena Bannett, Alexandra Bliss, Bernadette Corbie, Robert Dente, Anne-Michelle Gallero, Peter Harper, Suzanne Janso, Robert Marasco, Natalie McCrea, Brooke McGuire, Margarita Quiogue, Mary Jane Rigoroso, Steven Sandonato

Published by TIME Books
Time Inc.
1271 Avenue of the Americas
New York, New York 10020

ISBN: 1-931933-73-1

We welcome your comments and suggestions about Time Books. Please write to us at:
TIME Books
Attention: Book Editors
PO Box 11016
Des Moines, IA 50336-1016

If you would like to order any of our hardcover Collector's Edition books, please call us at 1-800-327-6388. (Monday through Friday, 7:00 a.m.- 8:00 p.m. or Saturday, 7:00 a.m.- 6:00 p.m. Central Time).

PICTURE CREDITS
FRONT COVER (TOP ROW): GEORGE MATTEI—ENVISON; JOHN KELLY—GETTY IMAGES; JOHN HENLEY—CORBIS
(MIDDLE ROW): LWA—JDC—CORBIS; JAMES CAVALLINI—PHOTO RESEARCHERS; STEVEN NEEDHAM—ENVISION; RICK GOMEZ—CORBIS
(BOTTOM ROW): ZEPHYR—PHOTO RESEARCHERS; CHRIS USHER; STOCKBYTE; STRYKER LEIBINGER

BACK COVER (TOP TO BOTTOM): ED RESCHKE—PETER ARNOLD; SPL—PHOTO RESEARCHERS; JEAN CLAUDE REVY—PHOTOTAKE

TIME

A to Z Health Guide

How to Live Better—and Longer

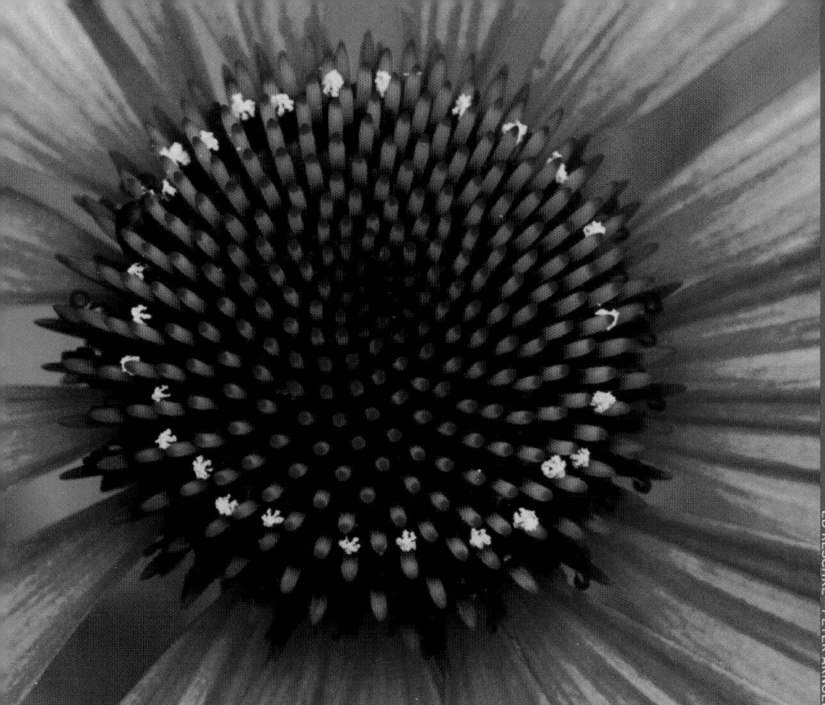

ED RESCHKE—PETER ARNOLD

Good Health

From A to Z, It's in Your Hands

"If you have your health, you have everything." It's hard to quarrel with that adage, for the pursuit of good health is a universal drive of mankind. And it's our good fortune to live in an age in which remarkable advances in medicine and health care are giving us potent new tools to help us live longer, happier lives. New scanning technologies are bringing us unparalleled views of the body's inner workings. Nutritionists are discovering how specific foods help foster good health. Research labs are creating drugs that not only fight the symptoms of disease but also help keep illness at bay.

Perhaps the most profound insight of modern health care is the increasing appreciation that each and every aspect of our lives—diet and exercise, friends and family, work and sexuality—has a role to play in maintaining our good health. Today we know that our moods are powerfully affected by chemicals in our brain. We understand that exercising and shedding excess pounds are great ways to help prevent a host of ailments from developing. We realize we can stave off the effects of aging every time we choose what to eat for dinner.

If there's a downside to all this good news, it is simply that there is too much of it for us to follow. And that's the purpose of this book. In its pages we've collected some of TIME's most helpful recent reporting—news you can use—from the frontiers of medicine, exercise, drugs and nutrition. We hope it finds you—and helps keep you—in the best of health.

INSIDE:

Frequently Used Terms

To avoid undue repetition, we have used acronyms for some health agencies, publications and other organizations throughout this book. They are:

AMA: American Medical Association
CDC: Centers for Disease Control and Prevention
FDA: U.S. Food and Drug Administration
NIH: National Institutes of Health
NIMH: National Institute of Mental Health
JAMA: *Journal of the American Medical Association*
NEJM: *New England Journal of Medicine*
USDA: U. S. Department of Agriculture
WHO: World Health Organization

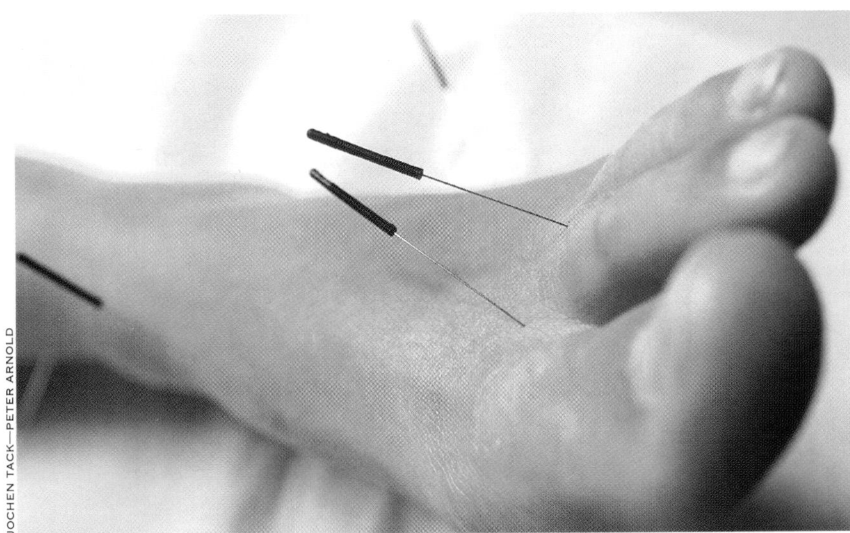

JOCHEN TACK—PETER ARNOLD

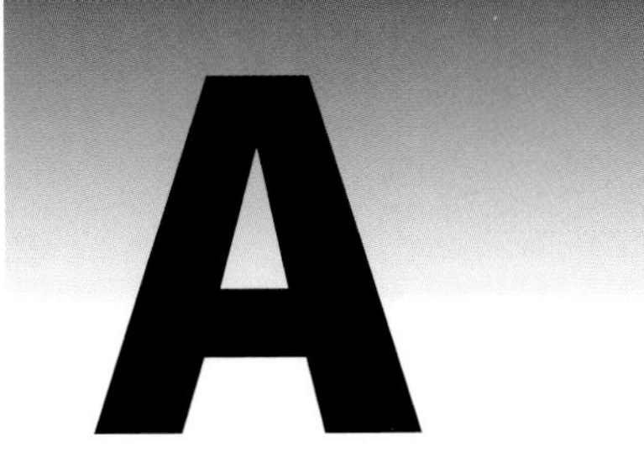

Acupuncture

The ancient Asian healing practice continues to infiltrate mainstream Western medicine, as scientists learn more about its workings

The Latest News One study cast new light on the question of how acupuncture works, while a second determined that acupuncture may be more helpful than drugs for some headache sufferers

Western scientists continue to explore how acupuncture's slim needles work, seeking insight into the pathways through the body that make the practice so effective in treating some maladies. Radiologist Bruce Rosen of Harvard Medical School set out to "connect the dots," using magnetic resonance imaging (MRI) to study how acupuncture changes the body's blood flow and the amount of oxygen in the blood. When Rosen's team applied needles to points on the hand linked to pain on acupuncture charts, blood flow decreased in certain areas of the brain within seconds. The brain areas affected are associated with mood, pain and cravings, perhaps explaining why acupuncture seems to help in treating depression, eating disorders and addiction. These areas in the brain are also rich in dopamine, a chemical in the body that increases when the brain is stimulated by positive associations, ranging from food to money to beauty to sex. The reduced blood flow in the brain, Rosen speculates, could lead to dopamine changes that trigger a "cascade" effect ending in the release of endorphins, the brain's natural pain-relieving chemicals.

More good news: scientists in Britain found signs indicating that acupuncture may help those who suffer chronic headaches and migraine. Their study found that the frequency of headaches among patients who had been treated with acupuncture dropped 34%, compared with a 16% drop among those who had used medication. The decline continued for at least nine months after the treatments had stopped. On average, those who had been suffering the most from headaches reported the greatest benefits from acupuncture.

■ Resources

WEBSITES: *nccam.nih.gov/health/acupuncture/*
www.nlm.nih.gov/medlineplus/acupuncture.html

ADHD

Scientists explore the causes of attention deficit/hyperactivity disorder (ADHD)—and implicate the fast pace of TV programming

Turn It Off How much TV should infants watch? The American Academy of Pediatrics recommends no TV before age 2

A groundbreaking study conducted at the Children's Hospital in Seattle concludes that frequent TV watching by infants and toddlers may shorten their attention span by age 7—making them more likely to have trouble concentrating and to become impulsive and restless. Although ADHD is believed to be primarily genetic in origin, environment can play a key role; the study indicates that heavy exposure to television can increase the likelihood that a child already at risk for ADHD will eventually develop the disorder.

A new study by the University of Pittsburgh finds that children with severe, persistent ADHD are more likely to drink, smoke cigarettes and use other drugs as teenagers. The good news, according to another study, is that if these children are treated with Ritalin, they are no more likely than their peers without ADHD to develop such problems.

■ Resources

WEBSITE: *www.nimh.nih.gov/healthinformation/adhdmenu.cfm*

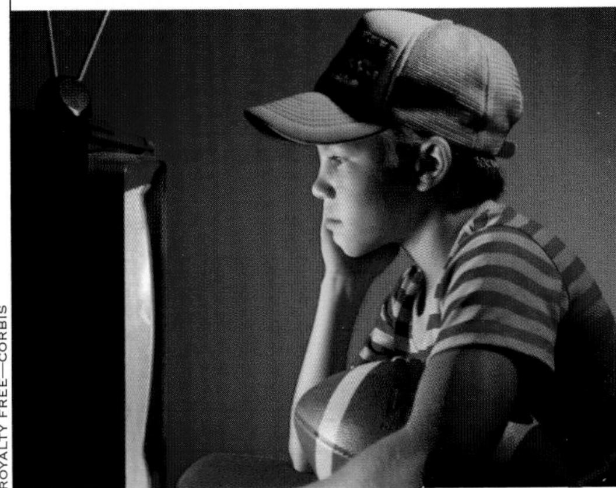

ROYALTY FREE—CORBIS

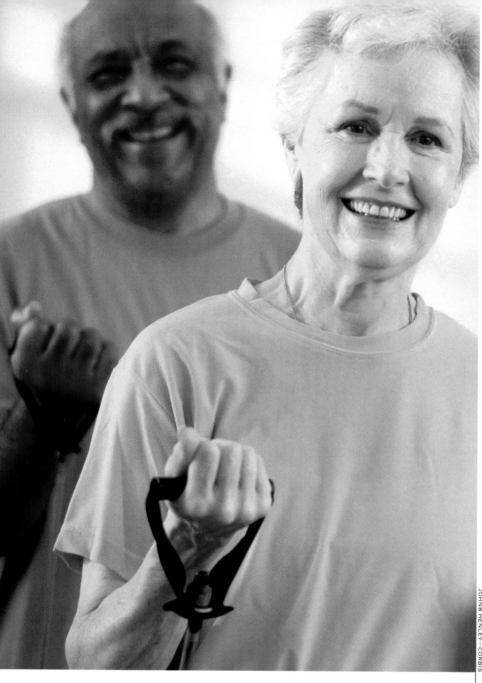
JOHNB HENLEY—CORBIS

Aging

The big news in aging gracefully doesn't involve drugs or surgery: studies show that an active body and robust social life are the best medicine for seniors

The Bottom Line Forty-five minutes of exercise twice a week can reduce or prevent age-related muscle loss

New insights into the aging process hold out the hope not only of extending life, but also of improving the quality of life for those who survive into old age. One finding that should surprise no one is that exercise, especially weight training, may be a magic bullet that staves off many of the more unpleasant effects of getting older. The huge payoff starts almost immediately: regular workouts may reduce or prevent many age-related illnesses, including heart disease, arthritis, osteoporosis, diabetes, depression, even mental decline.

LOOK OUT, VIAGRA!

"If exercise were a pill, it would be the best-selling medication in the world"

"If exercise were a pill, it would be the best-selling medication in the world," says Miriam Nelson, director of Tufts University's Center for Physical Activity and Nutrition. Twice weekly 45-minute sessions of strength training, she says, can reverse or prevent age-related muscle loss. In four weeks, grocery bags feel lighter, and in six weeks, arthritis pain may lessen. Women in Nelson's weight-training studies usually drop a dress size or two and gain the confidence to adopt a more active lifestyle.

➤**Diet** Better eating habits, almost always the partner of exercise for those seeking good health, may also play a role in mitigating the effects of getting older. One new study shows that anemia may contribute to physical disability in seniors, suggesting that routine hemoglobin tests and a diet containing the recommended amounts of iron, vitamin B12 and folic acid may help stave off some of the effects of aging. Separate research shows that enhanced intake of vitamin D, which aids in muscle function, may help prevent falls that sometimes lead to serious injury in seniors.

A March, 2004 study showed that, in mice at least, a low-calorie diet can help to extend life even if the change in eating habits doesn't begin until old age. Further testing is needed to verify that the same holds true for humans.

➤**Growth Hormone** One strategy for reversing the aging process has many health experts worried: a growing number of seniors are using human growth hormone (HGH) in hopes of remaining youthful. Approved by the FDA in 2003 as a therapy to spur growth in otherwise healthy children of "extremely short stature," HGH is increasingly being used "off-label" by seniors because it seems to confer a range of benefits, from increasing muscle mass and reducing body fat to enhancing energy. But researchers point to studies showing that these benefits might be temporary or even illusory: no study has documented an increased functional ability in elderly test subjects taking HGH. Moreover, HGH has serious side effects, including pain, swelling, and increased risk of diseases like high blood pressure, diabetes, and several forms of cancer.

➤**Relationships** Recent studies have bolstered the notion that interaction with a pet can offer significant health benefits to seniors. A 2003 study suggests that relating to pets may minimize or even reverse some of the damaging cell changes that occur naturally with aging. Levels of endorphins, serotonin and prolactin—substances that can enhance feelings of well-being—increased in study participants during interaction with pets, while cortisol levels (stress hormones) decreased. Another study reported dramatic decreases in ailments like bedsores and the necessity of confining patients to their beds when pets were present in nursing homes.

But man's best friend may be man. As part of the MacArthur Successful Aging Study, researchers examined more than 800 men and women in the context of their social networks and found that socially isolated men ages 70 to 79 appear to be at greater risk of heart disease than men with more robust social networks. Men with less active social lives also had much higher blood levels of C-reactive protein and interleukin-6, substances believed to be markers for cardiovascular disease. Curiously, no such link between sociability and these substance levels was found in women.

■ **Resources**

CDC WEBSITE ON HEALTHY AGING: *www.cdc.gov/aging*

NATIONAL INSTITUTE ON AGING: *www.nia.nih.gov.*
Phone: 301-496-1752

Why Do Asians Live So Long?

The people of Pinghan and surrounding Bama county, in the Guangxi province of China, are exceptionally long-lived. The county (pop. 238,000) has more than 74 centenarians and 237 residents who have reached their 90s. Elsewhere in Asia there are other, similarly fabled pockets of longevity, where, for reasons not fully understood, life expectancy exceeds global norms by wide margins. The Japanese, famously, live unusually long lives—an average of 81.6 years. By comparison, in the U.S. the average life expectancy in 2002 was 77.1 and only 74.5 for men, about the same as Cuba's. Okinawa, the southernmost prefecture in the Japanese archipelago, boasts the longest-lived population on the planet, with an average life expectancy of 81.8. Meanwhile, Japan is currently home to the world's oldest man (he's 113) and woman (she's 115).

Is it something in the water? Why do some communities, located in disparate places and harboring very different cultures, seem to be built atop a fountain of youth? You've heard some of the secrets of Asia's most senior citizens before: eschew an excess of meat, eat your vegetables and get plenty of exercise. Protein and animal fat typically play a minimal role in their diets. But it's not only the prevalence of fish and veggies on the table that makes a difference: many Asians say it's best to eat only until you are *hara hachi bu*, or "8 parts out of 10 full," as the Okinawan phrase puts it. An old wives' tale, perhaps, but scientific evidence has been steadily mounting for years that gives credence to this simple adage. A daily diet restricted to between half and three-quarters of the 2,100 calories recommended by the U.S. government appears to boost health in humans, and an equivalent reduction has extended the lives of lab rats. Indeed, dietary moderation is a consistent feature of the lives of the superwrinklies.

Also important is the avoidance of proven killers. Few of Asia's ancients smoke; if they once did, they kicked the vice long ago. Most will happily admit to taking a drink now and then, though, a habit whose benefits in moderation are well enough established that they are acknowledged even by such cautious institutions as the American Heart Association. ■

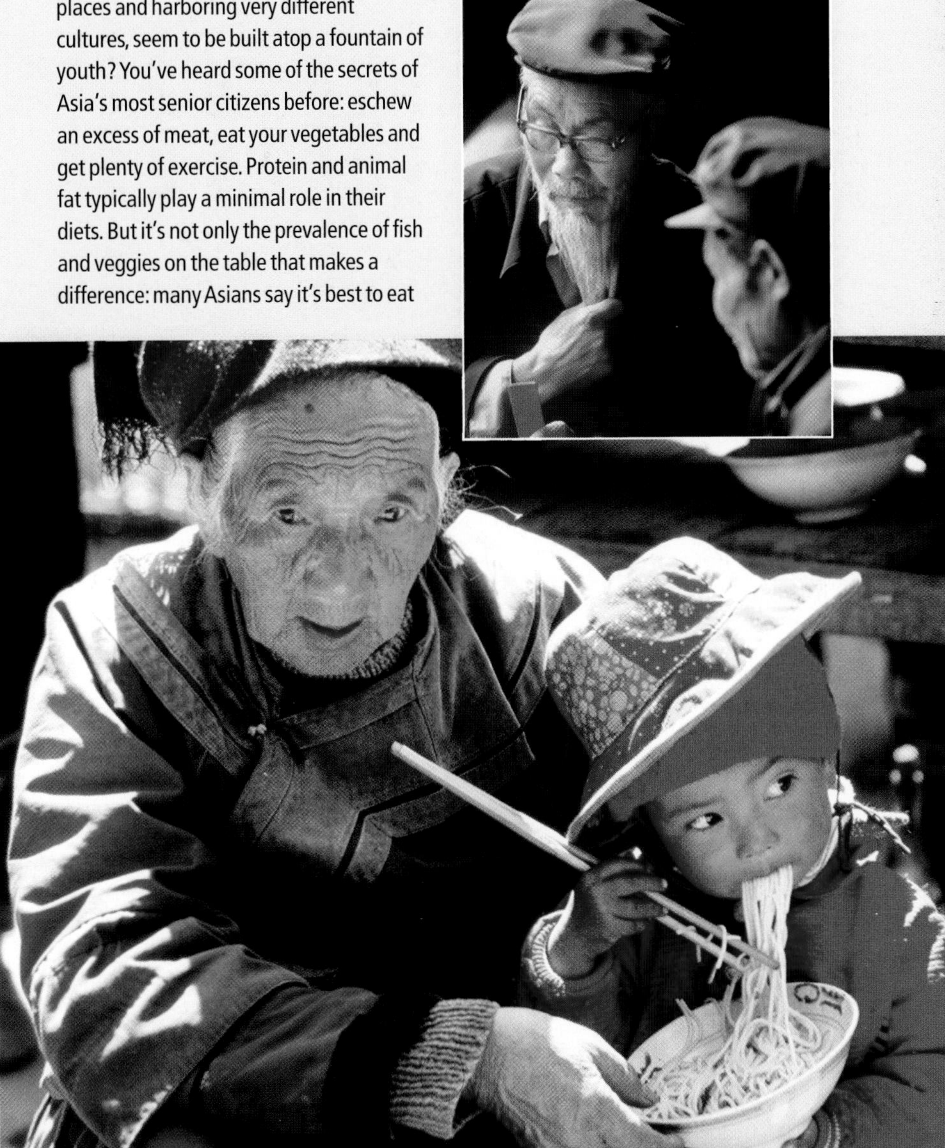

YANN LAYMA—STONE—GETTY; INSET: PAUL GREBLIUNAS—STONE—GETTY

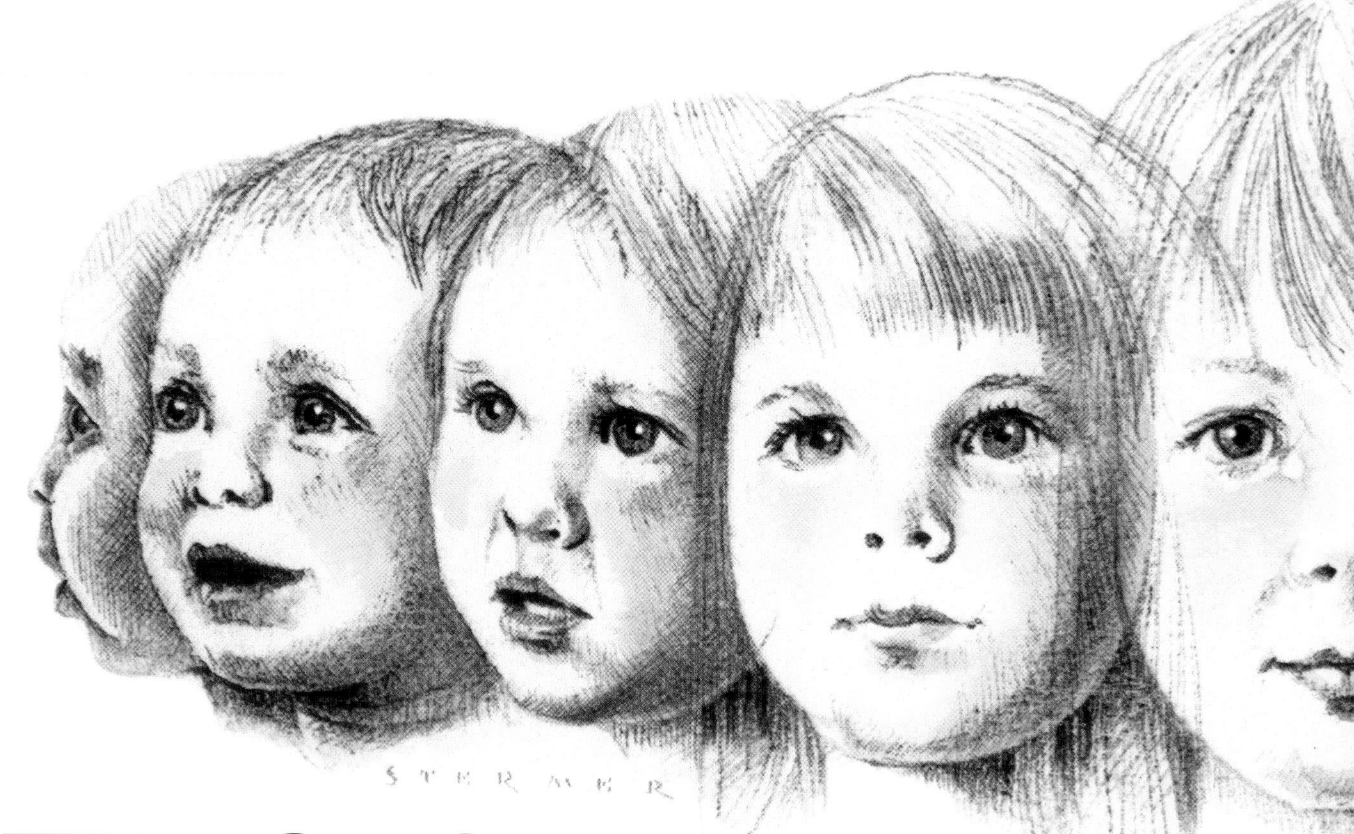

THROUGH THE AGES

CONCEPTION TO BIRTH

PRENATAL

The brain and nervous system develop and form an intricate network. But genetic errors and environmental factors like fetal exposure to alcohol or drugs can make this process go awry. Some common examples:

CEREBRAL PALSY

Affects about 10,000 U.S. babies a year. More than 80% show signs in the womb or before they are a month old. Usually diagnosed by age 3

FETAL ALCOHOL SYNDROME

Profound mental retardation caused by maternal alcohol abuse. Studies suggest that 1,200 to 8,800 FAS babies are born in the U.S. every year

NEURAL-TUBE DEFECTS

These include spina bifida and anencephaly, each of which affects 1 or 2 of every 10,000 live births

DOWN SYNDROME

The most common chromosome abnormality. Occurs in 1 of every 800 to 1,000 live births

INFANCY

0-5 yrs.

Excess neurons and synapses are pruned in the first 18 months, but the brain keeps growing, reaching 90% of adult size. Brain cells become more adept at communicating; babies learn to talk

AUTISM DISORDERS

Three to four times as common in boys

EPILEPSY

About 10% of Americans will have a seizure sometime during their life. By age 80, about 3% will have been found to have epilepsy

ATTENTION-DEFICIT/HYPERACTIVITY DISORDER

Tends to run in families and affects two to three times as many boys as girls. Between 3% and 5% of U.S. schoolchildren are thought to have ADHD

ANXIETY DISORDERS

Most prevalent group of psychiatric illnesses among children and adults

LATE CHILDHOOD

5-10 yrs.

Dramatic growth spurts in the temporal and parietal lobes, brain regions crucial to language and understanding of spatial relations, make this a prime time for learning new languages and music

DEPRESSION

In any given year, nearly 10% of adult Americans—two-thirds of them women—experience a depressive disorder. Up to 10% of children ages 6 to 12 have symptoms of major depression, but the typical age of onset is mid-20s

ANTISOCIAL BEHAVIOR

From lying and bullying to vandalism and homicide. More prevalent in boys, who tend to inflict physical harm on others

DYSLEXIA

Revealed when a child tries to learns to read

CONDUCT DISORDER

Various behaviors that show a persistent disregard for the norms and rules of society. Affects 6% to 16% of boys and 2% to 9% of girls under age 18

PUBERTY

10-13 yrs.

Just before puberty, the brain's gray matter thickens, especially in the frontal lobe, the seat of planning, impulse control and reasoning. This growth may be triggered by surges of sex hormones

EATING DISORDE

In the U.S., most common in teen girls and young women; on 5% to 15% of anorexic or bulimics and 35% o binge eaters are male

OBSESSIVE-COMPULSIV

Apparently caused by abnormally functioning brain circuitry. Neurotransmitter and hormone imbalances may also be involved

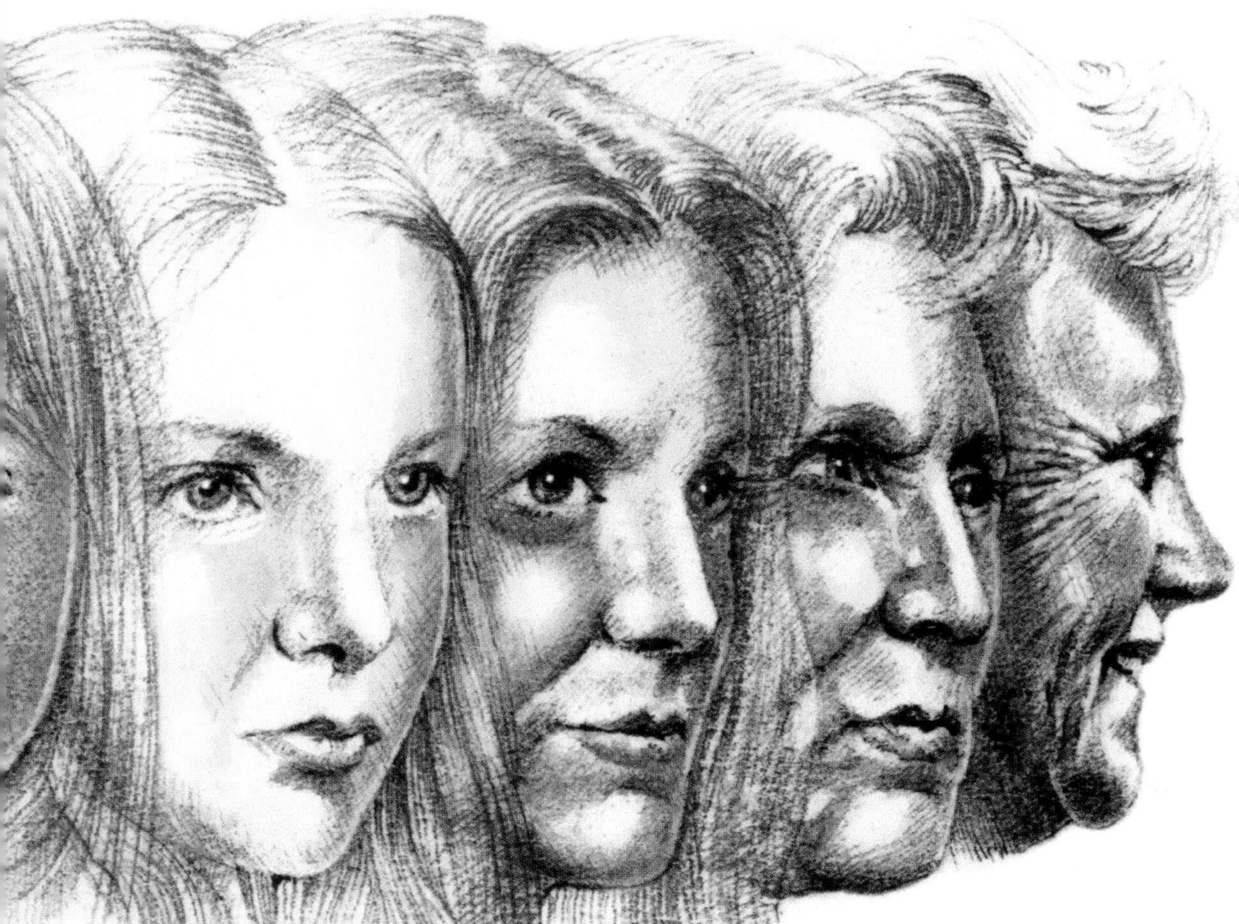

You become susceptible to different disorders as your brain develops, matures and ages. Here's a guide to the typical age of onset

ADOLESCENCE

13-20 yrs.

…e brain begins to shrink, …sing about 2% of its weight …d volume in each successive …cade. Abnormally high loss … gray matter during this …eriod may be a cause of …enage schizophrenia

EARLY ADULTHOOD

20-30 yrs.

By the late 20s, information processing begins to slow down. Memory centers in the hippocampus and frontal lobes seem most affected. However, this change is not usually noticeable until at least age 60

MIDDLE AGE

30-60 yrs.

Learning, memory, planning and other complex mental processes become more difficult, and reacting to stimuli takes longer. Plaques and tangles may form in certain brain regions

OLD AGE

60-100 yrs.

Aging, depression, anxiety disorders and Alzheimer's may alter sleep patterns. The decline in cognitive abilities becomes more pronounced. Coordination and dexterity are also affected

AGORAPHOBIA
Affects twice as many women as men

PANIC DISORDER
Afflicts 2.4 million Americans ages 18 to 54 in a given year. Twice as common in women

…SORDER

POSTPARTUM DEPRESSION
Hits 10% of new mothers

…CIAL PHOBIAS
…sistent fears of being watched, judged or embarrassed in situations … parties or performing in public. Affect men and women equally

BIPOLAR DISORDER
About 2.3 million adult Americans are manic-depressive

SEASONAL AFFECTIVE DISORDER
Most sufferers are women

PEAK SUICIDE YEARS
Third leading cause of death among people 15 to 24. White males are at greatest risk

SCHIZOPHRENIA
Affects about 1% of the U.S. population

PARKINSON'S DISEASE
More than 1 million Americans have it

HUNTINGTON'S DISEASE
More than 250,000 Americans have HD or are at risk of inheriting it

EARLY-ONSET ALZHEIMER'S
Just 5% to 10% of all Alzheimer's cases

MENOPAUSE
Sudden mood swings, irritability, inability to cope, memory lapses

STROKE
Risk rises sharply after age 65

ALZHEIMER'S DISEASE
Most common form of dementia among the elderly. Prevalence doubles every five years after age 65

PEAK SUICIDE YEARS
People age 65 and older have higher suicide rates than any other age group. The rate among U.S. white men 85 and older is six times the national average

Dr. Jay Giedd, National Institute of Mental Health; Centers for Disease Control; Natl. Center for Health Statistics; Natl. Institute on Aging; Natl. Institute of Child Health & Human Development; Natl. Institute of Neurological Disorders and Stroke; MEDLINEplus; infoaging.org; American Psychiatric Association; American Academy of Child & Adolescent Psychiatry; MayoClinic.com; NAMI; Natl. Mental Health Association

TIME Graphic; text by Andrea Dorfman

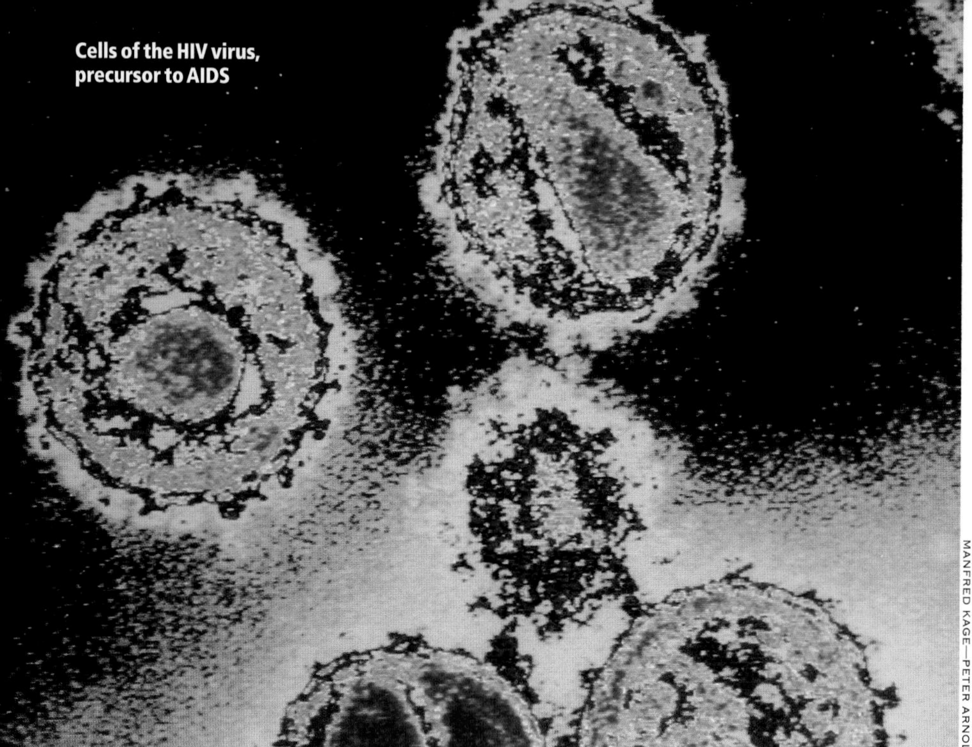

Cells of the HIV virus, precursor to AIDS

MANFRED KAGE—PETER ARNOLD

AIDS

While a few nations find success in fighting AIDS, Africa and China remain the focus of the global war against the killer epidemic

By the Numbers The number of those afflicted with AIDS is now so large that it has begun to reduce the rate at which the world's population is growing

Recent years have brought both good and bad news about AIDS, but there has been precious little of the former and a heartbreaking load of the latter.

➤Surging in Asia A long-standing lull in the rate of new HIV infections among gay and bisexual men in the U.S. may be coming to an end. Still incomplete data seem to show that in 2003, for the third year in a row, the number of new infections in this risk group rose substantially.

Internationally, the AIDS epidemic marked two grim milestones in 2003, the last year for which figures are available: approximately 5 million people worldwide were newly infected with HIV during the year, while 3 million people worldwide died of the disease. Both figures represent a jump of several hundred thousand cases over the 2002 figures, bringing the total number of deaths from AIDS since the epidemic began in the 1980s to more than 20 million, and the worldwide number of people living with HIV to some 38 million. If the disease remains uncured, most of these people are expected to die within 10 years. The numbers are so large that they have contributed to an overall slowing of the world's population growth. According to U.N. figures released in July 2004, about 1 in 4 new cases of HIV in 2003 was found in Asia, up from 1 in 5 in 2001.

Some genuine progress has been reported amid all the bad news. Even as new waves of HIV infection hit India, China and Eastern Europe, the epidemic may be receding in former hot spots like Senegal and Uganda, thanks to well-funded education and prevention measures.

A GLOBAL CRISIS

The U.N. estimates that 38 million people around the world are now living with HIV

➤Race for Drugs The small doses of encouragement in the AIDS battle include the news that the smallpox vaccine may be effective in preventing HIV infection. Early results from research at George Mason University in Virgnia indicate that blood cells from test subjects vaccinated against smallpox were one-fourth as likely to become infected with the AIDS virus as those not vaccinated.

A second study showed that a diabetes drug, Avandia, may help patients taking a "cocktail" of AIDS medications fight off some of the side effects of these drugs, including the abnormal redistribution of body fat than can endanger internal organs.

Two studies released in December 2003 have helped doctors refine the recipe for the AIDS cocktails. The conclusion: a mix of three widely used antiviral agents (AZT, 3TC and efavirenz) is more effective—and delays the inevitable onset of a patient's resistance to antiviral drugs—longer than any other combination.

But a third study dashed a hope long harbored by doctors and

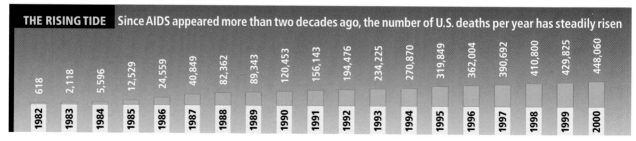

THE RISING TIDE Since AIDS appeared more than two decades ago, the number of U.S. deaths per year has steadily risen

Year	Deaths
1982	618
1983	2,118
1984	5,596
1985	12,529
1986	24,559
1987	40,849
1988	82,362
1989	89,343
1990	120,453
1991	156,143
1992	194,476
1993	234,225
1994	270,870
1995	319,849
1996	362,004
1997	390,692
1998	410,800
1999	429,825
2000	448,060

patients: taking "breaks" from AIDS medications does nothing to restore an antiviral agent's effectiveness once a patient has begun to develop a resistance to that drug.

➤**Pediatric AIDS** The dramatic progress made against pediatric AIDS continues, with infection rates among newborns down to about fewer than 100 cases among babies born in the U.S. each year, from rates more than 10 times as high a decade ago. Yet even as pediatric AIDS rates decline, new studies show that one-fifth of all pregnant women have never been tested for HIV and that almost half are unaware that treatment can prevent an HIV-positive mother from passing the virus to her baby.

Doctors themselves were caught unawares by a February 2004 study showing that nevirapine, a low-cost antiviral drug often used in poor nations to stop mother-to-baby transmission of HIV during childbirth actually stiffens drug resistance in large numbers of women and their infant children, perhaps leaving them vulnerable to AIDS later on.

A more welcome surprise came from the finding that two forms of a common (and generally harmless) bacteria found in the mouths of most infants can attach themselves to the AIDS virus and prevent it from infecting other cells. This surprising discovery offers the hope that babies of HIV-positive mothers, who are at risk of contracting HIV while breast feeding, can be protected.

➤**The Politics of AIDS** Controversy continued to shadow the area where AIDS meets public policy. In February 2004 President Bush sent Congress a $15 billion, five-year plan to fight AIDS worldwide. Three months later, the Administration unveiled plans for a fast-track program to quickly deliver low-price AIDS drugs to millions of patients in Africa and the Caribbean. Both these programs met with widespread approval.

But one effort to fight HIV and AIDS stirred up controversy. The Stop AIDS Project, a federally funded local initiative in San Francisco, ran afoul of Washington bureaucrats when it was deemed to violate a federal law against using public money to promote sexual activity. The group was ordered to tone down its presentations—which included discussions of safe-sex practices to use with male prostitutes and detailed precautions for anal and oral sex—or risk losing its federal grants.

NEXT FRONT: ASIA

AIDS is now growing fastest in Asia, where some 1.2 million new cases of HIV were reported in 2003

➤**Holding the Line** While the wait for a cure drags on, prevention remains the best defense against AIDS. But getting the message right isn't easy: HIV-prevention efforts, especially those targeting young people, often reflect the ideological dispute over whether public policy should promote sexual abstinence or condom use. Such campaigns often miss the middle ground: there would be no global AIDS pandemic if people had sex with fewer partners. Yet partner reduction, as scientists call it, is seldom emphasized in AIDS literature. Limiting sex partners, as an editorial in the *British Medical Journal* pointed out, is "good common sense—and good epidemiology."

■ Resources

NIH WEBSITE ON AIDS:
www.nlm.nih.gov/medlineplus/aids

Dr. Ho Goes to China

China is the world's most populous stronghold of AIDS. As many as 1 million Chinese are HIV positive, and that number could easily grow to 10 million by 2010, according to the Joint U.N. Program on AIDS. If current trends continue for another decade or so, China could overtake Africa, where 29 million people have been infected with the virus. These grim statistics led U.S. virologist Dr. David Ho, head of the Aaron Diamond AIDS Research Center in New York City (and TIME's 1996 Person of the Year, for his pioneering work on AIDS drug therapies) to journey more than a dozen times to China over the past three years, where he has set up labs, visited clinics, educated health workers and raised awareness of the crisis. Ho's efforts, along with those of other AIDS activists, led to a major public-awareness campaign across China, complete with posters, TV spots and a visit by Premier Wen Jiabao to a Beijing hospital, where he shook hands with AIDS patients.

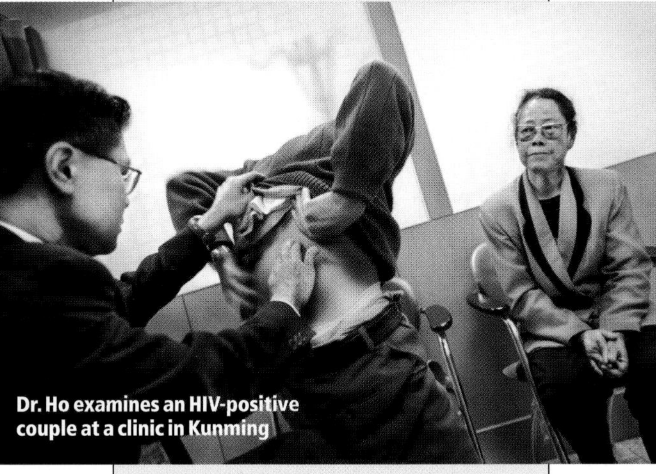

JOHN STANMEYER—VII FOR TIME

Dr. Ho examines an HIV-positive couple at a clinic in Kunming

Dr. Ho came to China to launch a vaccine-testing program, but the extent of the crisis led him to begin testing and treating patients. China's epidemic is compounded by the legacy of an ineptly run, government-sanctioned 1990s blood donation program that accidentally infected hundreds of thousands of people from China's mainstream who otherwise would have been at little risk of the disease. "The epidemic in China was bigger than our expectations," Ho said. "And the obstacles to convincing the government to take action remain considerable . . . But as AIDS researchers, we could not continue to be distant from the vast majority of patients."

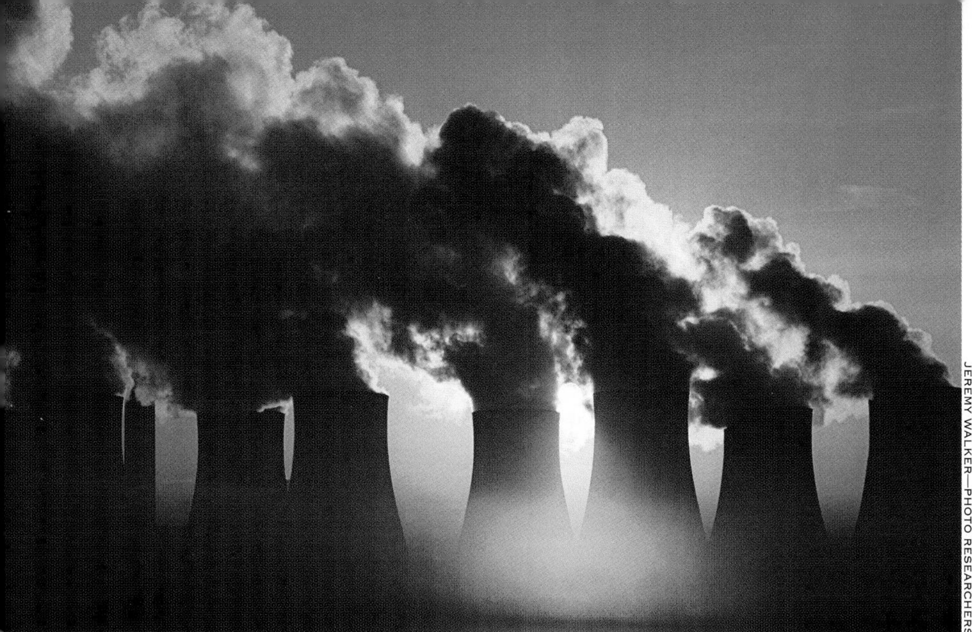

JEREMY WALKER—PHOTO RESEARCHERS

Air Pollution

A study on mice concludes that sooty air can cause genetic damage that is passed along in DNA; human research will follow

Cutbacks The U.S. Environmental Protection Agency ordered tougher curbs on ultrafine particulate pollution in 2004

Air pollution has been implicated in a growing list of maladies, including asthma and heart disease, but a 2004 study heightened scientists' concerns about the potential dangers of the tiny airborne particulates we call soot. Researchers in Ontario housed two groups of mice near particulate-spewing steel mills for 10 weeks. One group of mice breathed outside air, while the other was housed in a chamber equipped with HEPA filters—high-efficiency air filters designed to catch microscopic particles. Then the mice were bred and their offspring checked to determine whether specific DNA mutations had been passed along.

The researchers found that mice that breathed filtered air had mutation rates 52% lower than the mice exposed to full-strength steel mill pollution. The specific sperm changes measured were not linked to disease, but they were similar to a type of DNA damage that is. The research team stressed that major follow-up work will be required before it can be determined if people can inherit pollution-damaged DNA that harms their health. The good news to be found in the study: the HEPA air filters did their job, screening out damaging particulates.

■ Resources

EPA WEBSITE ON AIR POLLUTION: *www.epa.gov/airnow*

Alcohol

Upside: a study suggests that moderate alcohol use may help alleviate hypertension in men

Downside The National Highway Traffic Safety Administration announced that more than 1 in 5 teen drivers killed in accidents were intoxicated

Little is simple in the complicated interplay between alcohol and health. The social and health costs associated with excessive drinking—from fatalities caused by drunk drivers to deaths caused by liver damage—are well known. But there is another side to the story: science continues to find positive health benefits from moderate drinking. In this report, we'll begin by noting the latest positive findings about alcohol, then report on news of the perils associated with drinking.

➤The Benefits Heart experts agree: consumed moderately and steadily, red wine boosts the level of good cholesterol in the blood, cleansing the arteries and helping ward off heart disease. And the word is out: the number of people in the U.S. who drink wine at least once a week has soared since 2000.

A study released late in 2003—based on the experience of more than 14,000 doctors suffering from hypertension—suggested further benefits in alcohol: it found that drinking in moderation appears to reduce heart-related deaths in men with high blood pressure. The conclusion challenged the belief among heart experts that those with high blood pressure shouldn't drink, since heavy drinking can increase blood pressure.

TO YOUR GOOD HEALTH!

The number of people in the U.S. who drink wine at least once a week has climbed 32% since 2000

In the study, men with high blood pressure who reported having about one or two drinks a day were 44% less likely to die of cardiovascular causes like heart attacks than men with hypertension who rarely or never drank. But the results need to be confirmed before doctors will begin suggesting a moderate regimen of alcohol use for those with high blood pressure.

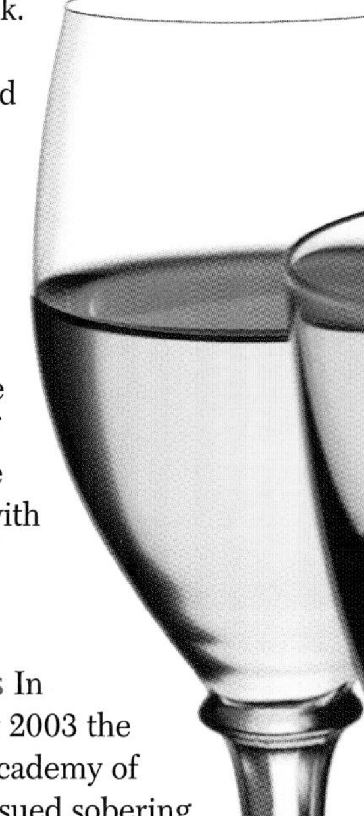

➤The Risks In September 2003 the National Academy of Sciences issued sobering

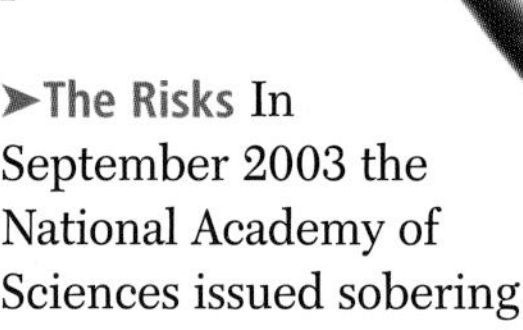

findings on underage drinking in America: 20% of eighth-graders and half of high school seniors surveyed in 2002 said they had had a drink in the past month. Nearly 30% of the seniors admitted to having had at least five drinks at a time within the previous two weeks.

Drunken behavior and violent crimes that result from adolescent drinking cost the U.S. $53 billion a year, according to the report, including $19 billion from traffic accidents alone. The academy called for such measures as cracking down on merchants who sell booze to kids, reining in glamorous depictions of drinking in movies and music and increasing excise taxes on liquor.

More bad news: the National Highway Traffic Safety Administration said in 2003 that 21% of young drivers killed in car crashes are intoxicated. Another study, however, suggests the greater statistical danger for teens is not drinking and driving but riding with a driver who is drinking. A survey of 1,534 Californians ages 15 to 20 found that nearly 50% had ridden in a car with a drunk driver in the previous 12 months.

ON TARGET?

Although alcohol use among U.S. teenagers is far more widespread than illegal-drug use at any age, the government spends 25 times as much on anti-drug campaigns as it does to stop underage drinking

➤Drinking Patterns Researchers have known for some time that alcohol consumption can increase a premenopausal woman's risk of someday developing breast cancer. But a 2003 study by researchers at the University at Buffalo suggests that a woman's drinking patterns may be as important as how much alcohol she consumes. A woman who regularly has three or four drinks one night a week appears to have an 80% higher risk of breast cancer than a woman who has three or four drinks over the course of a week. "It could be that the higher alcohol load at one time taxes the body's ability to handle alcohol's potentially toxic effects," said University of Buffalo epidemiologist Jo Freudenheim.

■ Resources

NIH ALCOHOL INFORMATION LINE:
800-729-6686

AMERICAN COUNCIL ON ALCOHOLISM HELP LINE:
800-527-5344

Allergies

A new study finds that man's best friend may be a child's best friend when it comes to warding off allergies at an early age

Outgrowing Peanut Perils Another study determined that peanut allergies need not be a lifelong affliction but may in some cases be outgrown

In recent years, doctors have begun to give parents some surprising advice about preventing allergies and asthma in children: let them cuddle up to family pets during the first year of life. The idea, supported by several studies, is to expose the infants to the microbes that make their home in animal fur. That would prime the baby's immune system, still under construction, to recognize common allergens as harmless and not to mount the sneezing, wheezing and red-eyed response. One caveat: whatever protection pets provide babies is erased if the parents smoke.

More surprising news: until recently, most doctors believed that peanut allergies, which affect some 1.5 million Americans and can be deadly, were a lifelong affliction. Now it turns out that some people outgrow them. Researchers gave 80 allergic children a "peanut challenge"—that is, they made them eat peanuts. More than half the kids passed the test, suffering no common allergy symptoms. The study looked at children with low levels (5 kilounits or less per liter of blood) of peanut-specific IgE—the antibodies that cause allergic reactions—and found that the lower the levels, the more likely the children were to outgrow their peanut sensitivities. These antibodies can be measured with widely available blood tests.

■ Resources

NIH ALLERGY CENTER:
www.nlm.nih.gov/medlineplus/allergy

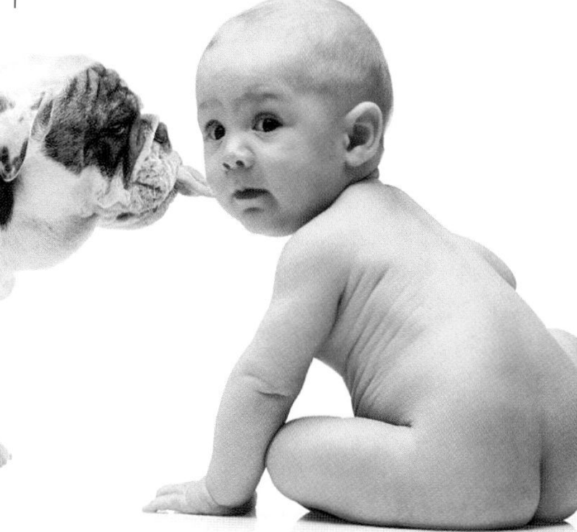

LWA-DANN TARDIF—CORBIS

Alternative Medicine

More and more Americans are embracing exotic botanical and probiotic supplements to ensure their good health, but a lack of regulation favors the sellers of supplements, not their consumers

The Bottom Line Let the buyer beware: supplement hawkers may fail to monitor the purity of their products and frequently omit government warnings of the specific dangers associated with their use

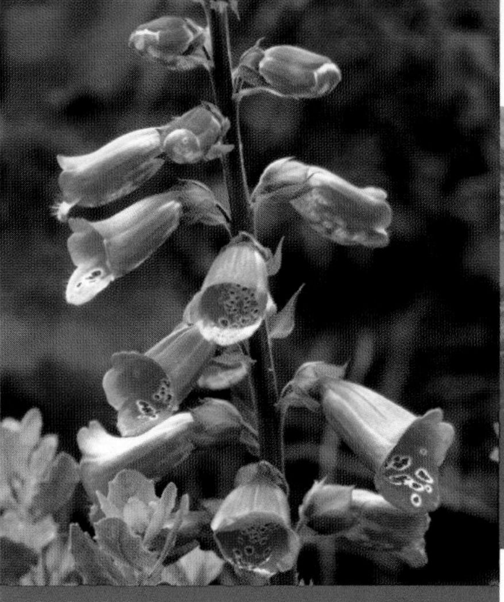

FOXGLOVE
Proved: Source of digitalis, used to treat heart disease
Unproved: Prevents heart disease

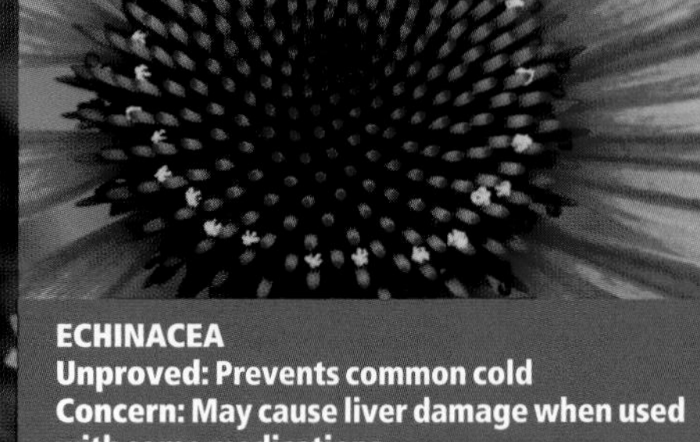

ECHINACEA
Unproved: Prevents common cold
Concern: May cause liver damage when used with some medications

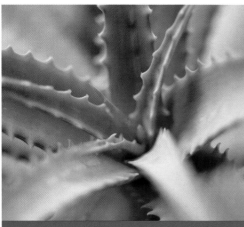

ALOE VERA
Proved: Relieves pain of burn and sunburn
Unproved: May relieve pain of irritable bowel syndrome and other digestive disorders

As the popularity of alternative and herbal medicines booms, concerns are rising that this largely unregulated sector of the healthcare market may, in some cases, be doing consumers more harm than good. An update on new findings:

➤**Ephedra** In December 2003, the FDA decided to ban ephedra, a Chinese herbal stimulant long used to fight colds and asthma but now popular as a weight-loss aid, athletic performance enhancer and energy booster. The FDA said it had received more than 16,000 reports of complications, ranging from dizziness to stroke, that may have been triggered by ephedra. The agency linked its use to as many as 155 deaths in the U.S.

Studies show that ephedra can indeed promote modest short-term weight loss (an extra pound per month), apparently by slightly suppressing appetite and boosting metabolism. Used in combination with caffeine, it may also jolt the muscles enough to enhance athletic performance for brief spurts.

The FDA had been trying to restrict ephedra supplements for the past six years, only to be beaten back by industry and political pressure. The 1994 Dietary Supplement Health and Education Act puts the burden of proof on the FDA to demonstrate that a supplement is harmful, rather than requiring a manufacturer to prove that it's safe. It also bars the FDA from restricting supplements until they have gone on the market. By contrast, the agency carefully vets prescription drugs long before they reach consumers.

GINKGO BILOBA
Unproved: Aids memory
Concern: Inhibits blood clotting

With ephedra banned, many enthusiasts have started taking other so-called natural stimulants—like synephrine and octopamine, found in bitter orange—which are not as potent as ephedra. But solid information on their safety and value remains sparse.

➤**Purity** Even supplements that are not harmful themselves can be of suspect purity. Sales of fish-oil supplements have boomed as evidence of the health benefits of omega-3 fatty acids mounts. But the same pollutants that contaminate fish—such as mercury, dioxins, DDT and PCBs—can be present in the fish oils extracted from them. A March 2004 study found rising levels of a flame retardant in samples of cod-liver oil. Given the lack of scientific oversight, it's up to consumers to keep up with potential contaminants in the oils.

Medical Marijuana

The controversy over the medical use of marijuana continues. In May 2004, Vermont joined eight other states (Alaska, California, Colorado, Hawaii, Maine, Nevada, Oregon and Washington) in allowing very sick patients to use pot, under a doctor's supervision, to alleviate symptoms like pain and nausea. The next month, the U.S. Supreme Court agreed to decide whether the federal government has the right to prohibit such use even in states where the voters or the legislature has approved it. (The Bush Administration claims it has this authority.) While this case is argued, more states seem poised to allow medicinal marijuana. And Canada has begun testing a plan to make government-certified pot available in local pharmacies, which would make it the second country in the world (after the Netherlands) to allow the direct sale of medical marijuana. ■

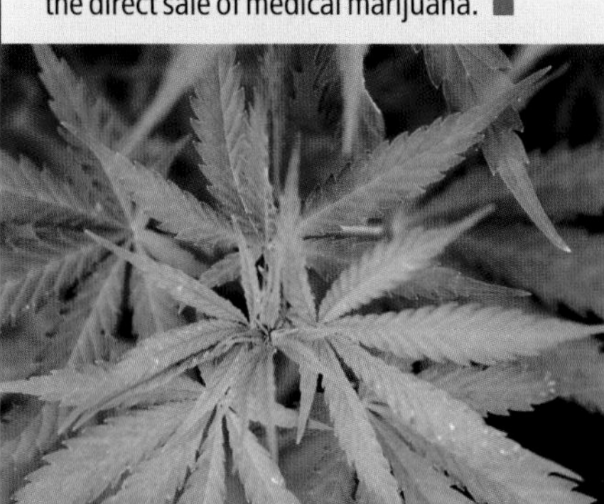

ALOE: MY NEUNSINGER—BOTANICA—CORBIS; FOXGLOVE: ED RESCHKE—PETER ARNOLD; ECHINACEA: ED RESCHKE—PETER ARNOLD; GINKGO BILOBA: KEN

➤**Web Warning** Another problem: the spurious claims being made by some Internet vendors. In one 2003 study, physicians searched popular websites for information about eight of the best-selling herbal products. They found that more than half of the sites made dubious health claims for their wares, while more than 1 in 4 "claimed to treat, prevent, diagnose or cure specific diseases," in violation of FDA regulations. Websites often sinned by omission: more than a third of those selling kava failed to

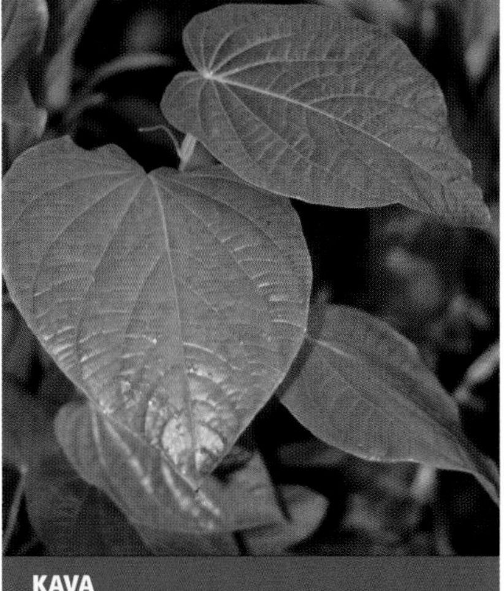

KAVA
Unproved: Provides energy
Concern: Can cause liver damage; subject of FDA warning in U.S.

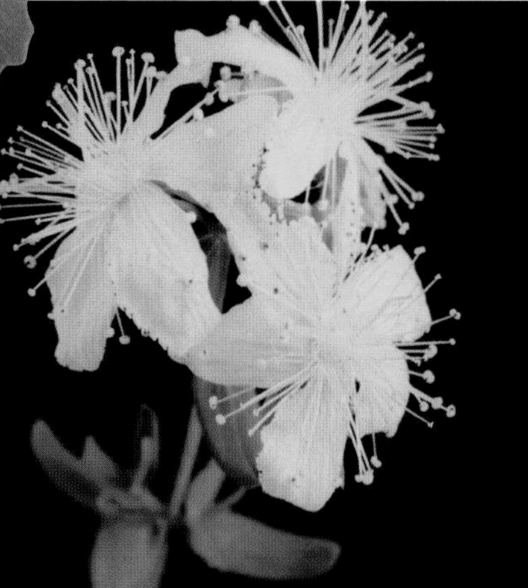

JOHN'S WORT
proved: Relieves depression
ncern: Reacts badly with some prescription drugs

disclose an FDA advisory linking it to serious liver problems.

But momentum may at last be turning in the consumer's favor. In January 2004, FDA commissioner Mark McClellan announced a policy shift that will focus heightened scrutiny on a range of suspect supplements, including bitter orange, aristolochic acid *(see sidebar)* and usnic acid, a lichen derivative linked to liver damage.

JUST SAY NO

Ephedra, now officially banned by the U.S. government, has been linked to 155 deaths

➤**Probiotics** Stars like Gwyneth Paltrow swear by them—and are making new stars out of the supplements known as probiotics. These health-giving bacteria that occur naturally in foods like yogurt and other dairy products can be made into pills and beverages. A mountain of evidence shows that certain "friendly" bacteria do indeed confer health benefits—but we don't yet know how.

One theory holds that probiotics produce natural antibiotics that kill harmful bacteria. But recent studies suggest that probiotics kick-start an anti-inflammatory response that wards off diseases. Other studies have shown that probiotics may be used to treat or help prevent a range of ailments, from irritable bowel syndrome and Crohn's disease to colon cancer and AIDS. But more study is needed before probiotics enter medicine's mainstream.

The real downside to probiotics: you may not be getting what you pay for. One small-scale study that analyzed 17 probiotic products found that more than half contained far less bacteria than the manufacturer claimed.

■ **Resources**

NIH CENTER FOR COMPLEMENTARY & ALTERNATIVE MEDICINE: *http://nccam.nih.gov*

The Dirty Dozen

A

The May 2004 issue of *Consumer Reports* cited a dozen herbal supplements that an investigation by the magazine's staff concluded were both dangerous and freely available to American consumers.

Definitely Hazardous

- **Aristolochic acid:** banned in 10 countries; known to have caused cancer, kidney failure and death

Very Likely Hazardous

- **Comfrey:** linked to irreversible liver damage and death; banned by various athletic associations
- **Androstenedione:** increases the risk of cancer and lowers levels of HDL (or "good") cholesterol
- **Chaparral:** linked to irreversible liver damage and death
- **Germander:** linked to irreversible liver damage and death; banned in France and Germany
- **Kava:** linked to liver damage and death; banned in six nations

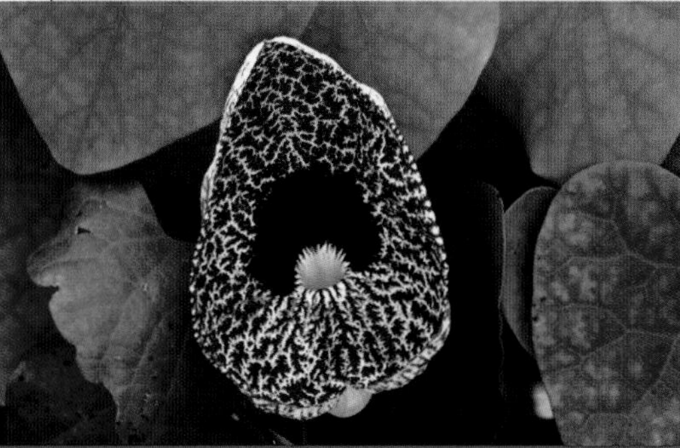

BIRTHWORT (ARISTOCHOLIC ACID):
Unproved: Fights obesity; aids bladder problems
Risk: Do not use—causes liver cancer and kidney failure

Likely Hazardous

- **Bitter orange:** linked to high blood pressure, increased risk of heart arrythmias, heart attack and stroke
- **Organ/Glandular extracts:** possible risk of mad cow disease; banned in France and Switzerland
- **Lobelia:** linked to low blood pressure, breathing difficulty, rapid heartbeat, diarrhea, dizziness and tremors
- **Pennyroyal oil:** linked to liver and kidney failure, nerve damage, convulsions, abdominal tenderness
- **Scullcap:** linked to abnormal liver function and liver damage
- **Yohimbe:** linked to respiratory distress, arrhythmias and heart attack ■

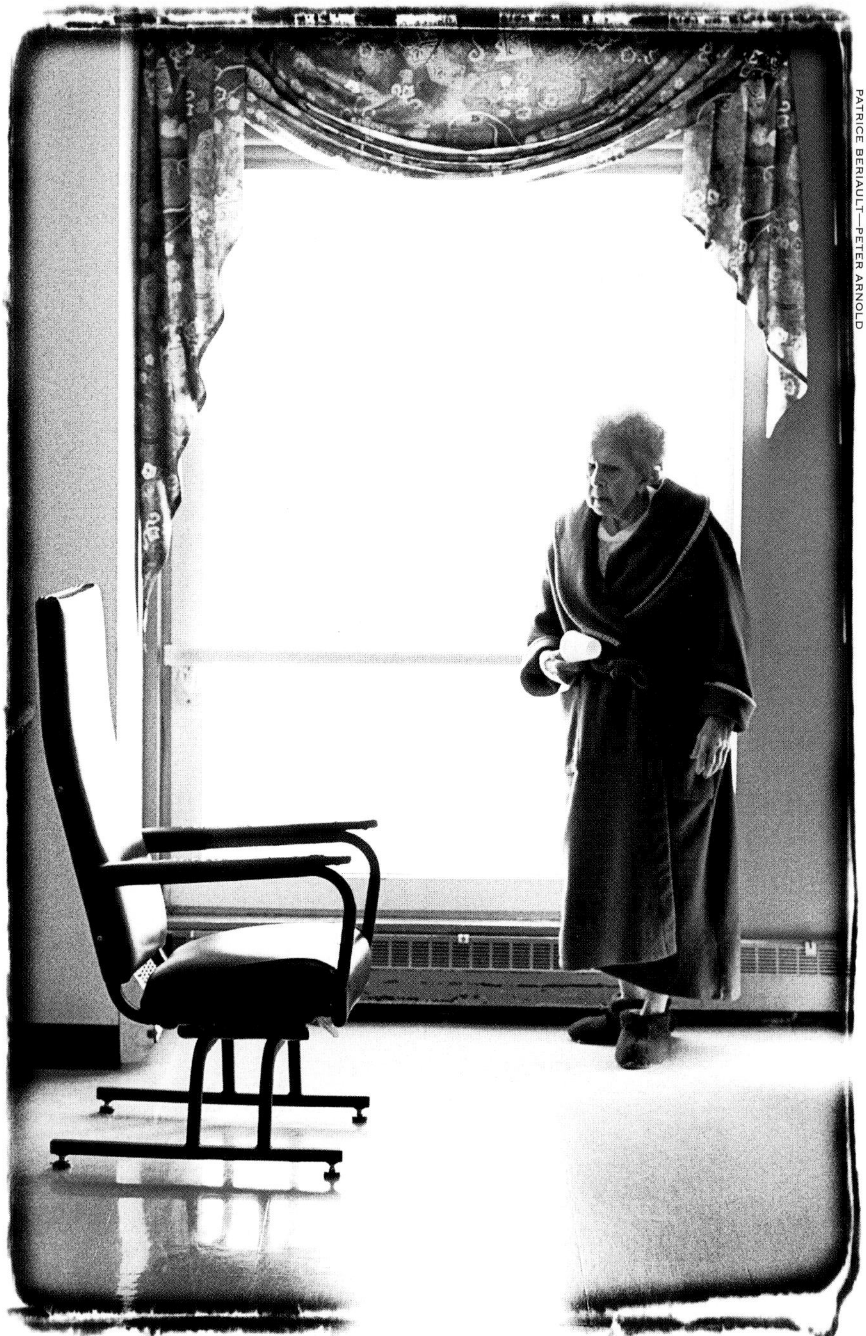

PATRICE BERIAULT—PETER ARNOLD

Alzheimer's Disease

Ronald Reagan's death in 2004 directed fresh attention to this brain ailment associated with aging that can spawn confusion, memory loss and depression

By the Numbers A study predicts a startling rise in the number of Americans who may contract Alzheimer's by 2050

A 2003 study offered a grim outlook for aging Americans: it tracked a diverse group of healthy seniors in Chicago over four years, and found that more of them developed Alzheimer's disease than previous models would have predicted. The study suggests that as many as 16 million people may be suffering from the disease by 2050, far higher than the 7.5 million to 14 million people estimated at risk in previous studies. A silver lining: the figures reflect the fact that Americans are living longer than ever before, and age is the single greatest risk factor for Alzheimer's.

➤Risk Factors: Diet and Weight Because those with Alzheimer's tend to waste away, obesity is not a condition we associate with the disease. But a new study from Sweden shows that women who are overweight and in their 70s have a significantly higher risk of developing the brain disorder by their late 80s—the first strong evidence linking the obesity epidemic to the growing incidence of Alzheimer's. It's also a good reason to stay trim. A 5-ft. 4-in. woman who weighs 145 lbs. increases her Alzheimer's risk 36% with every 7 lbs. she gains.

Another dietary tip: separate research shows that people who eat fish at least once a week have a 60% lower risk of contracting Alzheimer's than people who seldom or never eat fish.

➤Other Risk Factors Seniors who suffer from diabetes have a 65% greater risk of developing Alzheimer's than those who don't, one new study suggests. In a related finding, an eight-year study of 1,800 adults age 65 or older with no signs of dementia found that those who had a stroke before or during the investigation were 60% more likely to develop Alzheimer's. Researchers don't know whether an unidentified process contributes both to stroke and Alzheimer's, or if stroke damage hastens the progression of dementia. In either case, reducing risk factors for strokes—like diabetes, high blood pressure and smoking—may reduce the risk of Alzheimer's.

Scientists are also hunting for defective genes that may trigger Alzheimer's. Four have already been located, and several mutations on a gene associated

ALZHEIMER'S: RISK FACTORS

- Age
- Diabetes
- Obesity
- Stroke
- High blood pressure
- Smoking
- Defective genes

A Twilight Struggle

Former President Ronald Reagan's death in June 2004, 10 years after he announced he had contracted Alzheimer's, heightened our awareness of its debilitating cruelties. Shortly after his diagnosis, tears came to the eyes of the outdoorsman who once said, "There's nothing better for the insides of a man than the outside of a horse," on being told that it was no longer safe for him to ride. In 1998, his beloved Santa Barbara estate, Rancho del Cielo, was sold. In 1999 Reagan stopped going to his office in downtown Los Angeles. Still physically robust, he would rake leaves for hours on

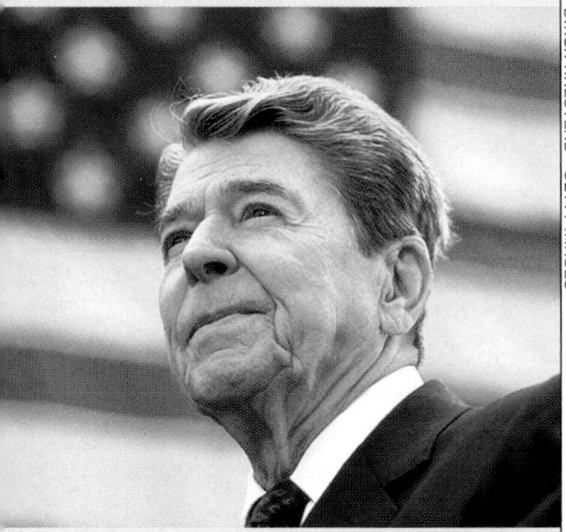

DIRCK HALSTEAD—GETTY IMAGES

end from the swimming pool of his Bel Air home. After his Secret Service agents quietly replaced the leaves, he would begin the task once more. But after falling and breaking his hip in 2001, Reagan never left the house.

In his final months, Reagan's mental deterioration robbed him of the balance and coordination necessary to perform basic tasks, like walking more than a few steps down a hall unaided. In the end, he succumbed to pneumonia, perhaps caused by food being inhaled into his lungs. Such "aspiration pneumonia" is among the most common causes of death among patients with advanced Alzheimer's disease. ■

with the much rarer early-onset Alzheimer's were tentatively identified late in 2003, but it's clear there are more genes to be found. The National Institute on Aging began to recruit families with multiple Alzheimer's victims in 2002, scanning their DNA to see how the genes of the healthy differ from those of the sick. Scientists hope that a genetic test for people most at risk for the disease may emerge from this research, but they cannot say when.

➤Prevention and Care How can those most at risk improve their chances of avoiding Alzheimer's? A study conducted at Johns Hopkins University indicates that people who take a regimen of the so-called antioxidant vitamins (a combination of vitamins C and E) may reduce their risk of getting Alzheimer's by 64% to 78%. Why this might be the case is not clear, but these vitamins may absorb damaging molecules called free radicals, which are produced along with the beta-amyloid plaque found in the brains of Alzheimer's patients, before these substances can injure brain cells.

The search for drugs to alleviate Alzheimer's symptoms continues. One large-scale study dimmed the hope (raised by earlier findings) that the painkillers Aleve and Vioxx may help. A Canadian study of the efficacy of three popular drugs often prescribed for Alzheimer's—Aricept, Exelon, Reminyl—also yielded poor results: fewer than 1 in 10 patients showed any improvement in cognition after treatment.

But there was also some good news: Namenda, the first in a new class of Alzheimer's drugs, has been linked to a lower rate of cognitive decline in patients who take this drug in conjunction with Aricept. And one therapy previously thought to be a dead end—a vaccine that seems to cure the disease in mice but was abandoned in 2002 because it caused deadly brain swelling in human tests—is being reformulated to avoid harmful side effects while still erasing the beta-amyloid deposits associated with Alzheimer's. Researchers say further study is needed before new trials can begin.

■ Resources

ALZHEIMER'S ASSOCIATION SUPPORT LINE: 800-272-3900
WEBSITE: *www.alz.org*

What Alzheimer's Does to the Brain

Spreading from the bottom to the top

The disease is characterized by the gradual spread of sticky plaques and clumps of tangled fibers that disrupt the delicate organization of nerve cells in the brain. As brain cells stop communicating with one another, they atrophy—causing memory and reasoning to fade

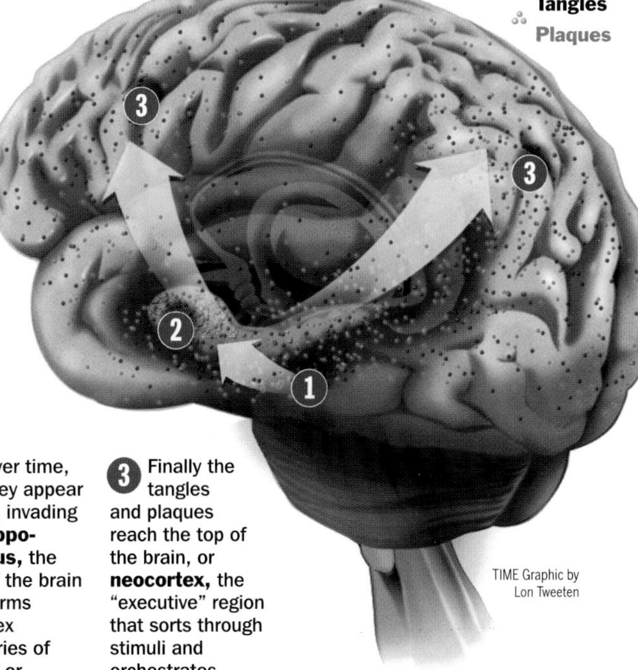

1 Tangles and plaques first develop in the **entorhinal cortex**, a memory-processing center essential for making new memories and retrieving old ones

2 Over time, they appear higher, invading the **hippocampus,** the part of the brain that forms complex memories of events or objects

3 Finally the tangles and plaques reach the top of the brain, or **neocortex,** the "executive" region that sorts through stimuli and orchestrates all behavior

TIME Graphic by Lon Tweeten

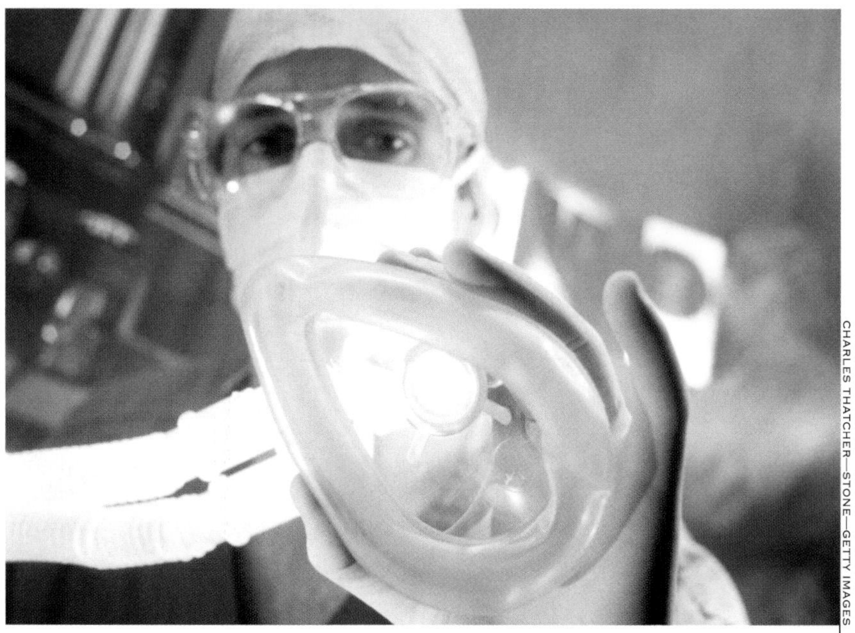
CHARLES THATCHER—STONE—GETTY IMAGES

Anesthesia

A new study of anesthesia failure, which leaves patients able to feel pain but unable to communicate it, leads to the use of monitors that can detect and report the problem

How Safe? The deaths of two women from complications of anesthesia while undergoing routine cosmetic surgery at a prestigious Manhattan hospital put both anesthesia and plastic surgery in the spotlight (*see* Body Alterations)

Anesthesia failure may sound like a leftover plot from an old *Twilight Zone* TV show, but it's for real. In this frightening event, a surgical patient under general anesthesia remains conscious on the operating table and able to feel pain, even as the sedative paralyzes him, rendering him unable to communicate his distress while surgeons cut him open. An October 2003 study concluded that anesthesia failure occurs more than 100 times a day in the U.S. The results of the study (the first U.S. research in more than 30 years to quantify "intraoperative awareness") contradict years of opinions by medical professionals who dismissed the phenomenon as myth. The findings are also in line with the last U.S. inquiry to examine the issue and are consistent with similar studies conducted abroad. This news led the FDA to approve the use of bispectral index (BIS) monitors by anesthesiologists to track the brain waves of surgical patients and reveal how deeply a patient is sleeping. One study has shown that the use of BIS monitors can reduce anesthesia failure as much as 82%.

KNOCKED OUT—NOT

In anesthesia failure, patients are awake during surgery, but unable to tell doctors they are conscious

There is also some encouraging news on the anesthesia front: a genetic test has been developed (and is now in clinical trials) to screen for a rare condition known as malignant hyperthermia, in which even minor anesthesia can throw a patient's metabolism into a life-threatening state of overdrive, breaking down muscles and raising body temperature as high as 110°. The test is expected to be available for widespread use in the fall of 2004.

■ **Resources**

NIH ANESTHESIA WEBSITE: *www.nlm.nih.gov/medlineplus/anesthesia.gov*

Antibiotics

Antibiotics are wonder drugs, but our bodies become tolerant to them if we use them too often. Doctors are right to think twice before writing a prescription

Down on the Farm The World Health Organization has reported that the common practice of feeding antibiotics to livestock to prevent disease can promote antibiotic resistance

If you have a sore throat that is accompanied by a fever but not a cough, your lymph nodes are swollen, and there are yellow or white patches on your tonsils or the back of your throat, chances are, the problem is a kind of bacteria called Group A *Streptococcus*—or strep, for short. That's when antibiotics like penicillin or erythromycin come in handy.

The trouble is, most sore throats, even those with a runny nose and cough, are usually just a cold. Most of the time, colds are caused by viruses and can be treated with chicken soup and a painkiller like acetaminophen.

It's not always easy, even for doctors, to tell the difference between viral and bacterial infections on the basis of symptoms alone.

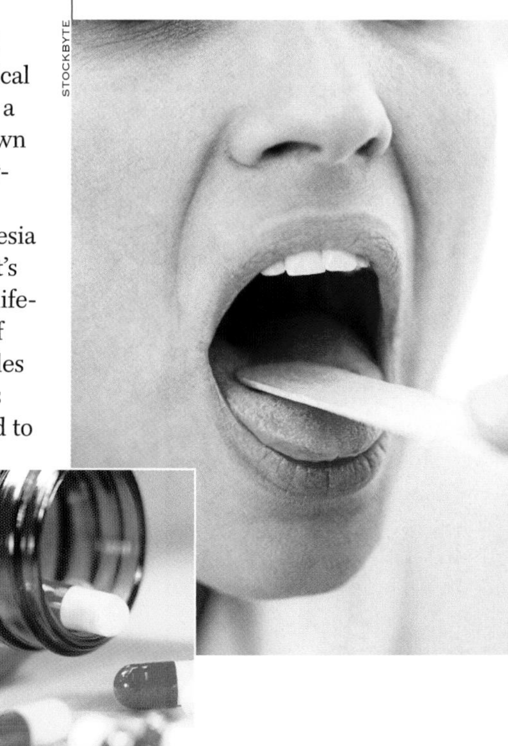
STOCKBYTE

DAVID AUBREY—CORBIS

A new study has shown that doctors guess wrong about these symptoms as often as 40% of the time. This leads to the widespread overuse of antibiotics, which reduces their effectiveness, rendering some varieties of strep (and other potentially serious bacterial infections) resistant to most known antibiotics.

For decades, the main reason to treat strep throat was to make sure it didn't get a chance to turn into rheumatic fever, a serious illness that can damage the heart. But for reasons that are not clear, the incidence of the disease has dropped dramatically in most of the U.S. since the 1930s. And studies have shown that many adults get over mild strep infections without taking antibiotics. Children, who are more susceptible to strep and rheumatic fever, are usually treated more aggressively.

The study showed that doctors get the best results if they rely on a microbiologic lab test—either a two-day throat culture or a somewhat less accurate 20-min. rapid-response test. So be patient if your doctor swabs your sore throat or your child's instead of immediately prescribing antibiotics. That will increase the chances that the drugs will still work when you really need them.

➤Livestock Farmers also overuse antibiotics, often dosing the feed given to livestock in the belief that the drugs will ward off infection and promote growth. But a new study released by the World Health Organization seemed to show just the opposite, concluding that farm animals not fed antibiotics suffer no significant health consequences and their bodies are host to far fewer drug-resistant bacteria. Whether the findings will change the practices of the farming industry remains to be seen.

■ Resources

NIH WEBSITE: *www.nlm.nih.gov/medlineplus/antibiotics*

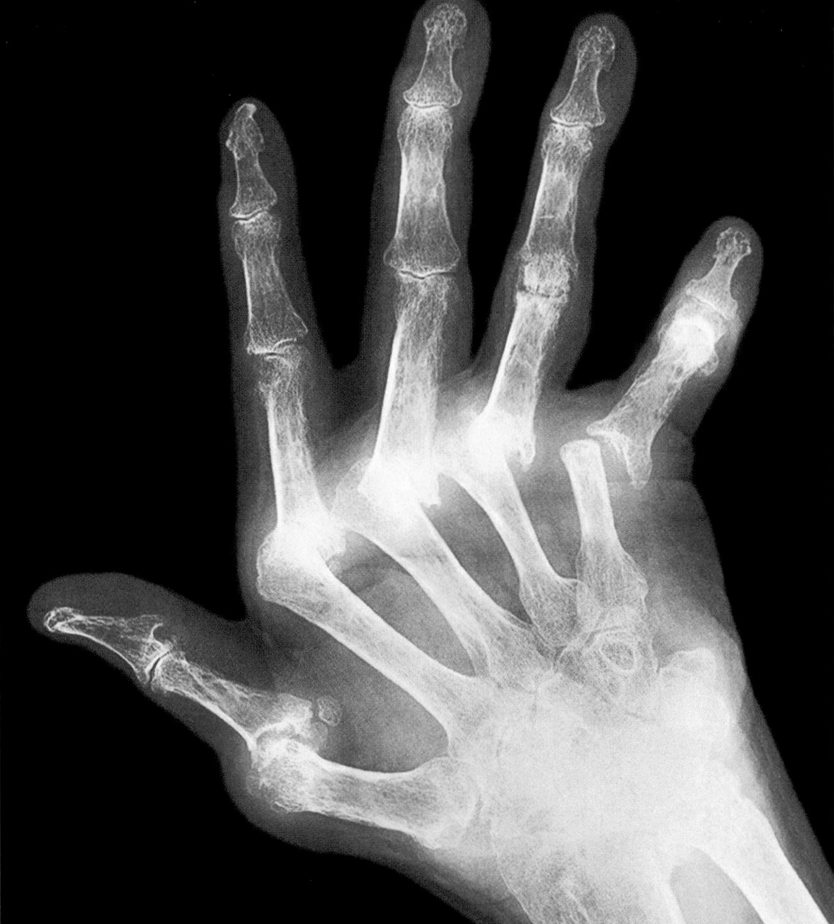

CNRI—PHOTO RESEARCHERS

Arthritis

New therapies, new technologies and new insights into treatment for osteoarthritis are emerging. We're also learning to manage rheumatoid arthritis better

By the Numbers 1 in 4 U.S. adults has been diagnosed with some form of arthritis, while an additional 17% may have the disease without knowing it

Arthritis is currently the leading cause of disability in the U.S., yet the number of those afflicted by its most common form, osteoarthritis, is expected to increase dramatically in coming years as the baby boomer generation reaches the condition's peak range.

There are two distinct forms of arthritis. Osteoarthritis is a degenerative disease that attacks the cartilage in the body's joints and often afflicts older people. The ailment is proving to be far more complex in origin and progression than we had previously believed.

Rheumatoid arthritis, which is much less common, is considered a disease of the immune system, and is characterized by inflammation of the joints. Affecting some 1% of the world's population, it is two to three times more likely to strike women than men.

➤Treating Osteoarthritis Modern medicine still has a way to go in understanding the origin and development of osteoarthritis. The process of discovery is complex, for the disease can apparently be set off by a number of factors, including changes in the tendons and ligaments that support our joints by anchoring muscle to bone. Inflammation, the immune system's response to many ailments—whose side effects are currently being implicated as an agent in many diseases (*see* Inflammation)—also seems to play a role in causing the swelling that accompanies some cases of osteoarthritis.

Until we better understand the origins of osteoarthritis and can

ANATOMY OF A BREAKDOWN

Doctors used to think that failing cartilage caused osteoarthritis. Now they know it is a complex process involving muscles, tendons, bones—even genes

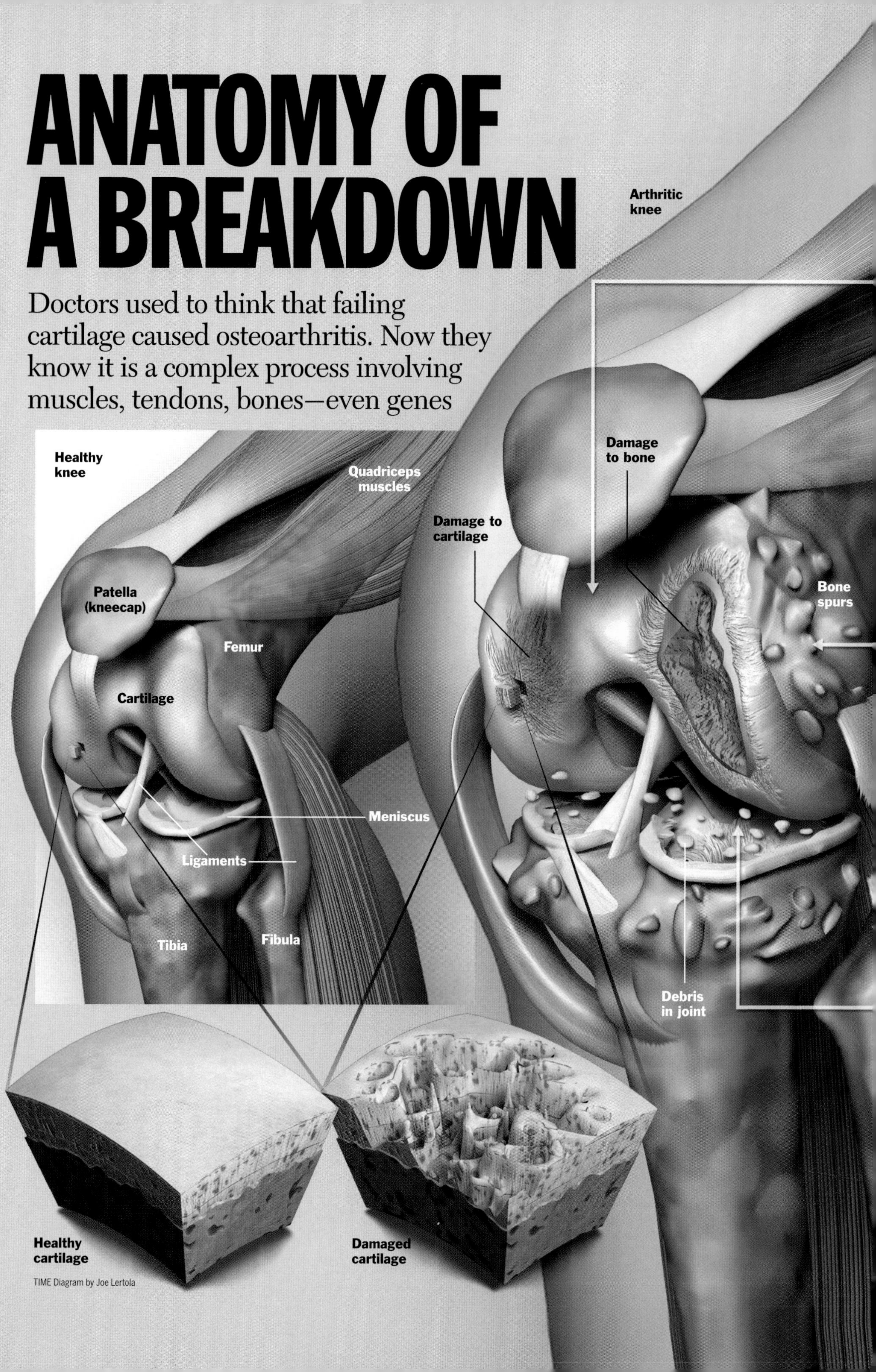

TIME Diagram by Joe Lertola

A HOST OF CULPRITS

CARTILAGE: Made up of water, proteins and sugars, cartilage is the body's shock absorber. Injury, age and many other factors can cause cartilage to break down, but the end result is the same: without its cushion, bones start to grind against one another

MUSCLES: These support the joints. The quadriceps, for example, are responsible for holding up the knee and relieving some of the stress of walking and running. Weak quads can put too much strain on the joint, leading to tears in the tendons

BONE: While bone normally responds to eroding cartilage by sending out spurs and other odd growths, sometimes it's the other way around: changes in bone structure that affect the shape of a joint can trigger a breakdown in the cartilage

TENDONS AND LIGAMENTS: By connecting and anchoring muscles and bones, these provide support for the joint. If they are torn in an injury or weakened from lack of use, the cartilage in the knee is forced to bear more weight, hastening its collapse

INFLAMMATION: As cartilage degrades, immune cells swoop in to engulf and destroy the dying tissue. In their zeal, they even attack healthy tissue. The debris, including toxic enzymes, can build up in the fluid of the joint, causing painful swelling

GENES: More than half of arthritis sufferers are born with mutations in their genes that control cartilage formation and destruction. These aberrations can result in cartilage that is weaker to begin with or that degrades faster than it should

thus hope to prevent it, doctors and health-care professionals are doing their best to find the optimal combination of diet, exercise and drugs to alleviate its symptoms.

Some of the most promising treatments for osteoarthritis don't directly treat the body's joints. For older patients, a new study has shown that receiving care for depression can significantly lessen the impact of pain associated with osteoarthritis of the knee.

A second study found that overweight seniors who suffer from osteoarthritis may be able to improve their quality of life significantly by losing weight through a routine of diet or exercise or (ideally) both. Losing weight reduces the pressure on those painful joints.

What kind of exercise is best for elderly patients suffering from osteoarthritis? A study of both hip and knee patients found that hydrotherapy (exercising in a swimming pool) improves mobility about as much as exercising in a gym, but with a much greater reduction in joint pain.

In 2003 the *New England Journal of Medicine* published the results of a clinical trial showing that Celebrex, a long-used drug for treating the pain of degrading cartilage, does not protect patients against bleeding ulcers (a common side effect of arthritis medications) as well as previously believed. On the other hand, a different study found Celebrex may help combat heart disease by improving blood-vessel flexibility and lessening inflammation.

➤Treating Rheumatoid Arthritis

For years, many doctors have advised those suffering from rheumatoid arthritis to avoid physical activity, concerned that exercise might further aggravate their patients' already inflamed joints. But a recent study has shown that while regular exercise doesn't appear to yield the same benefits in pain reduction to victims of rheumatoid arthritis that it does for those with osteoarthritis, neither does it increase pain or joint swelling in rheumatoid arthritis sufferers. In the meantime, exercise can improve mobility and reduce the psychological stress that is a serious byproduct of this irritating, unrelenting disease.

On the pharmaceutical front, in 2003 the FDA gave fast-track approval to Humira, a new drug that helps relieve the symptoms of rheumatoid arthritis.

High Heels: Not Guilty

Women who can't bear to give up their Manolos can breathe a bit easier. Although osteoarthritis afflicts the knees of twice as many women as men, tottering around in high heels is apparently not the cause. A new study found that the rates of osteoarthritis of the knee in a group of 111 women between ages 50 and 70 were not affected by their heels, no matter how often they wore them or how high the heels were.

Factors that did increase risk: previous knee injury, heavy smoking, osteoarthritis of the feet and, most important, having been overweight (with a BMI of 25 or higher). ■

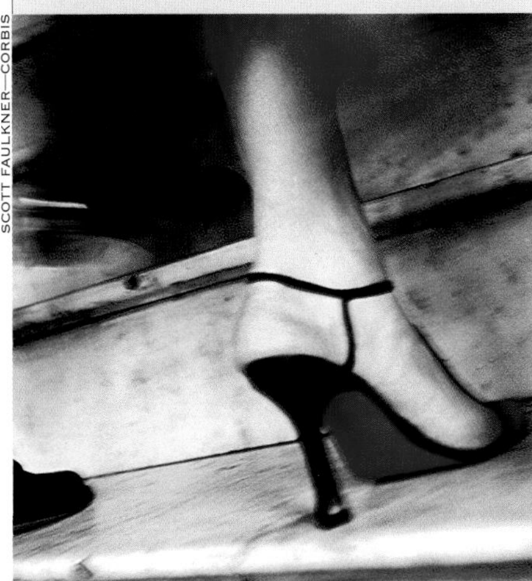

SCOTT FAULKNER—CORBIS

■ Resources

ARTHRITIS FOUNDATION:
www.arthritis.org; 800-283-7800
ARTHRITIS SOCIETY:
www.arthritis.ca; 800-321-1433
HUMIRA WEBSITE:
www.humira.com

Aspirin

Research continues to reveal the benefits of aspirin: studies show that it may help ward off the most common form of breast cancer and that it lowers the risk of developing the polyps that precede colorectal cancer

Hold Off, for Now Despite the good news on breast cancer, doctors do not yet recommend that all women take aspirin daily, as it may lead to internal bleeding

Talk about second acts! Aspirin, which humans have been taking for more than 100 years now to fight headaches and other pains, is turning out to be a sort of all-purpose wonder drug that helps prevent a number of major ailments, including heart attacks and strokes, when consumed in moderate amounts. In 2004 alone, studies showed that aspirin may help ward off breast cancer and colorectal cancer. Aspirin use carries the possibility, however, of such side effects as internal gastric bleeding, so you should consult a doctor before beginning a regimen of aspirin use.

➤Breast Cancer In a Columbia University study released in May 2004, researchers tracked more than 2,800 women—about half of whom had breast cancer—and found that those who took aspirin seven or more times a week had a 26% lower risk of

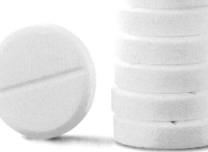

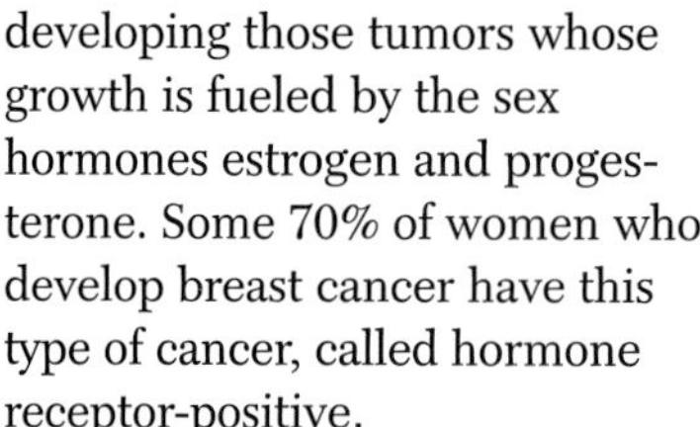

developing those tumors whose growth is fueled by the sex hormones estrogen and progesterone. Some 70% of women who develop breast cancer have this type of cancer, called hormone receptor-positive.

Women in the study who used aspirin at least four times a week for at least three months were almost 30% less likely to develop hormone-fueled breast cancer than women who used no aspirin. The effect was strongest in older, post-menopausal women. Aspirin had no effect on the risk of developing the other type of tumor, hormone receptor-negative. The study did not yield conclusive results as to whether ibuprofen and acetaminophen offer a similar preventive value.

Doctors say it's too early to recommend aspirin to all women, but those already using the drug may have another reason to keep taking it.

➤Colorectal Cancer A study of more than 27,000 female nurses found that those who used two or more 325-mg aspirin tablets a week had a 25% lower risk of developing adenomas—pre-cancerous polyps in the colon—than those who used aspirin less frequently. Those participants who used more than 14 tablets a week had half the risk of those nurses who used no aspirin at all.

■ Resources

FDA ADVISORY ON ASPIRIN THERAPY: *w.fda.gov/fdac/features/2003/503_aspirin*

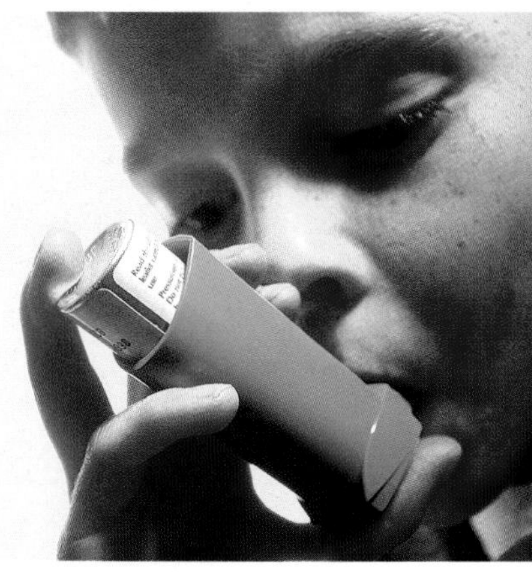

JOHN MILLER—STONE—GETTY

Asthma

More Americans are suffering from asthma—the number is up from 6.7 million in 1980 to close to 20 million today. The FDA has approved a new drug that fights the disease, but it's expensive

The Bottom Line Each year, asthma sufferers account for 500,000 hospital admissions and 2 million emergency room visits. Asthma's total cost to the U.S. economy every year: $11 billion

ASTHMA HOT SPOTS

Here is the list of the 10 worst cities in the U.S. for asthmatics, from the Allergy and Asthma Foundation of America

1. Knoxville, Tenn.
2. Little Rock, Ark.
3. St. Louis, Mo.
4. Madison, Wis.
5. Louisville, Ky.
6. Memphis, Tenn.
7. Toledo, Ohio
8. Kansas City, Mo.
9. Nashville, Tenn.
10. Hartford, Conn.

As the number of America's asthmatics grows, researchers are heightening their efforts to understand and treat the disease. Here's the latest from the asthma front:

➤Treatment In 2003 the FDA approved sale of a new drug, Xolair, that in a study of more than 6,000 asthma sufferers reduced the number of attacks by one-half. The drug is a synthetic antibody, a custom-made version of the thousands of antibodies the immune system produces to knock out blood-borne microbes. It is specially designed to wipe out another antibody, IgE, the root cause of all allergic disease.

The new drug also promises to radically reduce the number of medications asthmatics must take. But it is costly: Xolair's price ranges from about $8,000 to $10,000 a year. While the drug will probably cut the overall cost of treating asthma, its expense will limit its use to patients with severe disease. The drug's developers are exploring its effect on hay fever and on those with peanut allergies.

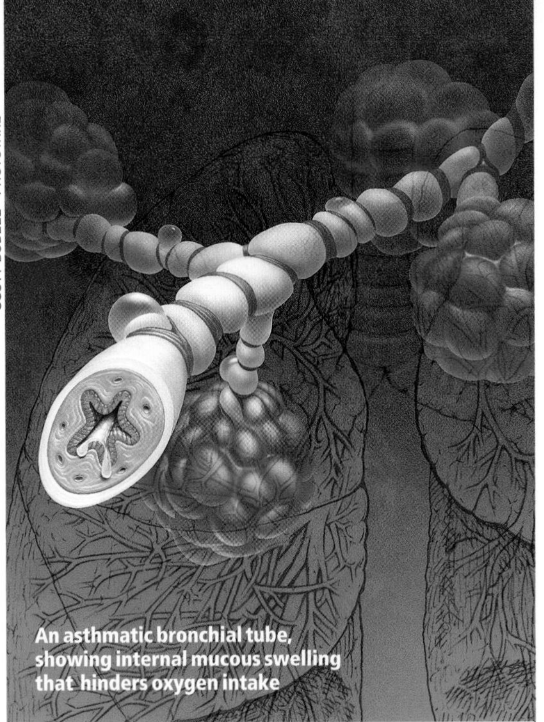

SCOTT BODELL—PHOTOTAKE

An asthmatic bronchial tube, showing internal mucous swelling that hinders oxygen intake

➤A Link to Ear Infections Children's ear infections can be quickly cured and are generally regarded as minor ailments, but one new study found that such infections may be linked to asthma. In a study of more than 7,500 kids ages 2 to 11, University of Illinois at Chicago scientists found that children who suffered three or more ear infections in their lifetime were twice as likely as children with no ear problems to have asthma.

It's not clear what the two diseases have in common; one possibility is that the bacteria that cause ear infections may play a role in the development of asthma. It could also be that the antibiotics used to clear up ear infections somehow increase a child's asthma risk. The study also showed that children's ear-infection rates go up as their parents' education level increases. A possible explanation: those kids tend to spend more time in day care, where more social contact breeds more risk.

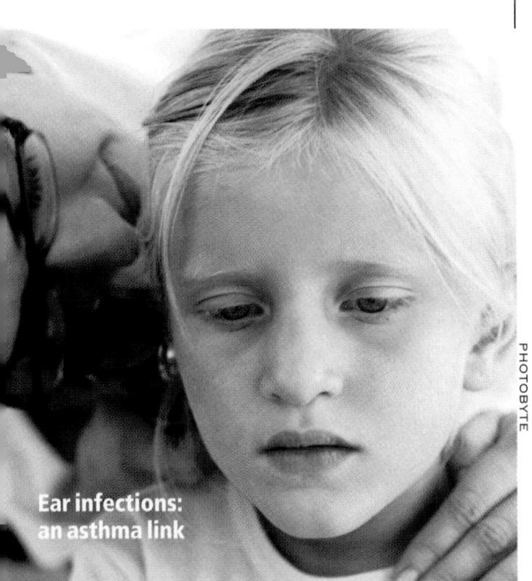

PHOTOBYTE

Ear infections: an asthma link

➤Other Recent Findings Many chronic asthma sufferers inhale corticosteroids to reduce their wheezing symptoms, but high doses of steroids have such side effects as increasing one's susceptibility to bruising, cataracts and glaucoma. Earlier studies suggested that people with mild asthma might be able to reduce their dose of steroids while still enjoying the benefits of the drug. A 2003 study confirmed this finding, and that's good news for asthmatics.

Another 2003 study found that parent-administered oral steroids—which are sometimes recommended to aid the wheezing symptoms of children under 5—are not particularly effective. Researchers found little difference in symptoms between a group taking the steroid prednisolone and a group that took a regimen of placebos.

■ **Resources**

XOLAIR: *www.xolair.com*

NIH ASTHMA CENTER: *www.nlm.nih.gov/medlineplus/asthma*

ASTHMA & ALLERGY FOUNDATION: *www.aafa.org*

Autism

British researchers retract a controversial report that linked autism to childhood vaccinations, and the search for clues to the mystery of autism goes on

The Cost Children with autism and its milder cousin, Asperger's syndrome—neurologically based developmental disorders—have trouble communicating; lack appropriate social skills; and display, unusual, repetitive behavior

British researchers caused a furor in 1998 when they published a controversial report suggesting a link between the growing number of autism cases and the standard childhood vaccine for measles, mumps and rubella (MMR). The report touched off a firestorm: although other physicians criticized the authors for jumping to conclusions, many worried parents stopped immunizing their children. Early in 2004, 10 of the 13 original authors decided to retract the paper, acknowledging that their data were not strong enough to support their incendiary conclusion.

PROBING THE ENIGMA

Scientists are hoping a study of 100,000 infants in Norway may help unlock the mysteries of autism

In February 2004 the National Institutes of Health announced it would help fund a long-term study of 100,000 infants in Norway to probe the causes of autism. The research will measure diet, vaccination, birth weight and head circumference, as well as exposures to toxins (including mercury, long suspected as a factor in autism). Scientists now believe that some children have a strong genetic predisposition to the disease that may be set off by environmental exposure—but they cannot identify the triggers.

■ **Resources**

WEBSITES: NATIONAL ALLIANCE FOR AUTISM RESEARCH: *www.naar.org*

THE AUTISM SOCIETY OF AMERICA: *www.autism-society.org*

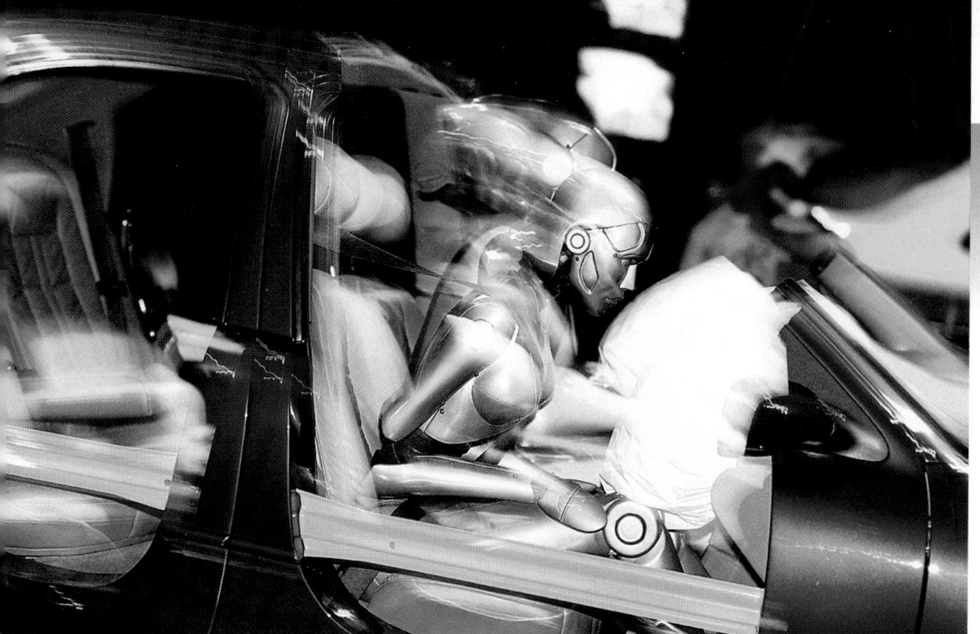

Auto Safety

When should older drivers give up their keys? Concerned seniors—and their relatives—shouldn't wait to ask some tough questions

Side Effects Statistics show that side air bags in cars save lives and may ultimately be as vital as seat belts, especially when they offer head protection to travelers

It's dangerous out on the roads, so a new report from the Insurance Institute for Highway Safety suggests car buyers invest in side air bags with head protection. Drivers whose vehicles had such devices were 53% less likely to die in a crash than those without them, according to government figures.

Sometimes air bags aren't the issue: when Russell Weller, 86, lost control of his 1992 Buick at a California farmers' market in July 2003, he injured 40 people and killed 10. With 16% of all drivers 65 or older and with that figure expected to rise to 25% by 2030, families are worried anew about when it's safe for seniors to drive and when it may be time to take away the keys.

No one denies that the skills necessary for good driving decline with age, even if they decline at different rates for different people. One way to make sure that older family members are not road hazards is to ride with or follow the driver during an outing. Checking the car for dents can help too.

Concerned seniors should ask themselves some tough questions: Do traffic distractions at intersections confuse me? Does glare bother me? Do I get lost a lot? Am I taking any medications that could affect my alertness? For drivers over 55, some organizations offer quizzes to help determine driving fitness; one address is below.

Ultimately, family members may have to confiscate the keys—perhaps with the help of a doctor. If necessary, you can secretly call the police department and ask an officer to dissuade your elderly relative from taking to the road, at least for that day. In some states, you or a doctor can contact the department of motor vehicles and request a re-examination of an older driver—which can lead to license suspension or even revocation. Loss of mobility is tough for seniors, but loss of control behind the wheel is worse.

CRASH COURSE

Drivers whose vehicles had side air bags with head protection were 53% less likely to die in a crash than those in cars without them

---

■ Resources

WEBSITES: *Seniordrivers.org*

AAA WEB QUIZ: *aaafoundation.org/quizzes*

B

Bipolar Disorder

Once known as manic depression, bipolar disorder leads to ferocious mood swings. The disease runs in families, and now family therapy is promising to help relieve it

In Brief A 2004 study probed the efficacy of lithium, the standard medication to control bipolar disorder, against two newer drugs, divalproex and carbamazepine. Lithium proved more effective in preventing suicide than the newer drugs

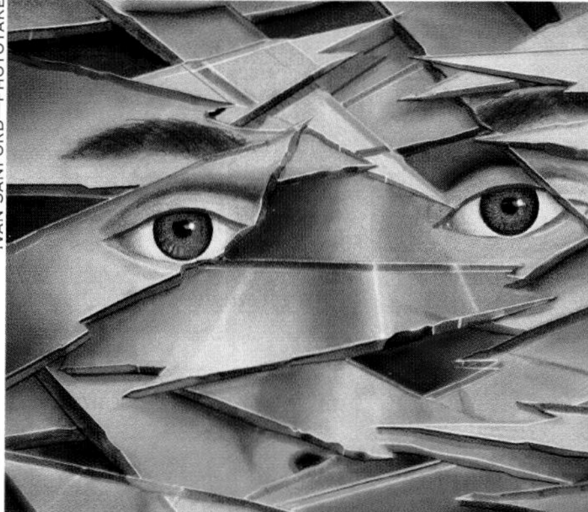

IVAN SANFORD—PHOTOTAKE

Bipoloar disorder is a family affair; according to one expert, it is "hugely familial." Children with one bipolar parent have a 10% to 30% chance of developing the condition; a bipolar sibling means a 20% risk; if both parents are bipolar, the danger rises as high as 75%. Now there is hope that family action in the form of therapy may help alleviate some of the symptoms of the ailment.

In recent years, mood-controlling drugs like lithium have helped doctors balance the intense mood swings associated with the disease. But some 60% of patients on medications relapse within two years and can experience some of the typical swings between euphoria and depression even earlier than that. In a new study, bipolar patients took part in intensive courses of family-based therapy with spouses, parents and siblings to learn about symptoms and strategies for preventing a relapse. Some 35% of those who received family therapy suffered a relapse, compared with 54% of those who had no therapy. The family groups also prolonged the intervals between relapses.

Resources

NIMH WEBSITE: *www.nimh.nih.gov/healthinformation/bipolarmenu.cfmov*

Birth Control

A male birth control pill may be on the horizon, say researchers in Australia, but it involves implants to regulate testosterone levels

Monthly Reprieve A new birth control pill works on a 91-day cycle, allowing women to exercise more control over the timing of their menstrual periods

A PILL FOR MEN?

Researchers Down Under believe they will bring a male birth-control pill to market within five years

The sexual revolution, Part 2, has begun at last, according to a 2003 study out of Australia. For one year, 55 men took an experimental birth control drug. All of them had fertile partners; none of the women got pregnant. The men reported no serious side effects, other than a slightly elevated libido (which some people pay good money for).

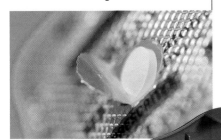

While women ovulate only once a month, men produce millions of sperm every day, which poses big challenges for a male "pill." Birth control pills for women are effective almost immediately. For men, it takes longer for a drug to start working and to wear off—about three months. Researchers used a dose of the hormone progestin to turn off sperm production. The problem is that this also suppresses testosterone production. So in order to avoid unpleasant side effects like lethargy and sexual dysfunction, most recent trials also gave men testosterone supplements via implants. The bad news: it will take at least five years and many more studies before a male birth control drug hits the market.

➤Regulating Menstruation And lest we forget the ladies: a new birth control pill called Seasonale helps women control menstrual periods. Approved in the fall of 2003 by the FDA, the pill contains the same ingredients found in the original Pill but works on a 91-day cycle instead of the traditional 28. Women take active-ingredient pills 84 days in a row, then placebos for the final week, reducing the number of periods from 13 a year to just four. One caveat: test subjects using Seasonale experienced nearly two weeks of bleeding during their first cycle. The abnormal flow, however, diminished over time.

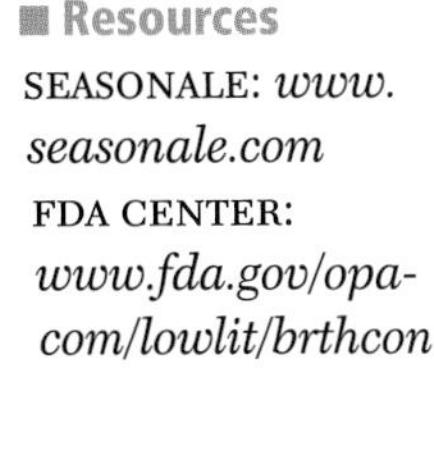

Resources

SEASONALE: *www.seasonale.com*

FDA CENTER: *www.fda.gov/opacom/lowlit/brthcon*

Blood

Experimental tests put in place in 2003 screen the U.S. blood supply, keeping West Nile virus at bay

Warning Deep vein thrombosis, a blood-clotting risk for airline passengers, is also a danger for patients confined in hospitals

Americans got a scare in 2003 when it was reported that West Nile virus had entered the U.S. blood supply. However, nearly 1,000 units of blood infected with West Nile virus were kept out of the blood supply in 2004 because of new, experimental tests that screened virtually all blood donated since July 1, 2003.

➤Deep Vein Thrombosis New research shows that nearly a third of all adults have a hard-to-detect heart defect called patent fora-

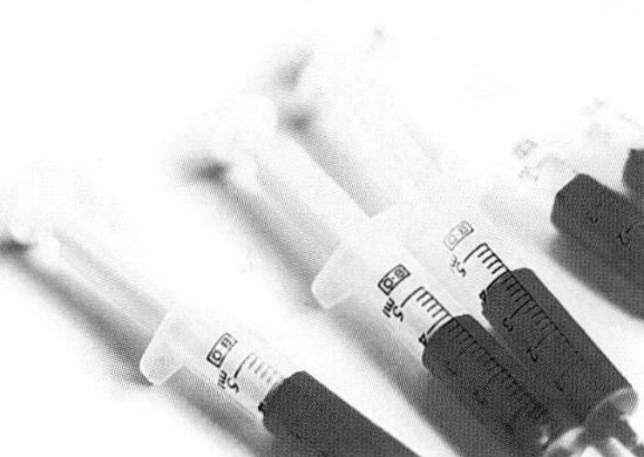

NICK DAVID—PHOTONICA

men ovale (PFO), which may contribute to deep vein thrombosis (DVT, a.k.a. "economy-class syndrome")—clots that form in the legs after long periods of inactivity. Yet while airlines take care to warn passengers about the signs of DVT and take steps to prevent it, a 2004 study found that hospitals, where patients sometimes remain sedentary for days after surgery, are among the most dangerous places for people at risk of DVT—and that hospitals do less than airlines to prevent it.

Resources

NIH DVT WEBSITE: *www.nhlbi.nih.gov/health/dci/Diseases/Dvt/DVT_WhatIs*

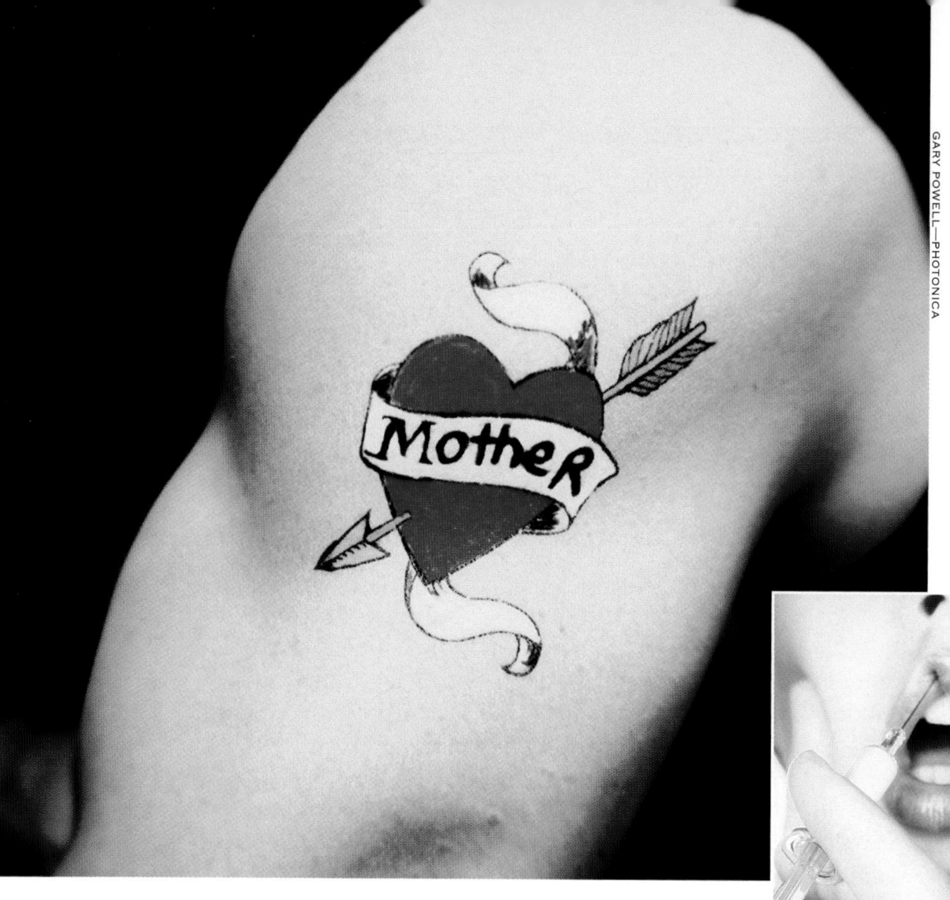

GARY POWELL—PHOTONICA

Body Alterations and Cosmetic Surgery

Cosmetic surgery is booming, but patients are not taking the proper precautions to assure their safety

By the Numbers Cosmetic procedures by plastic surgeons have increased 293% since 1997. Some 8.3 million Americans underwent cosmetic surgery in 2003

Once upon a time, tattoos were for troublemakers and piercing was for punks. But in the 1990s body modifications entered the mainstream, at least for young people. The end isn't in sight: the latest fad in the Netherlands is a tiny charm that is surgically inserted under the mucus membrane of the eye. At the same time, cosmetic surgery lost its taint. With such reality TV shows as Fox's *The Swan* now promoting plastic surgery as routine—even in cases involving extreme transformations requiring multiple procedures—interest in body alterations is exploding. The term makeover once suggested little more than a new eye shadow or a dye job. Now it is just as likely to result in a straighter nose, leaner thighs and a brow in no danger of furrowing. Stomach stapling, which should be a last-resort, radical treatment for obesity, is becoming more common, even among children. That these procedures involve anesthesia, injections, and all the risks of major surgery, is a distinction increasingly lost on the general population.

➤How Safe Is the Surgery? Plastic surgery does mean going under the knife, and lately there have been plenty of reminders of the risks involved. From May 2003 to January 2004, five people in Florida died following cosmetic plastic surgery performed in doctors' offices. Early in 2004, two women died of complications from anesthesia after plastic surgery at a prestigious Manhattan hospital. One of them—*The First Wives Club* author Olivia Goldsmith, whose work often satirized the plastic-surgery lifestyle—died in a seemingly routine chin-tuck procedure.

In fact, the vast majority of cosmetic procedures succeed without incident. But with the number of these operations skyrocketing, and with the increasing popularity of so-called extreme makeovers, in which doctors perform many procedures over a short period of time, things can end badly more often. One problem: it is not legally necessary for a person to train as a plastic surgeon to practice the surgery; a medical degree suffices. So it's up to the patient to monitor the surgeon and decide whether he or she is comfortable with their training. A patient should also investigate the facility where a procedure is to be performed.

CONEYL JAY—STONE—GETTY

➤Stomach Stapling Perhaps fueled by the

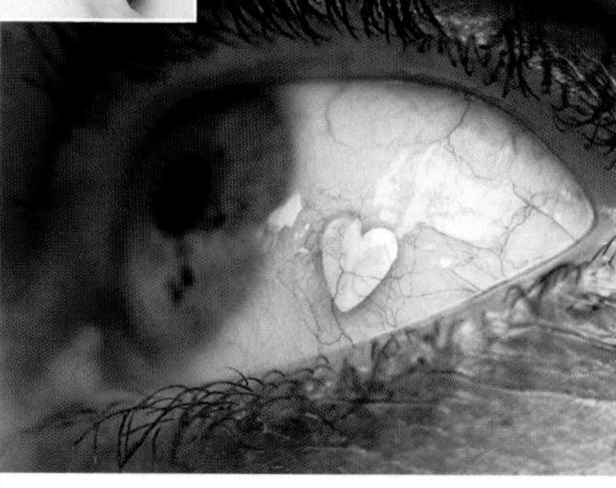

MICHEL PORRO—GETTY IMAGES

HOW THE SURGERY WORKS

1 NORMAL DIGESTION

Food is chewed and descends through the **esophagus** into the **stomach,** where a strong acid further breaks it up. Then it travels through the **small intestine,** where nutrients are absorbed. Whatever cannot be digested is stored in the **large intestine** until it is eliminated

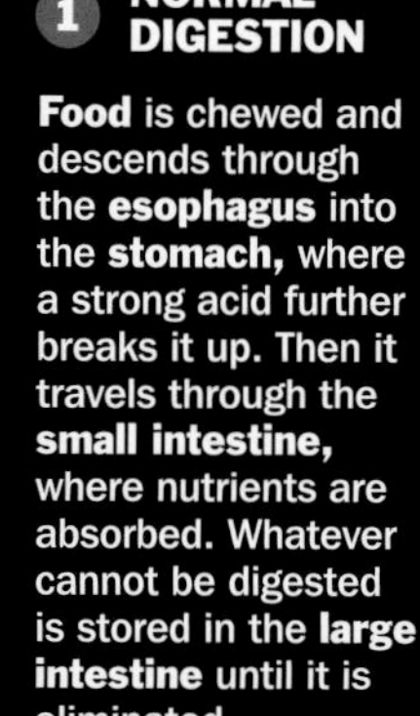

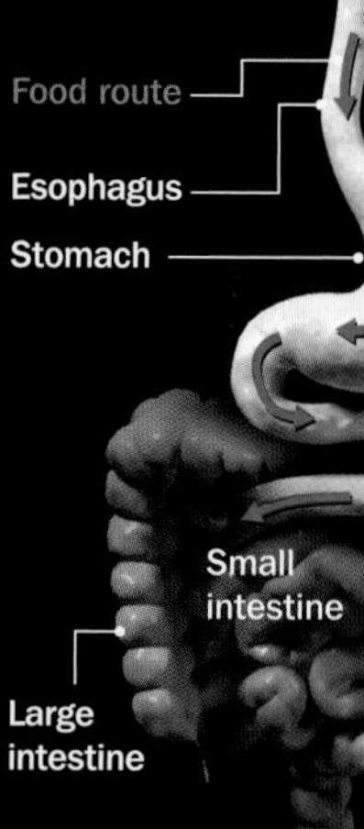

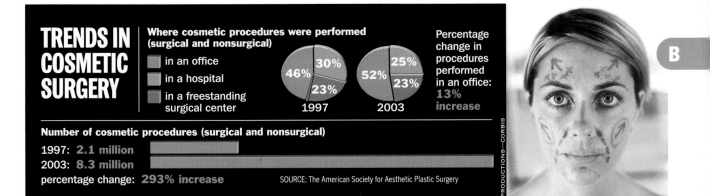

TRENDS IN COSMETIC SURGERY

Where cosmetic procedures were performed (surgical and nonsurgical)

- in an office
- in a hospital
- in a freestanding surgical center

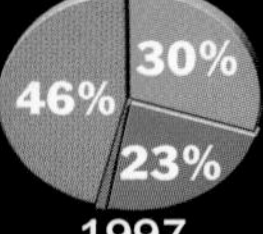

	in an office	in a hospital	in a freestanding surgical center
1997	46%	30%	23%
2003	52%	25%	23%

Percentage change in procedures performed in an office: 13% increase

Number of cosmetic procedures (surgical and nonsurgical)

1997: 2.1 million

2003: 8.3 million

percentage change: 293% increase

SOURCE: The American Society for Aesthetic Plastic Surgery

ER PRODUCTIONS—CORBIS

successful operation performed on NBC's popular *Today Show* weatherman Al Roker, gastric bypass surgery, also known as stomach stapling, has boomed in popularity. The procedure radically alters the size and shape of the stomach and shortens the length of the small intestine so that the body can no longer take in normal amounts of food. Eat more than five or six bites, and you will feel the same nauseous sensation you get when you overeat. Patients must take supplements for the rest of their lives to avoid serious nutritional deficiencies.

The operation should not be undertaken lightly. Yet now a dozen hospitals around the U.S. either have started doing gastric bypasses on obese teens or are planning to, though no one knows what the life-altering surgery may do to someone who is still growing. Even under the best circumstances, there are substantial risks: as many as 1 in 100 obese adult patients dies from the procedure. "This is a treatment of last resort," says Dr. Thomas Inge of Cincinnati Children's Hospital. "The bar should be higher for adolescents than it is for adults." Experts are strongly urging teens and their parents to explore alternatives to gastric bypass surgery before teens undergo the life-altering surgery.

Silicone Bounces Back

After a lengthy review process, the F.D.A. ruled in November 2003 that silicone breast implants, banned since 1992, could return to the market. Their sale was halted in 1992 because of concerns that leaking implants could cause serious illness. Later studies could not directly link the implants to the myriad chronic diseases that had been attributed to them. The FDA ordered manufacturers of the implants to follow patients for 10 years, to inform potential subjects about scarring, ruptures and other complications, and to advise implantees to have annual exams to check for slow leaks.

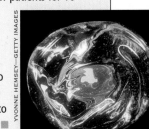

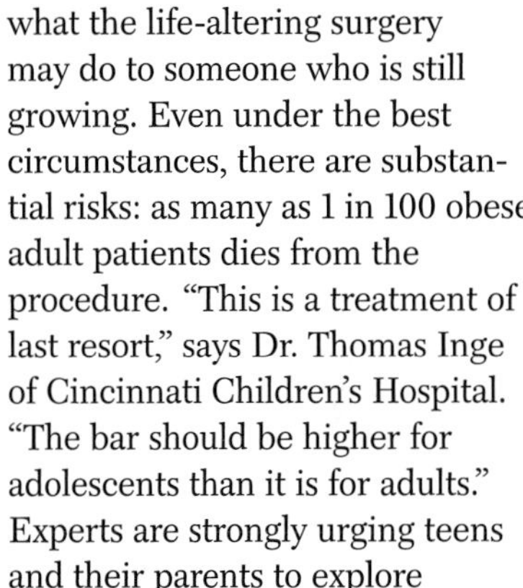

YVONNE HEMSEY—GETTY IMAGES

Resources

NIEH WEBSITE: *www.niehs.nih.gov/multimedia/qt/diversity/2004/duwlp/home*

WHAT CAN GO WRONG

2 STOMACH IS STAPLED

Surgeons divide and **staple** the stomach so that only a **pouch** the size of an egg can receive food. After the operation, meals consist of a few small bites that must be chewed extremely well (recommended: at least 30 times per morsel)

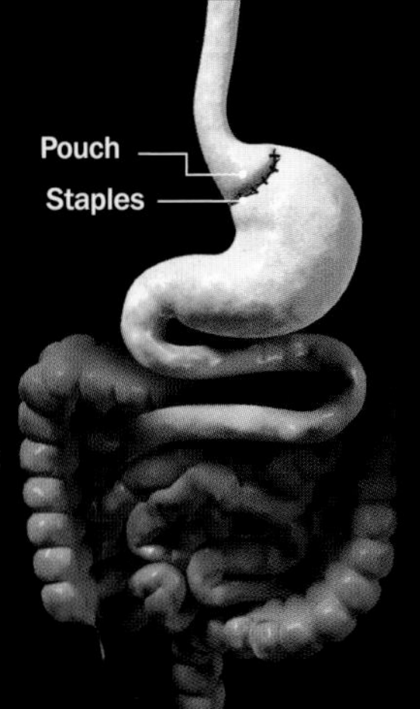

3 GASTRIC TRACT IS REROUTED

The stomach **pouch** is attached to the **small intestine.** Surgeons fashion the **new connection** about a third of the way down the small intestine, greatly reducing the number of calories and nutrients the body can absorb

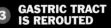

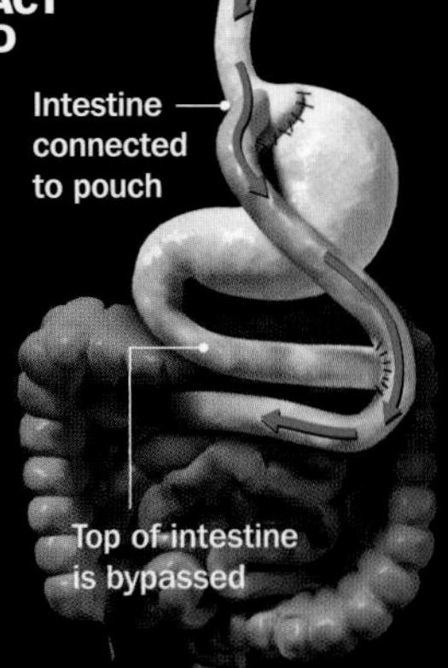

- **Death** About 1 in 100 patients undergoing gastric bypass dies as a result of the operation
- **Sugar dumping** Once the top third of the small intestine has been bypassed, the body can no longer easily handle sugars and other refined foods. Ingesting them can lead to violent vomiting and/or diarrhea
- **Osteoporosis** Bones don't mature completely until our 20s, and gastric bypass makes it harder for the body to absorb calcium
- **Anemia** The body also has trouble absorbing iron

Source: The National Institute of Diabetes and Digestive and Kidney Diseases
Time Diagram by Ed Gabel

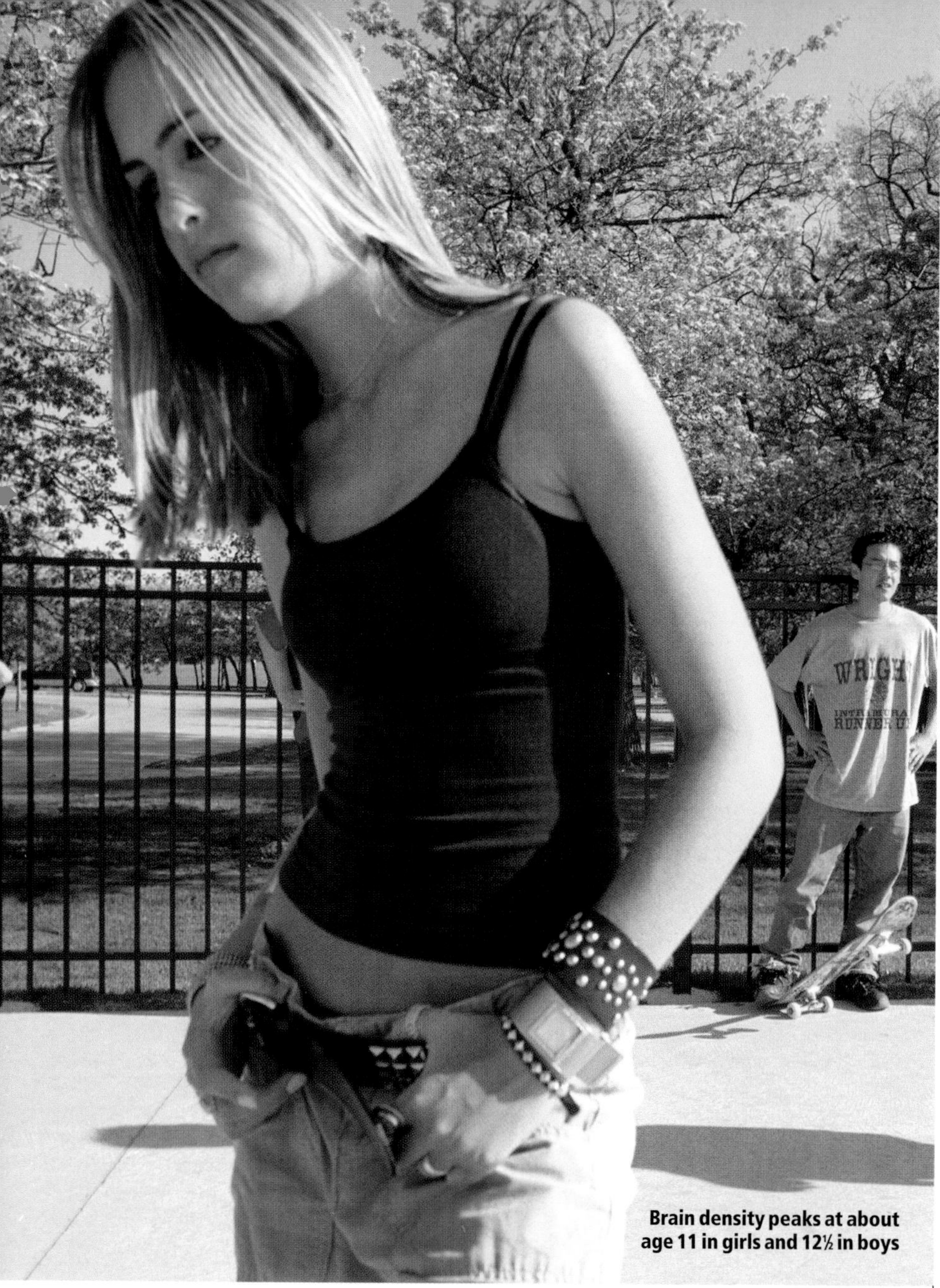

Brain density peaks at about age 11 in girls and 12½ in boys

KATRINA WITTKAMP

Brain

What makes teenagers act ... like teenagers? As new technology reveals the brain at work, we're finding that your rebel may indeed have a cause: a physiological one

Unfinished Symphony The big news: our brains do not fully form until well after the years of adolescence—and that helps explain the conflicts and cares of teens

Every parent knows that adolescence is a tempestuous period, and now science is illuminating why. Magnetic resonance imaging (MRI) scanning technologies are detailing how our brains grow and mature over time. And scientists are finding that not only is the brain of the adolescent far from mature but both its gray and white matter undergo extensive structural changes well past puberty.

The new images have opened surprising vistas on the developing brain, and the newly detected physiological changes help account for the adolescent behaviors so familiar to parents: emotional outbursts, reckless risk taking and rule breaking, and the impassioned pursuit of sex, drugs and rock 'n' roll. Increasingly, the wild conduct once blamed on "raging hormones" is being seen as the by-product of two factors: a surfeit of hormones, yes, but also a paucity of the cognitive controls needed for mature behavior.

➤Construction Ahead One reason scientists have been surprised by the ferment in the teen brain is that the organ grows very little over the course of childhood. By the time a child is 6, it is 90% to 95% of its adult size. In fact, we are born equipped with most of the neurons our brain will ever have—and that's fewer than we have in utero. Humans achieve maximum brain-cell density between the third and sixth month of gestation, the culmination of an explosive period of prenatal neural growth.

During the final months before birth, our brains undergo a dramatic pruning in which unnecessary brain cells are eliminated. New long-term studies have documented that there is a second wave of proliferation and pruning that occurs later in childhood and that the final, critical part of this second wave, affecting some of our highest mental functions, occurs in the late teens.

Unlike the prenatal changes, this neural waxing and waning alters not the number of nerve cells but the number of connections, or synapses, between them. When a child is between the ages of 6 and 12, the neurons grow bushier, each making dozens of connections to other neurons and creating new pathways for nerve signals. The thickening of all this gray matter—the neurons and their branchlike dendrites—peaks when girls are about 11 and boys 12½, at which point a serious round of pruning is under way.

Gray matter is thinned at a rate of about 0.7% a year, tapering off in the early 20s. As a result, the brain becomes a more efficient machine, but there is a trade-off: it is probably losing some of its raw potential for learning and its ability to recover from trauma.

However a particular brain turns

out, its development proceeds in stages, generally from back to front. The very last part of the brain to be pruned and shaped to its adult dimensions is the prefrontal cortex, home of the so-called executive functions: planning, setting priorities, organizing thoughts, suppressing impulses, weighing the consequences of one's actions. In other words, the final part of the brain to grow up is the part capable of deciding, I'll finish my homework and take out the garbage, and *then* I'll IM my friends about seeing a movie.

PRUNING BRAIN CELLS

We are born with most of the brain neurons we will ever have—and that's fewer than we have in utero

"Scientists and the general public had attributed the bad decisions teens make to hormonal changes," says Elizabeth Sowell, a UCLA neuroscientist. "But once we started mapping where and when the brain changes were happening, we could say, Aha, the part of the brain that makes teenagers more responsible is not finished maturing yet."

➤**Raging Hormones** Hormones, however, remain an important part of the teen-brain story. Right about the time the brain switches from proliferating to pruning, the body comes under the hormonal assault of puberty. For years, psychologists attributed the intense, combustible emotions and unpredictable deeds of teens to this biochemical onslaught. And new research adds fresh support. At puberty, the ovaries and testes begin to pour estrogen and testosterone into the bloodstream, spurring the development of the reproductive system, causing hair to sprout in the armpits and groin, wreaking havoc with the skin and shaping the body to its adult contours.

The sex hormones are especially active in the brain's emotional center—the limbic system. This creates a tinderbox of emotions. Not only do feelings reach a flashpoint more easily, but adolescents tend to seek out situations where they can allow their emotions and passions to run wild. This thrill seeking may have evolved to promote exploration, an eagerness to leave the nest and seek one's own path and partner. But in a world in which fast cars, illicit drugs, gangs and dangerous liaisons beckon, it also puts the teenager at risk, since the brain regions that help us question risky, impulsive behavior are still under construction.

CHRIS USHER—APIX

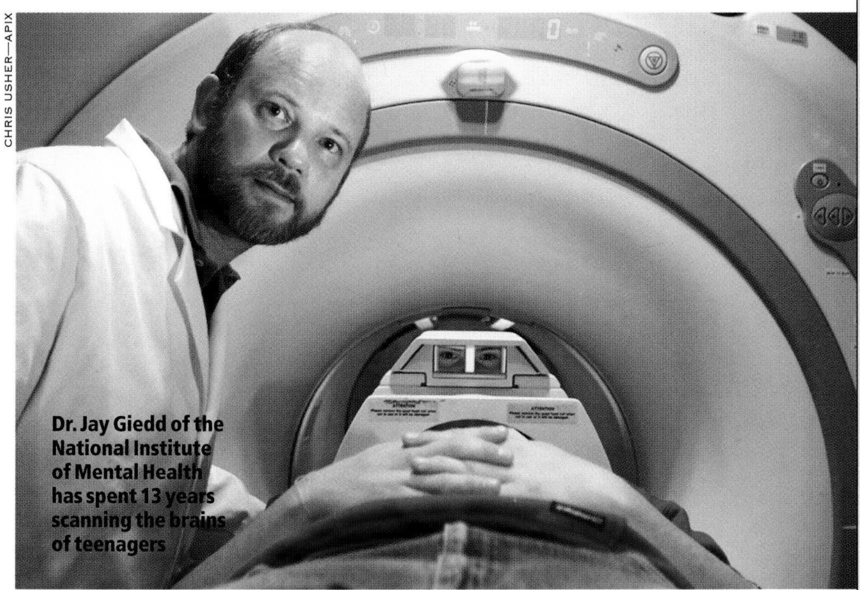

Dr. Jay Giedd of the National Institute of Mental Health has spent 13 years scanning the brains of teenagers

DONNA DAY—CORBIS

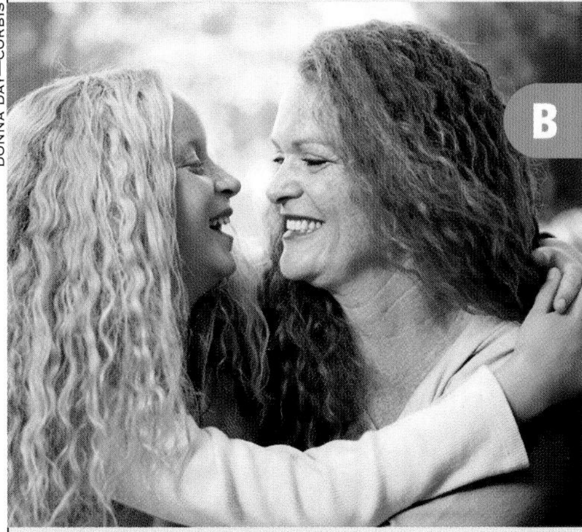

B

Rules for Parents

Drawing on the latest scientific studies of adolescents, Laurence Steinberg, a professor of psychology at Temple University and the author of *The 10 Basic Principles of Good Parenting* (Simon & Schuster), offers this advice for the parents of teens:

1. What you do matters Many parents believe that by the time children have become teenagers, there's nothing more a parent can do. Wrong. Good parenting helps teenagers develop in healthy ways, stay out of trouble and do well in school.

2. You can't be too loving Don't hold back when it comes to pouring on the praise and showing physical affection—just don't embarrass your teens in front of their friends.

3. Stay involved Don't withdraw when your child becomes a teenager. It's just as important for you to be involved now—maybe even more so.

4. Adapt your parenting As children age, their ability to reason improves dramatically, and they will challenge you if what you are asking doesn't make sense.

5. Set limits Teenagers need rules and limits. Be firm but fair. Relax your rules bit by bit as your child demonstrates more maturity.

6. Foster independence Give your children the psychological space they need to learn to be self-reliant, and resist the temptation to micromanage.

7. Explain your decisions Your rules and decisions have to be clear and appropriate. It's not good enough to say "Because I said so."

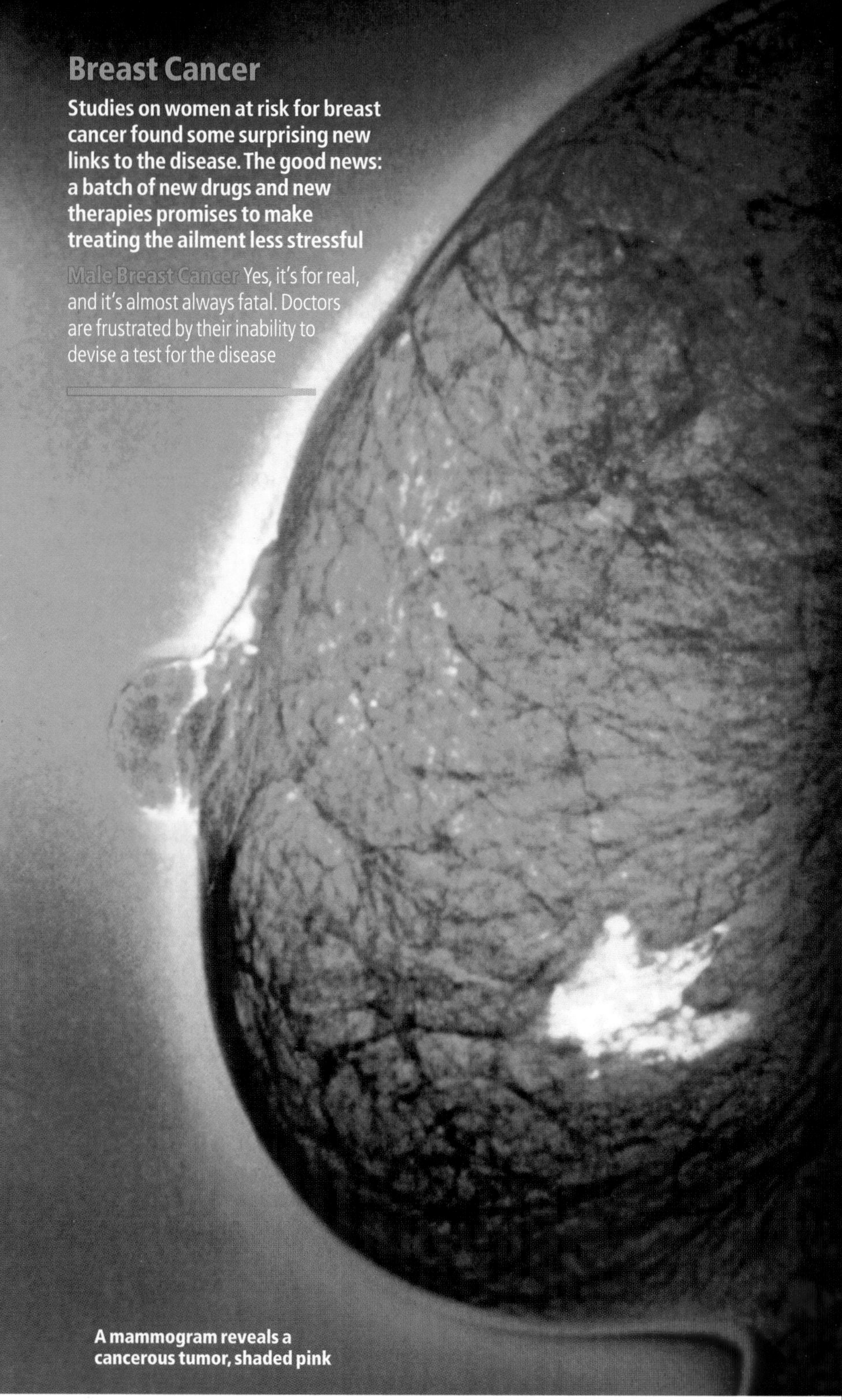

Breast Cancer
Studies on women at risk for breast cancer found some surprising new links to the disease. The good news: a batch of new drugs and new therapies promises to make treating the ailment less stressful
Male Breast Cancer Yes, it's for real, and it's almost always fatal. Doctors are frustrated by their inability to devise a test for the disease

A mammogram reveals a cancerous tumor, shaded pink

COLLECTION CNRI—PHOTOTAKE

A barrage of sobering reports in 2003 and '04 altered the categories of women potentially at risk for breast cancer in complex ways, narrowing the range in some cases and expanding it in others. In this entry, we will first describe the newfound risk factors for breast cancer, then discuss the treatment and prevention of the disease. But we'll begin with some very good news about the best way to fight breast cancer: preventing it in the first place.

➤Prevention: Aspirin and Statins In major news of 2004, aspirin was found to help prevent certain types of breast cancer (*see* Aspirin). In a study of 2,800 women—about half of whom had breast cancer—those who took aspirin seven or more times a week had a 26% lower risk of developing those tumors whose growth is fueled by the sex hormones estrogen and progesterone.

Women in the study who used aspirin at least four times a week for at least three months were almost 30% less likely to develop hormone-fueled breast cancer than women who used no aspirin. The effect was strongest in older, postmenopausal women. Aspirin had no effect on the risk of developing the other type of tumor, hormone receptor-negative.

Statins, the new cholesterol-reducing drugs, also appear to have a beneficial effect on breast cancer risk. A new analysis of data from the ongoing Women's Health Initiative study shows that women who take these cholesterol-lowering medications may be as much as 75% less likely to develop breast cancer than those who do not.

➤Prevention: Exercise Although the benefits of exercise in preventing invasive breast cancer have been long established, it has not been clear whether physical activity also helps prevent breast carcinoma in situ (BCIS, an early form of cancer that may be a precursor to invasive breast cancer). Now, new research indicates that women who do even minimal exercise also have a 35% lower risk of BCIS. A separate study also shows that older women can help reduce their risk of breast cancer (or a recurrence of earlier breast cancer) by lowering their estrogen levels through exercise.

Women who exercise moderately for 75 to 150 minutes a week, a study found, were 18% less likely than inactive women to develop breast cancer. The more the women exercised, the more their risk declined, but once again the incremental difference was small.

➤Risk: Family History One surpris-

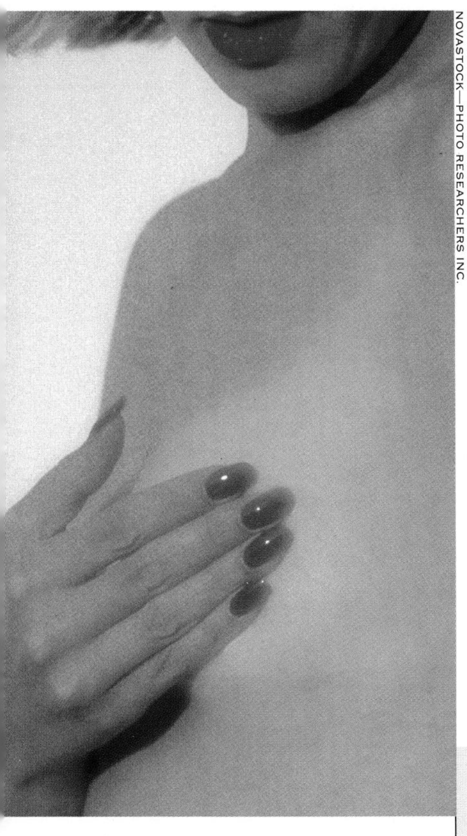

NOVASTOCK—PHOTO RESEARCHERS INC.

ing study showed that even though a family history of breast cancer continues to be a leading predictor of the disease, women whose families have little or no history of the ailment can still carry an inherited genetic mutation that makes it almost certain they will eventually develop breast cancer. Women who carry this mutation on their BRCA1 or BRCA2 genes have a lifetime risk of the disease that tops 80%. The good news: these mutations account for less than 10% of U.S. cases of breast cancer.

➤**Risk: Antibiotics?** More disturbing news sprang from research that reviewed the medical records of more than 10,000 women in a Seattle-area health plan. The study compared pharmacy and breast-cancer-screening records and found that women who filled 25 or more prescriptions for antibiotics over a 17-year period developed breast cancer at twice the rate of those who took no antibiotics. Moreover, there seemed to be what scientists call a dosage-response trend: among women who took more antibiotics, the death rate from cancer was even higher, as much as 3.5 times as great.

While some headlines left the impression that taking antibiotics doubles a woman's risk of getting breast cancer, a closer reading shows that this study raised more questions than it answered. It is entirely possible that breast cancer was creating the women's need for antibiotics—rather than the other way around—by undermining the immune system, for example. Or perhaps an underlying problem like chronic inflammation was making the women's bodies a breeding ground for both bacterial infections and tumors. It's worth noting that the antibiotics users were, on average, older and heavier, had stronger family histories of cancer and were more likely to use hormone-replacement therapy (HRT)—all risk factors for breast cancer. But there are risks in taking antibiotics, and further study is needed to determine whether breast cancer is one of them.

OBESITY: A RISK FACTOR

Obese women have a 31% greater risk of developing breast cancer than women who are not obese

➤**Risk: Pregnancy and HRT** Women with a history of breast cancer have long been discouraged from taking hormone replacement therapy. But until recently, the jury was still out on whether women newly diagnosed with breast cancer should

Good Tidings from the Laboratory Front

It was major news in 2004 when a study found that **aspirin** may help ward off certain types of breast cancer (*see* Aspirin). The little white pill overshadowed the good news about other drugs coming through the pipeline to fight breast cancer.

The benefits of **tamoxifen**, a drug that decreases estrogen levels, have been clarified in recent years, but it is also known to increase the risks of endometrial tumors, uterine sarcoma and dangerous blood clots. A new study found that lower doses of the drug (which decrease the risk of side effects) do not lessen its effectiveness.

A separate study showed that the chemotherapy drug **letrozole** can pick up where tamoxifen leaves off, after tumors develop resistance to the latter, usually five years after surgery. Among the caveats: no one can say how long women should remain on letrozole. While bone density loss is a known side effect, other long-term effects are unclear.

Nor is letrozole the only alternative to tamoxifen. New research shows that women who switch from tamoxifen to another estrogen inhibitor, **exemestane**, about midway through their five-year course of treatment have a lower risk of breast-cancer recurrence and a higher overall rate of long-term survival.

More good news appears to be on the way. A large-scale study of a new drug, **anastrozole**, has begun to test preliminary findings that it may cut breast-cancer rates in post-menopausal women as much as 70%. And trials of a promising vaccine designed to prevent a recurrence of the disease in breast cancer survivors are being monitored by the FDA. Also being tested is a new class of chemo drugs known as **aromatase inhibitors**, which are intended to act as replacements for tamoxifen when a patient develops resistance to it. Researchers hope they may slash recurrence of breast cancer as much as 50%. ■

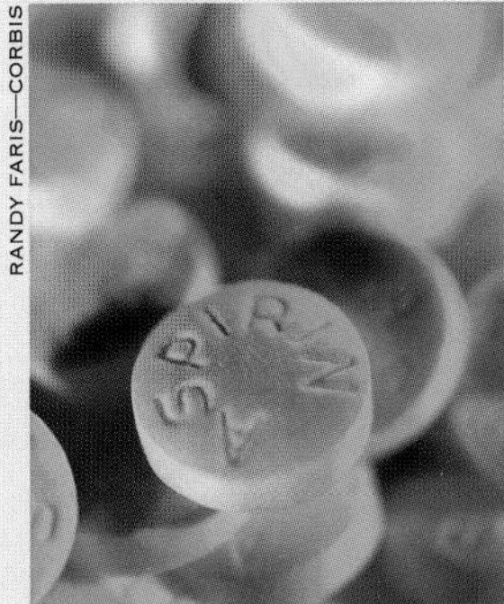

RANDY FARIS—CORBIS

THE CUTTING EDGE OF CANCER TREATMENT

Surgery, radiation and chemotherapy are still the first line of defense against breast cancer. But exciting new techniques are entering clinical trials and, if they work, may eventually replace the old standards with kinder, gentler treatments

TIME Graphic by Ed Gabel

Sources: Acueity, Proxima Therapeutics, M. D. Anderson Cancer Center, Rosetta Inpharmatics

TUMOR ABLATION

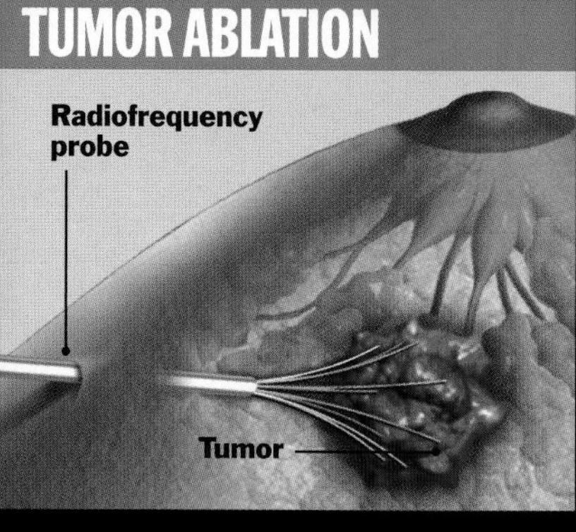

■ **HOW IT'S DONE**
Cancers can be frozen or vaporized with lasers or high-energy radiowaves delivered by a probe through a tiny incision. In one technique, the probe opens like an umbrella inside the breast

■ **AVAILABILITY**
Already used for liver tumors. Clinical trials for breast cancer are under way, but could take five years to complete

ENDOSCOPY

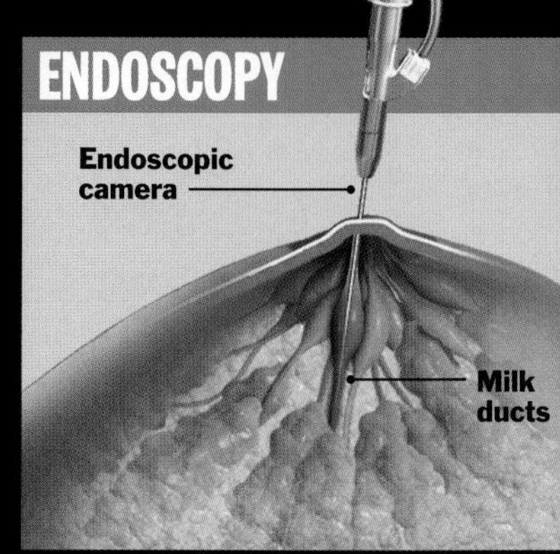

■ **HOW IT'S DONE**
Tumors can be examined with a miniature fiber-optic camera that is inserted through the nipple and into a milk duct. Eventually surgeons may be able to treat tumors through the same tiny probe

■ **AVAILABILITY**
The fiber-optic scope was okayed by the FDA in 2002. Using it for treatment may be less than five years away

powerful enough to spot them, these growths are at the heart of a raging debate in the cancer community. Doctors know what to do when they find tumors the size of marbles or plums: apply surgery, radiation or chemotherapy. But what do you do with cancers the size of pencil points? Do you treat them as you would a massive tumor? Do you leave them alone? Should you even look for them to begin with?

Thirty years ago, these miniature tumors, which usually don't spread into the rest of the body, were diagnosed in some 6% of breast-cancer patients. Today the ratio is closer to 20%, due to advances in detection techniques. Yet the treatment of choice is still surgery, then radiation. "We may be far overtreating our patients," says one oncologist. "We've now got women being diagnosed with tumors that probably never would have been treated if we didn't have mammography. They probably would have lived long, natural, healthy lives never knowing they had breast cancer."

That's what makes DCIS treatment so controversial. What if most of the tiny tumors that show up in high-resolution mammograms are the ones that grow the slowest or maybe even disappear of their own accord, thus posing no real danger? And if that's the case, wouldn't it make sense to leave those tumors alone until you could figure out whether they are going to grow?

In one 1988 trial, about 1,200 women whose tumors were less than 2 cm across with no evidence of malignancy in their lymph nodes

Mammograms: Why the Shortfall?

Two reports issued in June 2004 summed up all that's right and all that's wrong with mammograms. The first found that fewer than 1 in 20 American women follows the recommendation to get an annual mammogram to screen for breast cancer. The noncompliance cut across lines of age, race, education and even personal medical history.

The second finding : even though mammograms miss up to 17% of tumors in women who have breast cancer and sound a large number of false alarms in women who don't, they are still the most reliable means of detecting breast cancer in its earliest stages. The report noted some of the reasons women forgo the procedure: insurers don't want to cover it; doctors don't want to perform it (misdiagnosis of breast cancer is the most common cause of malpractice suits); and women don't enjoy sweating out the wait for results , which can take several months, because of a lack of qualified radiologists. ■

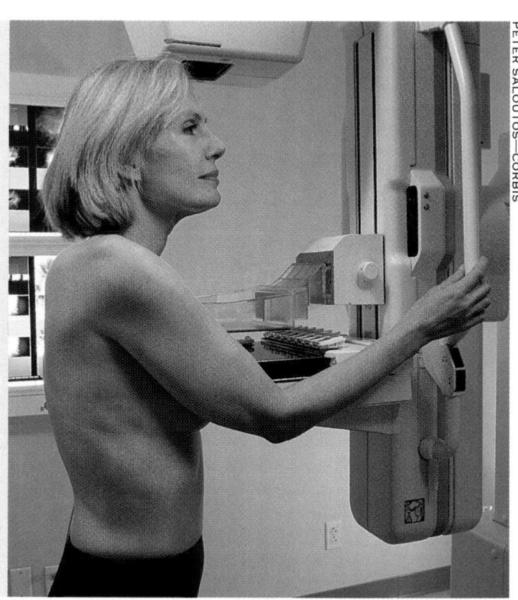

PETER SALOUTOS—CORBIS

TARGETED RADIATION

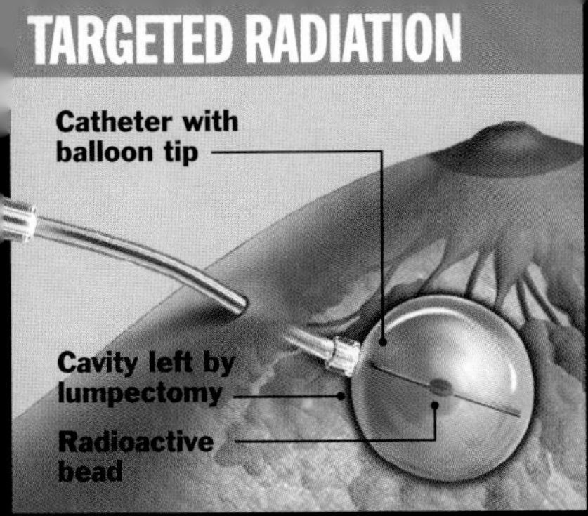

■ HOW IT'S DONE
After a lumpectomy, a tiny radioactive bead is delivered directly into the tumor site through a small balloon-tipped catheter. Treatment takes a matter of days, not weeks

■ AVAILABILITY
Clinical trials on 70 patients nationwide have been completed. The procedure is awaiting FDA approval

MOLECULAR FORECASTING

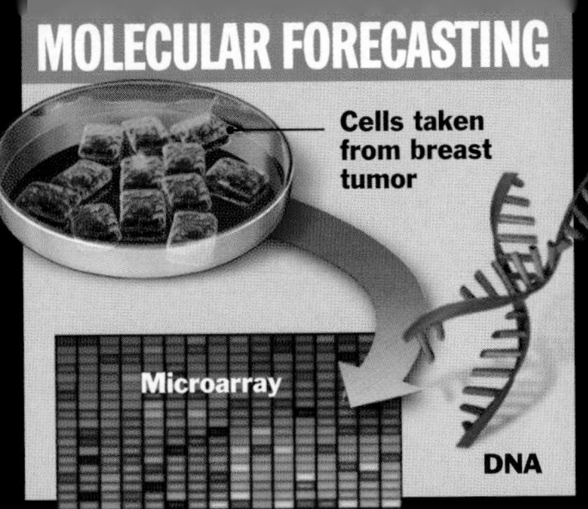

■ HOW IT'S DONE
With microarrays, scientists can study patterns of gene activity using strands of cancer DNA and predict which tumors are likely to spread. The technique may someday be used to design customized treatments

■ AVAILABILITY
Clinical trials for breast cancer are starting this year; treatment may be widely available within the decade

SMART DRUGS

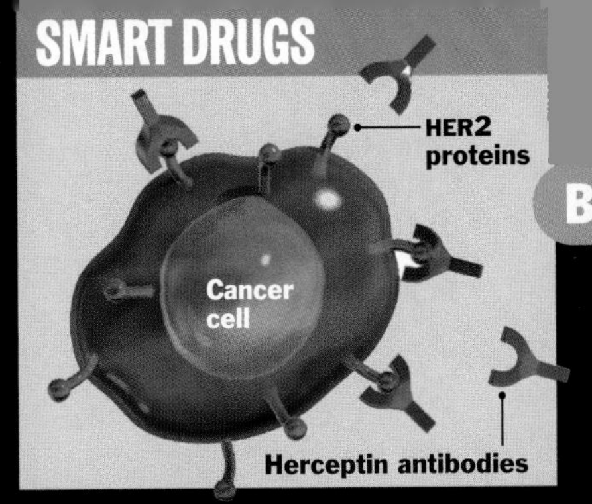

■ HOW IT'S DONE
As scientists come to understand at the molecular level precisely how tumors form, they are designing a new generation of smart drugs that bind to specific receptors or block particular proteins

■ AVAILABILITY
Herceptin, the first of these smart drugs for breast cancer, is available for certain advanced cancers

B

weren't treated as aggressively as they might have been: no follow-up chemo was done. For five years after their tumors were surgically removed, doctors did nothing more unless there was a recurrence. Though 11% of the women did in fact develop a second cancer, their survival rate was comparable to that of another group of women who had undergone chemotherapy at the time of their surgery.

Still, no one is recommending a wholesale "cut and wait" approach for DCIS lesions (though this method has been proved effective for men with prostate cancer, on the basis of a single study). For one thing, waiting to see how aggressive a cancer truly is makes a lot more sense for men in their 80s than for women in their 40s.

➤Treatment: Mastectomy A new study shows that the painful choice to have the breasts removed before cancer develops may benefit women at the highest risk for the disease. Among almost 500 women who carry the abnormalities in the brca1 and brca2 genes that are thought to predict breast cancer, almost half of the 384 who chose not to undergo preventive surgery developed breast cancer within six years, while only two of the 105 women who opted for a mastectomy were similarly afflicted.

In one area, at least, the choices have become clearer, rather than less so: a lumpectomy followed by radiation, it has been shown, is just as effective as a full mastectomy. Doctors and patients had long been concerned that simply removing a tumor instead of an entire breast might increase the chances of a relapse. But two recent studies found no difference in survival rates between those who had undergone mastectomies and those who had chosen the less drastic route, lumpectomy with radiation.

TO BEAT CANCER, GET FIT

Women who exercise even moderately—as little as 75 to 150 minutes a week—are 18% less likely than inactive women to develop breast cancer

➤Treatment: Stem Cell Therapy
The emerging science of stem-cell therapy offers hope as a supplement to chemotherapy: new research indicates that women who undergo chemotherapy along with transplantation of their own stem cells have a higher survival rate (and a greater chance of avoiding a recurrence of breast cancer) than those who opt for chemo alone. However, stem-cell transplantation surgery carries the risk of serious side effects, and there have been cases where it resulted in death.

➤Treatment: Radiation Therapy
The majority of breast-cancer patients undergo radiation therapy as part of their treatment, but radiotherapy still puts healthy tissue at risk—even though lower doses have made it safer than it once was. But a new study suggests that targeted radiotherapy can work just as well as whole-breast radiation therapy in preventing cancer recurrences. The approach, called partial breast irradiation, treats only areas nearest to the tumor, minimizing exposure of healthy tissues to X rays. It can also mean a shorter treatment and recovery period.

■ Resources

NIH BREAST CANCER INFORMATION: *www.nlm.nih.gov/medlineplus/breastcancer*

AMERICAN BREAST CANCER FOUNDATION HOTLINE: 877-539-2543

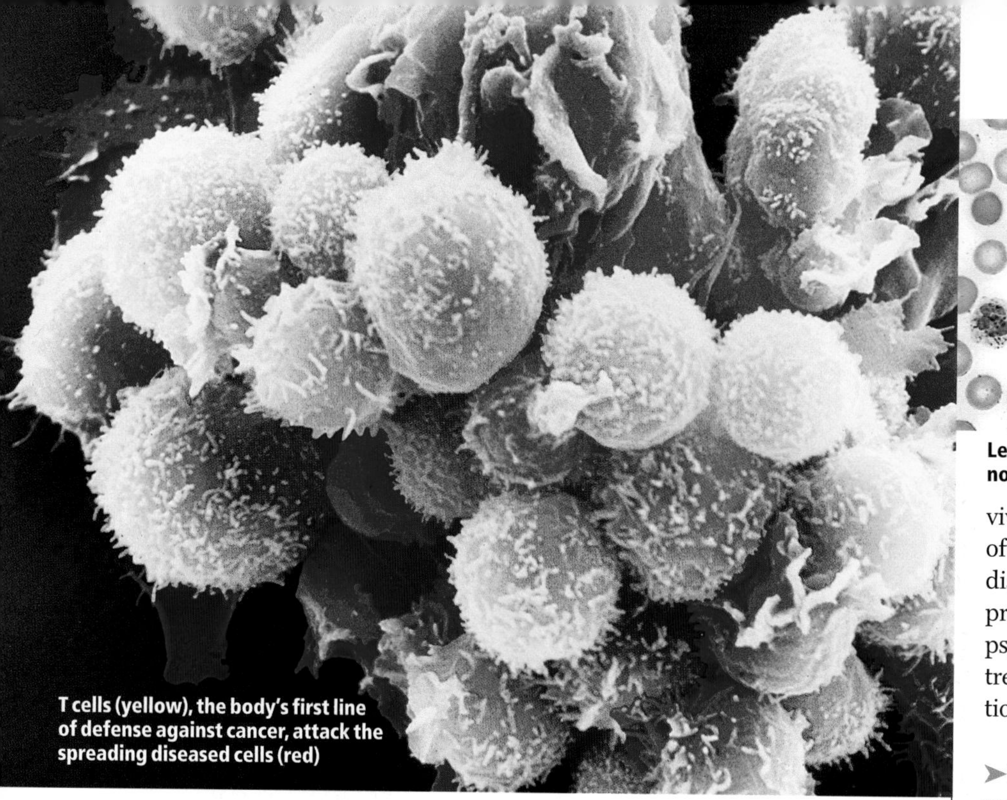

T cells (yellow), the body's first line of defense against cancer, attack the spreading diseased cells (red)

Leukemia cells (red) circulate among normal blood cells (brown)

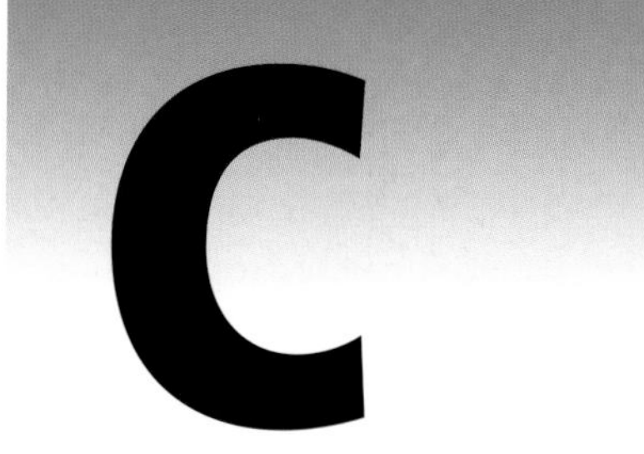

Cancer

The good news: cancer rates are still on the decline in America, and at the same time, the probability that victims will survive an attack of cancer continues to climb

Contents This entry reports on cancer news in general and also covers specific cancers that occur less frequently. The forms of the disease that afflict the most patients—breast, colorectal, lung and skin cancers—are treated in separate entries

Here's a statement many of us once thought we would never read: there's good news in the war on cancer. The average American's risk of developing or dying from this disease that spawns uncontrolled cell growth has kept up a decade-long trend and continues to recede ever so slightly each year. Since 1993, overall death rates from cancer have dropped 1.1% a year, while rates of new cases of all kinds of cancers are dropping about half a percent a year. The total number of U.S. cancer survivors has more than tripled over the past 30 years, to almost 10 million. And patients whose cancer was diagnosed between 1995 and 2000 have an estimated 64% chance of surviving five years, compared with a 50% chance of five-year survival for the same patients in the early 1970s.

Even lung cancer is retreating, if only a bit. Among women, new diagnoses have dropped about 2% a year since 1998, finally catching up with a similar trend among men that began years earlier (*for more, see* Lung Cancer).

> **THE FORCE IS WITH YOU**
>
> Almost two-thirds of patients with cancer diagnosed between 1995 and 2000 will survive. Only one-half of those stricken in the early 1970s survived

These encouraging trends are particularly pronounced among the disease's youngest victims. In the 1970s, the five-year average survival rate for all kinds of cancer among children was about 50%. Now it hovers around 80%. The satisfaction about this advance is tempered, though, by a new study suggesting that survivors of childhood cancers are often plagued by neurological disorders, heart and lung diseases, problems with growth and fertility, psychological stress related to treatment, and ongoing complications related to the original cancer.

➤Goal: 70% Survival All this good news is largely due to advances in cancer detection and prevention. Unfortunately, the benefits have not been apportioned evenly throughout the population. Minorities still are more likely than whites to die from cancer, with black men 26% more at risk of death from a malignancy than white men, while Hispanic men are 16% more at risk than non-Hispanic whites. For women, the disparity is even greater: black females are 52% likelier to die of cancer than whites, while Hispanic women are 20% more likely. Researchers theorize that many of these disparities may be attributable to the poor access to high-quality health care and the lack of health insurance that is common among minorities and poorer Americans.

Even among the more fortunate, the statistics are still far short of the aggressive goal that government cancer experts have set for themselves: they hope to increase the overall five-year survival rate to 70% by 2010. Indeed, the American Cancer

Eat As the Greeks Do?

Can your diet help shield you from cancer? For decades, doctors have been intrigued by the apparent health benefits of the so-called Mediterranean diet, a group of eating patterns that has existed around the Mediterranean basin for centuries. These regimens emphasize lots of fruits, cooked vegetables and legumes, grains (whole, not refined) and, in moderation, wine, nuts, fish and dairy products, in particular yogurt and cheese. But most Americans tend to focus on one

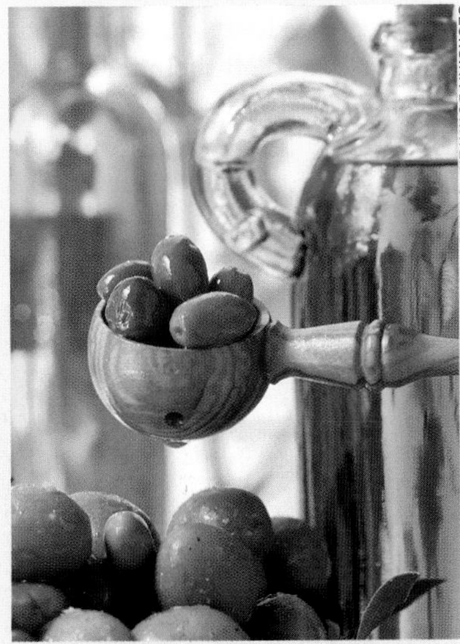

GEORGINA BOWATER—CORBIS

component of these diets—olive oil—as if it were a magical potion that could be drizzled over any meal to make it healthy.

Life should be so easy. According to the most rigorous study of such diets ever conducted, people who follow a Mediterranean diet do seem to reduce their risk of dying from cancer by 24%. But the study was unable to link the cancer-preventing benefits to any one ingredient, not even olive oil, suggesting that the health benefits of the diet stem from the interaction of all its components.

So what about olive oil? Its main benefit may be that it encourages the eating of vegetables—which simply seem to taste better when sautéed in olive oil, with a dash of herbs and garlic, than when steamed. Perhaps that's the secret of the Mediterranean diet: it treats food as food, not medicine. ■

Society estimates that 156 people an hour will learn they have cancer throughout 2004, and by year's end, more than 563,000 people will have died from it.

GOING TO THE SOURCE

New drugs fight the spread of cancer by cutting off the blood supply that helps tumors keep growing

➤Halting Angiogenesis There may be more good news in the near future. One source of this optimism is a new class of medications that starve tumors by choking off their blood supply. In the past year, the FDA approved the first of a new generation of drugs that prevent a process called angiogenesis, in which tumors grow new blood vessels to create their own supply of nourishment. (Adults do not ordinarily grow new circulatory tissue, except during pregnancy, ovulation or after an injury to aid in healing.) The first of these new drugs, Avastin, when taken in combination with standard chemotherapy, has helped patients with advanced cancer live 30% longer (about five months) than those who underwent only chemotherapy—and some of these patients survived for several years.

➤The Sleeping Cure A good night's sleep competes with chicken soup as a traditional cure-all. But can it help someone beat cancer? New studies show that shift workers have higher rates of breast cancer than women who are able to sleep normal hours.

Two possible culprits are the hormones melatonin and cortisol. Melatonin is an antioxidant that mops up damaging free radicals, but the body produces less of it when sleep cycles are disrupted. Cortisol, which helps regulate the immune system, may also be compromised by troubled sleep. Said an expert: "Cancer might be something to lose sleep over, but we'd rather help people regain the sleep and lose the cancer."

A separate study found that relaxation techniques like yoga are every bit as effective as sleep-inducing drugs in helping cancer patients (especially those undergoing chemotherapy) for whom sleeplessness is an issue.

HOW TO STARVE A TUMOR

1 **As a cancer tumor grows, it builds its own network of capillaries that tap into the body's blood supply and draw on the oxygen and nutrients the tumor needs to survive**

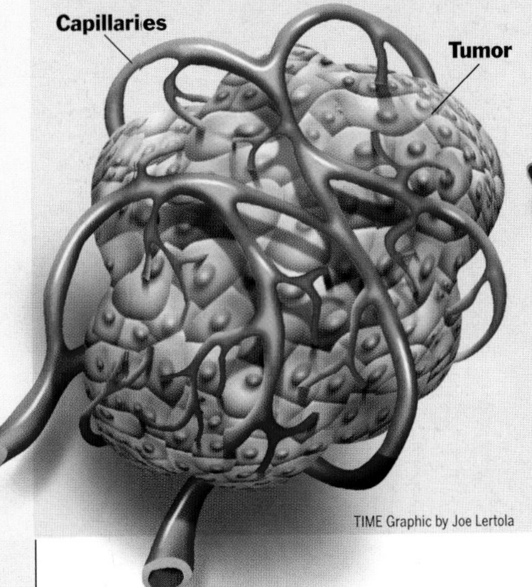

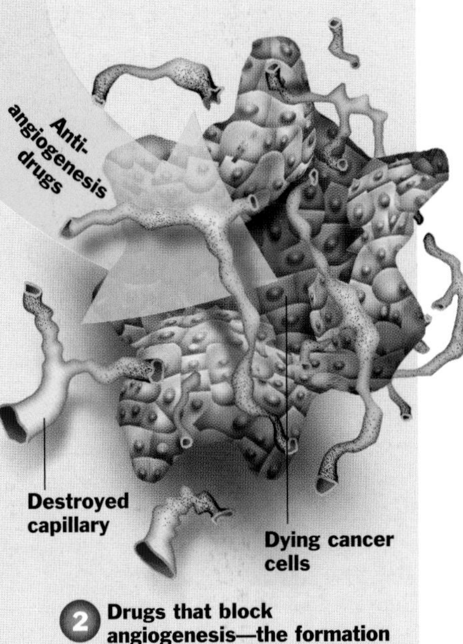

2 **Drugs that block angiogenesis—the formation of new vessels—cut the tumor off from its blood supply. Gradually, malignant cells die and the tumor starts to shrink**

TIME Graphic by Joe Lertola

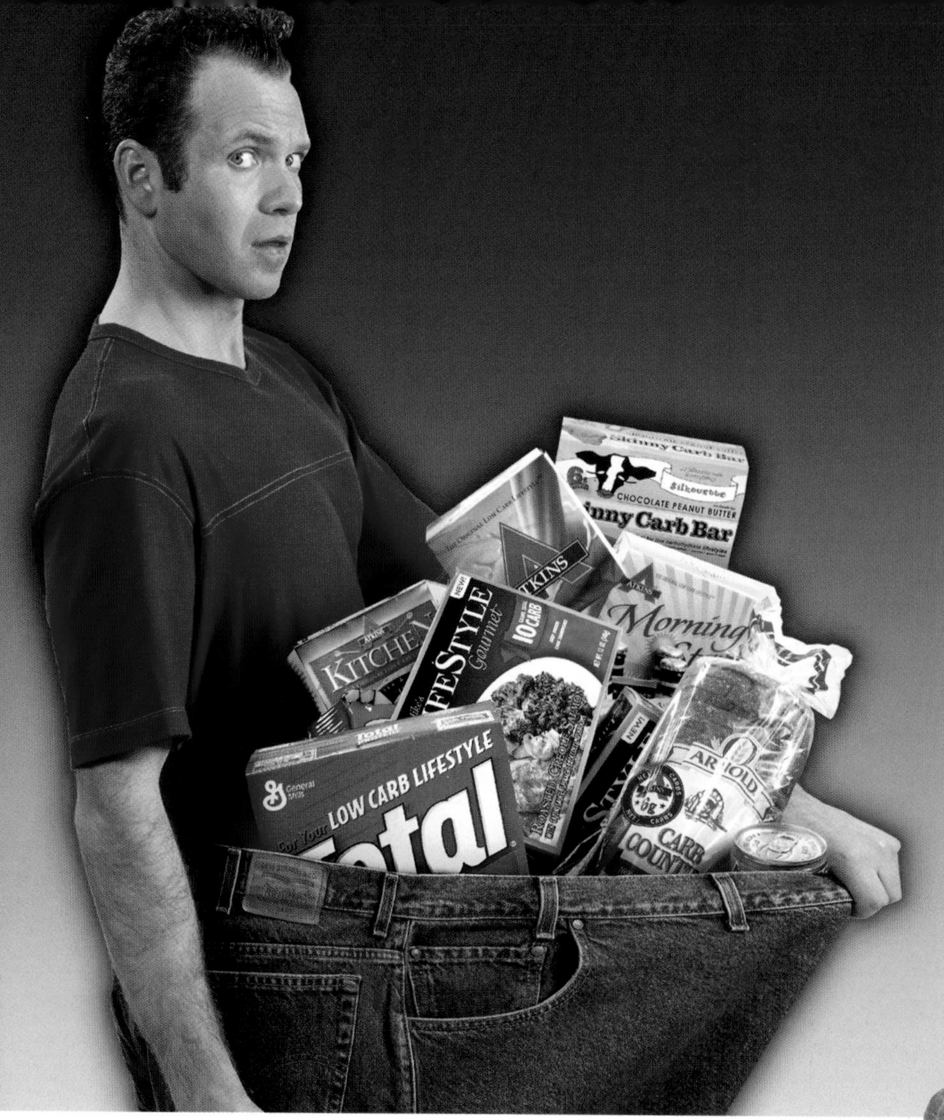

Carbohydrates

It's official: the low-carb trend is the hottest diet craze in decades. Beyond the hype, here are the real benefits (and real risks) of hopping aboard the low-carb bandwagon

Definition Carbohydrates are compounds of carbon, hydrogen and oxygen (hence their compound name) that form sugars, starches, and fiber. They are one of the three principal types of nutrients used by the body as sources of energy

Welcome to Low-Carb America! The nation's latest diet fad promises two things Americans just can't resist—pounds to drop and profits to crop—so it seems as if everyone is giving the low-carb culture a whirl. Whoopi Goldberg does it. So do Jennifer Aniston and Bill Clinton. What's good enough for the famed is, of course, appealing to the rest of us. Some 26 million Americans were on a hard-core low-carb diet in 2004. And 70 million more were limiting their carb intake without formally dieting, according to a poll by Opinion Dynamics Corp.

Counting carbs has become as powerful a fixture in the economy as it has in society. Some 586 distinct new low-carb foods and beverages hit the grocery shelves in the first quarter of 2004, up from 633 in all of 2003 and 339 in 2002, bringing the total over just two years to 1,558 new entries. Low-carb-related sales from such consumables as Michelob Ultra beer and books like *Dr. Atkins' New Diet Revolution* are expected to hit $30 billion in 2004, reported *LowCarbiz*, a trade publication that owes its existence to carbophobia.

GOING DOWN

After six consecutive years of gains, the number of overweight Americans fell 1 percentage point in '03

➤A Brief Weight Loss Still, not everyone is convinced: critics of the carb counters' revolution claim that Atkins, South Beach, Zone and other protein-packed eating regimens are part of a fad that will soon run its course, like low-fat diets in the 1980s. But they can't deny that hundreds of thousands of Americans have dropped 20 or 50 or 100 lbs. after cutting carbs from their meals.

Both sides found support for their arguments in recent studies. New research showed that the low-carb Atkins diet really does melt the pounds away—at least in the short run. Subjects in two trials ate either a low-carb diet or a conventional low-calorie, high-carb menu. At the end of six months, the carb cutters lost twice as many pounds as the calorie counters. The pounds, however, quickly reappeared after the first part of the study was completed. By the end of the next six months, the two test groups showed no difference in the amount of weight they'd lost.

IN

The studies also found that those who ate the low-carb way enjoyed higher levels of HDL, or "good" cholesterol, but it's not yet clear whether this boost offers enough benefit to the heart to compensate for the extra fat consumed in protein-rich diets.

Exactly why all those pounds melt away when we give up pota-

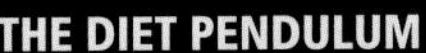

toes and bread remains something of a mystery to the dieting public. Is it mostly the temporary loss of water weight? Do low-carb fanatics lose weight while consuming more calories, as a Harvard study suggests, or do they end up eating less because they simply get bored with the high-protein life? Or is there some sort of metabolic magic when steak, eggs and cheese replace the starches in our diet?

Dr. Robert Atkins, who got the ball rolling in 1972, controversially ascribed the weight loss to ketosis, the fat-burning state a body reaches when deprived of carbs. His critics have bordered on fanatic, their stridency growing in proportion to the diet's increase in popularity.

Yet there are signs that carb counting may be working. One market-research firm, NPD, found that after six consecutive years of weight gain, the number of overweight adult Americans fell 1 percentage point, to 55%. Was it carb counting? No one really knows. But at fast-food restaurants, salad orders (low in carbs) rose 12%, while French-fry (carb mountain) consumption fell 10%.

➤The Nutritionists Speak The more carb counting becomes ingrained in our lives, the more worried many nutritionists grow. They argue that low-carb weight loss, while real, will not last for many folks, who once they stop dieting will obey their taste buds and return to the junk foods they love.

What if they stay off carbs indefinitely? This is where the jury is out. A growing body of medical evidence supports the notion that in the short term, low-carbing can work for weight loss and that getting slimmer is beneficial in fighting heart disease and diabetes. The study of long-term effects is only now getting under way, and one worry is the higher cholesterol counts that can accompany a diet rich in fatty meats. Without question, high cholesterol levels contribute to heart disease.

➤Good Carbs, Bad Carbs How does carb counting work? In simple terms, carbs are digested or broken down into sugars, which then circulate in the bloodstream. As sugar levels in the blood rise, so does insulin. Peaks of insulin push the body to store excess sugar as fat. By cutting carbs, you effectively cut sugar surges and thus not only store less fat but also start to burn off more of the fat you have.

If this were the whole story, of course, there would be little controversy and none of the colossal food frenzy being waged among companies desperate to get on the right side of the carb culture.

But there is a second front in carb wars: good carbs vs. bad carbs. The good ones are found in whole-grain breads, beans, fruits and vegetables. They contain fiber and break down slowly when digested, avoiding those damaging sugar and insulin spikes. The bad ones are found in white rice, potatoes, most commercial breads and all manner of processed crackers, cookies, chips, soda and candy bars. Bad carbs break down more quickly and cause sugar overload.

THE DIET PENDULUM

Studies show that low-carb dieters shed pounds much faster than low-calorie dieters, but they often gain them right back

As you might imagine, those in the carb business are trying to claim that their carbs are the benevolent ones. All this spin can make the low-carb universe difficult to navigate. But there are a few simple things to keep in mind:

■ First, watch out for bald-faced low-carb claims—they might be "carbage." That's because the Food and Drug Administration has yet to define what constitutes a low- or light- or reduced-carb anything. Hence the proliferation of fuzzier labeling terms like carb smart, carb conscious, carb aware and carb fit. Russell Stover, for example, received a warning letter from the agency about the name of its Low Carb line of chocolates. The company has offered to change the name but hopes it won't have to since the FDA announced in 2004 that the agency will come up with a definition for low carb.

■ Second, there is the confusing notion of net carbs. Some manufacturers subtract the good carbs from the bad ones and advertise the difference. This is a slippery slope because the FDA insists that a carb is a carb is a carb. Just remember: net carbs are not the same as fewer carbs.

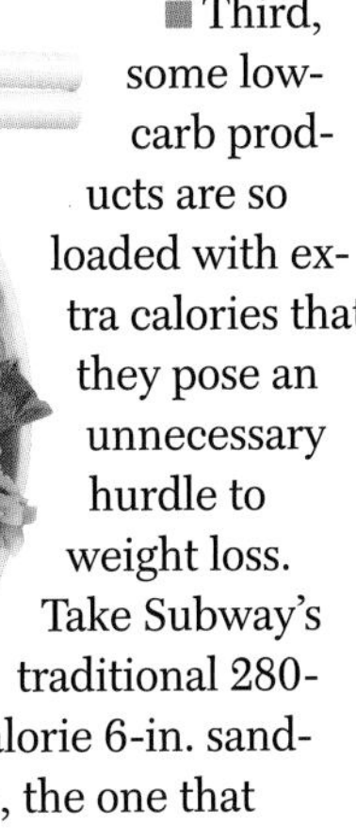

■ Third, some low-carb products are so loaded with extra calories that they pose an unnecessary hurdle to weight loss. Take Subway's traditional 280-calorie 6-in. sandwich, the one that

Cholesterol

A federal health agency revises its guidelines for cholesterol levels, lowering them significantly for those most at risk of heart disease

On the Horizon Statins, the wonder drugs that have revolutionized the way we fight the buildup of harmful cholesterol, may soon be replaced by a more potent drug

After five different clinical trials over a three-year period concluded that lower cholesterol levels would better protect people at greatest risk of heart attack, the experts at the NIH's National Cholesterol Education Program (NCEP) changed their guidelines, setting aggressive new target levels that will take some getting used to.

The revised guidelines focus on low-density lipoprotein (LDL)—the so-called bad cholesterol. Four years ago, the NCEP recommendations called for patients at high risk of heart attack, including those who have diabetes or already have heart disease, to try to get their LDL level under 100 mg/dL (milligrams per deciliter). (For those without these risk factors, the guidelines allow some wiggle room, up to 129 mg/dL.) But the guidelines create an additional category of patients at "very high" risk—a group that includes heart patients who smoke, diabetics with heart problems and people who are in the hospital for a heart condition. For these people, the new guidelines give doctors the option of being more aggressive in lowering their LDL cholesterol to less than 70 mg/dL.

MEET APOA-1 MILANO

A new drug based on a rare, mutant form of cholesterol promises to be the best plaque fighter yet discovered

Some cardiologists argued that for very-high-risk patients, the lower figure should have been made mandatory. It very nearly was, says Dr. James Cleeman, the NCEP coordinator, but the evidence supporting such a move was "just short of conclusive." He expects the results of three more clinical trials, due to be completed in the next couple of years, to settle the matter.

The new recommendations are likely to increase sharply the use of statin drugs. It's almost impossible to achieve such low LDL levels without these cholesterol-cutting medications, although even the NCEP says the best ways to lower cholesterol are to get more exercise, eat less saturated and trans fats and maintain a healthy weight.

The policy change came on the heels of the first head-to-head comparison of two of the most popular statins: Lipitor (made by Pfizer) and Pravachol (Bristol-Myers Squibb). The results were a big win for Lipitor, which not only lowered LDL levels more than Pravachol did (from an average of 150 to 79, vs. 110 for Pravachol) but appeared to have a measurable effect on the buildup of plaque in patients' arteries. Pravachol merely slowed the progression of those fatty deposits, whereas Lipitor stopped them cold and may have even shrunk them a bit. It's not yet clear whether Lipitor's protective benefits are due to its power to reduce LDL levels or to its ability to fight inflammation, a major cause of heart disease.

In other promising news for those at risk for cardiac problems, ApoA-1 Milano, an experimental drug based on a mutant form of HDL cholesterol, shows signs of being up to 10 times more effective than statins at reducing the arterial plaque that triggers most heart attacks (*see* Heart).

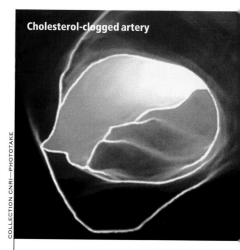

Cholesterol-clogged artery

COLLECTION CNRI—PHOTOTAKE

DAMAGE CONTROL

Arterial disease, the main cause of heart attacks, can be reversed by a drug that mimics a rare form of HDL—the so-called good cholesterol—found naturally in a handful of lucky Italians

1 THE DRUG IS INJECTED ... The artificial HDL is given to a patient whose arteries are lined with fatty, cholesterol-laden deposits called plaque

2 ... ATTACKS THE PLAQUE ... Like ordinary HDL but more effective, the artificial HDL binds to cholesterol and wrenches it from the plaque

3 ... AND FLUSHES IT AWAY The plaque shrinks and stabilizes, and cholesterol is carried to the liver for disposal

Sources: Esperion Therapeutics; *J.A.M.A.*

TIME Graphic by Lon Tweeten

Resources

NATIONAL CHOLESTEROL EDUCATION PROGRAM: *www.nhlbi.nih.gov/about/ncep*

Colds

Scientists have identified a new virus as a cause of the common cold, but they're not much farther along in stopping your sneezes

Coming Soon The makers of Kleenex plan to market an antiviral tissue they claim will help stop contagion. Some scientists say the product may hasten the spread of bugs that resist antiviral agents

Researchers have added a new villain to the list of viruses that will give you a cold: metapneumovirus, discovered only in 2001, is now believed to cause as many as 15% of all colds in children and is so ubiquitous that all human beings are thought to have been exposed to it by age 5. Why has it taken scientists so long to find a virus this common? Because the virus is difficult to cultivate in laboratory cell cultures, the standard method for indexing viruses.

One product that consumers (and the FDA) may be thinking twice about is the over-the-counter zinc nasal spray. Often used to ease symptoms and shorten the duration of the common cold, these sprays have been alleged in several consumer complaints (and at least five lawsuits) to cause a severe burning sensation, followed by a loss of smell and taste. The FDA is reviewing these complaints and considering further action.

■ Resources

NIH WEBSITE: *www.nlm.nih.gov/medlineplus/commoncold*

CRISTINA PEDRAZZINI—PHOTO RESEARCHERS

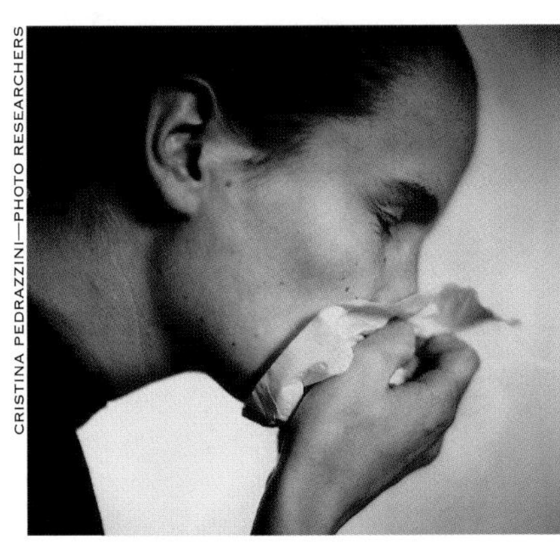

GOPAL MURTI—PHOTOTAKE

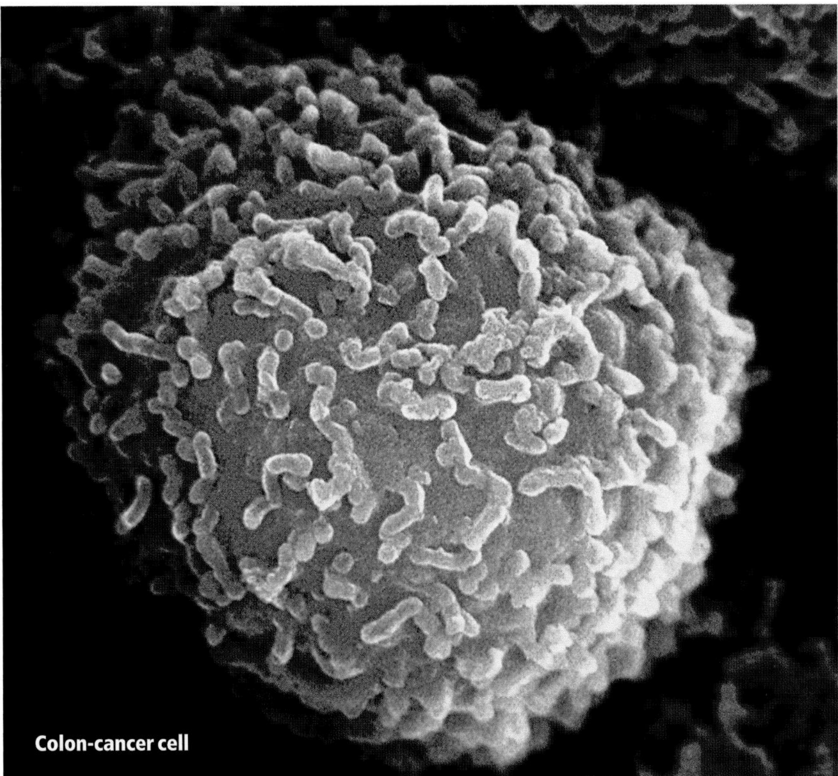

Colon-cancer cell

Colorectal Cancer

Researchers are discovering new ways to prevent the onset of this fast-moving, stealthy disease, the No. 2 killer among types of cancer

In the Spotlight Thanks to TV star Katie Couric's attention-getting live colonoscopy on NBC in 2000, awareness of the need to screen for the disease is at an all-time high

Colorectal cancer is an especially deadly form of the disease: it ranks second only to lung cancer in the number of Americans it kills each year. It's also insidiously stealthy, but new drugs, new technology, new approaches to surgery and heightened public awareness offer much encouragement to those at risk for the disease. Yet when all is said and done, your best chance of beating colon cancer isn't new at all: it involves early detection through aggressive screening.

ASPIRIN TO THE RESCUE

The drug seems to be an effective fighter of colorectal cancer, helping prevent the polyps that lead to it

➤Prevention A new study suggested that having a bowl of high-fiber cereal for breakfast may lower your chances of developing colon cancer. The research, which focused on men, found that test subjects who ate the most cereal fiber were half as likely to develop precancerous colon polyps as those who had the least.

A separate study found that female test subjects who had diets heavy with certain processed carbohydrates, like those used in cookies and cakes, increased their risk of colon cancer. Subjects whose diets skewed more to carbohydrates that the body takes longer to digest, such as those in brown rice and wheat breads, were deemed to be less at risk. The study gauged the chance of developing colon cancer for the let-them-eat-cake group to be more than double the risk of those in the second group.

Two other studies examined the possible role of aspirin in preventing colon cancer and found that, at least for patients deemed to be at

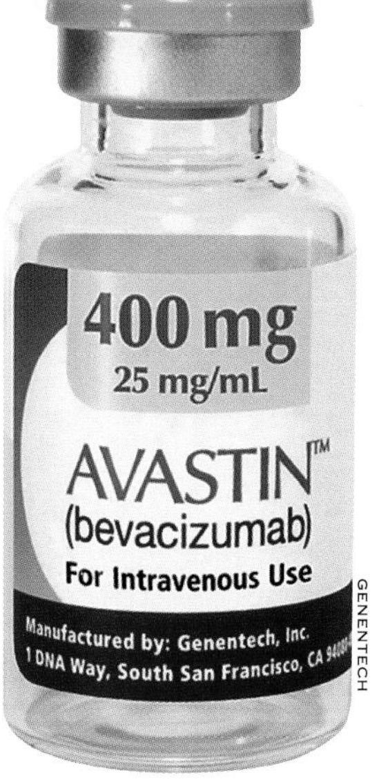

GENENTECH

high risk of developing the disease, the white pill in your medicine cabinet can significantly reduce your chances of developing pre-cancerous polyps.

➤Treatment: Drugs When the FDA approved Genentech's colorectal cancer drug Avastin in February 2004, it validated a cancer-fighting strategy proposed more than 30 years ago. Avastin is the first in what researchers hope will be a whole new class of drugs called angiogenesis inhibitors, which attack tumors by thwarting their ability to create blood vessels, thus starving cancer cells of oxygen and nutrients (*see* Cancer).

Another encouraging development: the recently approved chemotherapy drug oxaliplatin (Eloxatin) may increase the length of time a patient with advanced colon cancer is expected to survive. Studies of more than 700 patients found that those taking oxaliplatin lived almost one-third longer (19.5 months, compared with 15 months) than patients receiving standard chemotherapy treatment. What's more, oxaliplatin seems to be associated with fewer side effects, such as infection and diarrhea.

➤Treatment: Surgery While minimal invasiveness has become increasingly common for operations such as coronary bypass, it is still a relatively new approach for colon-cancer patients. But a seven-year study found that laparoscopic surgery (in which doctors cut three small holes in the abdomen and operate with the help of a small video camera) can offer significant rewards: less pain, smaller incisions and a quicker recovery time. Laparoscopic surgery appears to be as safe and effective as a traditional operation, which requires that surgeons open the abdomen with an 8-in. incision, instead of the 2-in. cut used in this newer, "keyhole" approach.

➤Risk Factors The graveyard shift has always been lonely, but a recent study suggested it may be unhealthy as well. In new results from the continuing Nurses' Health Study of more than 78,500 women, those who worked overnight shifts at least three times a month for 15 years were 35% more likely to develop colon cancer than those who worked only days.

Researchers think the increased risk may be linked to lowered levels of melatonin, which usually reaches peak production in the body in the middle of the night; nighttime exposure to light can dramatically reduce that output. The hormone is believed to have anti-cancer properties, but researchers say more study is needed before a link can be confirmed.

GRAVEYARD SHIFT

Women who worked during the night were 35% more likely to develop colon cancer than daytime workers

■ Resources

NIH WEBSITE: *www.nlm.nih.gov/medlineplus/colorectalcancer.h.gov*
NATIONAL CANCER INSTITUTE: *www.cancer.gov/cancertopics/types/colon-and-rectal*

Virtual Colonoscopy

If you've ever had a colonoscopy—that much dreaded procedure in which a physician inserts a lighted tube into your rectum and snakes it up your large intestine, looking for abnormal growths that could lead to colon cancer—it's easy to see the appeal of the so-called virtual colonoscopy. The procedure is far less invasive: a small device blows air into the rectum to inflate the bowel while a CT scanner takes X rays. Unfortunately, when the process was first tested, the results were poor. In some cases, half the polyps that needed to be caught were missed.

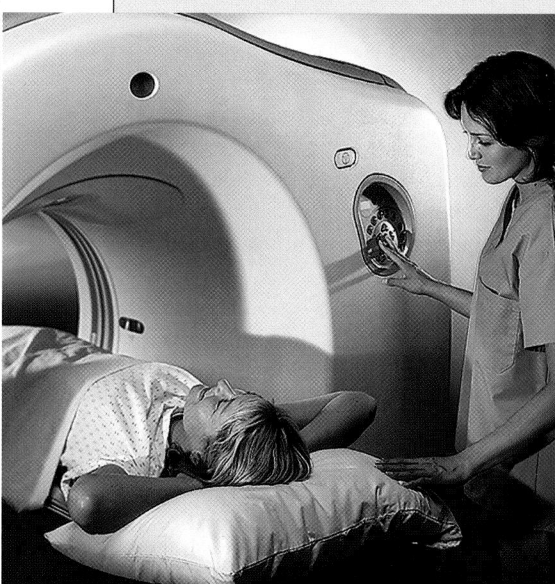
GENERAL ELECTRIC CO.

So there was great interest when a December 2003 report suggested that a new, 3-D virtual colonoscopy (using a special marking potion consumed in advance) might be as good as a traditional colonoscopy. The patient-friendly approach promised to encourage more screenings and save lives. Currently, only about half the folks who ought to be screened for colorectal cancer undergo the available tests for the disease.

But researchers' hopes were dashed again: an April 2004 study deemed virtual 3-D colonoscopies significantly less effective at finding polyps than the standard procedure. The disparity prompted the *Journal of the American Medical Association* to editorialize that the difference between virtual colonoscopy's potential and its results is "so great that physicians must be cautious." ■

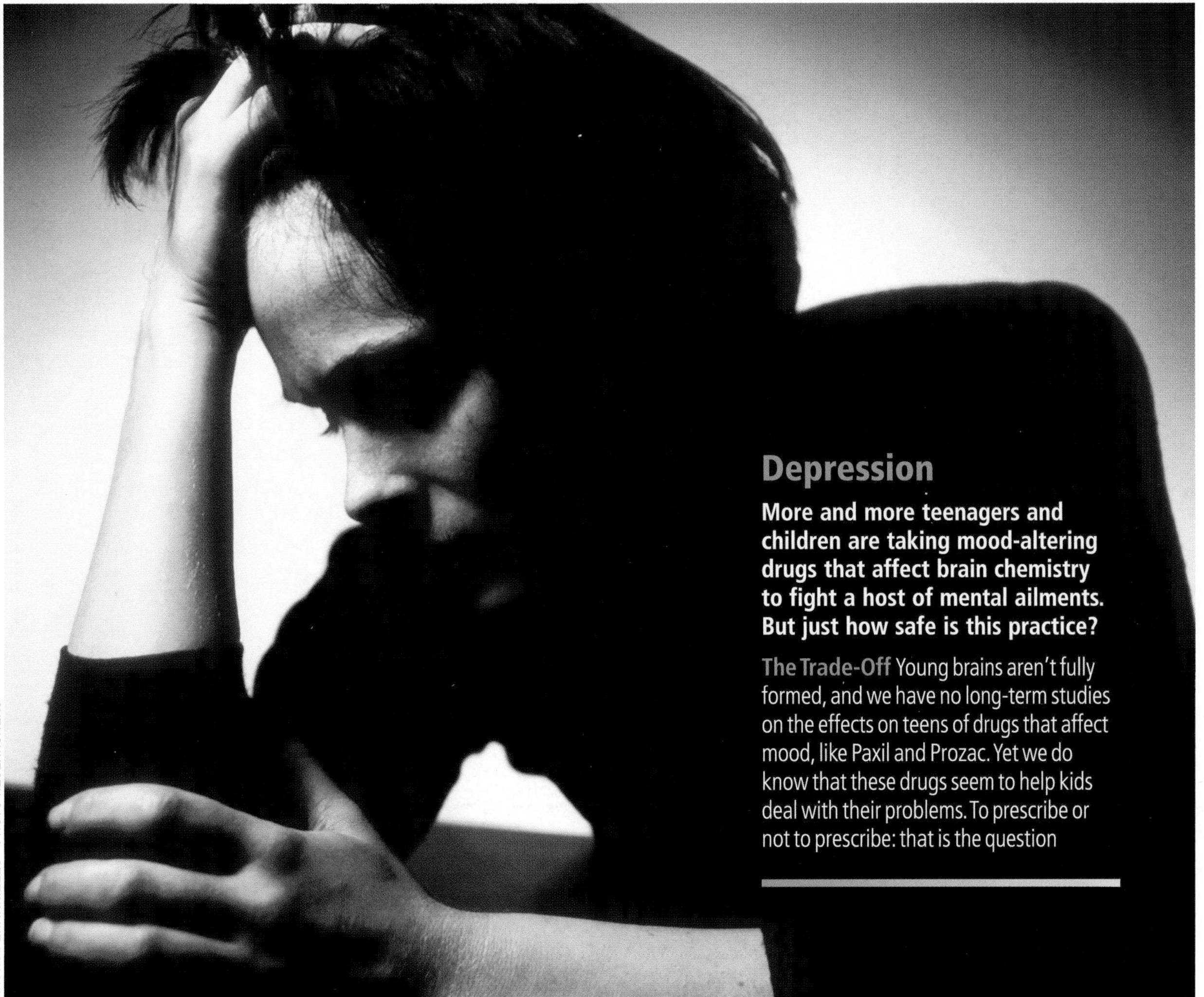

MAURO FERMARIELLO—PHOTO RESEARCHERS

C

D

Depression
Diabetes
Diet & Nutrition
Dyslexia

Depression

More and more teenagers and children are taking mood-altering drugs that affect brain chemistry to fight a host of mental ailments. But just how safe is this practice?

The Trade-Off Young brains aren't fully formed, and we have no long-term studies on the effects on teens of drugs that affect mood, like Paxil and Prozac. Yet we do know that these drugs seem to help kids deal with their problems. To prescribe or not to prescribe: that is the question

D

A generation of American kids is growing up with quick, medicated fixes for their problems with depression and behavior. And that has many doctors—and parents—concerned. Here is a look at the benefits and risks of prescribing antidepressant drugs to youngsters whose brains are still developing.

➤A Medicated Generation Just a few years ago, psychologists couldn't say with certainty that kids were even capable of suffering from depression the same way adults do. Now, according to PhRMA, a pharmaceutical trade group, as many as 10% of all American kids may suffer from some mental illness. Perhaps twice that many have exhibited some symptoms of depression. Up to a million others may suffer from the alternately depressive and manic mood swings of bipolar disorder (BPD), one more condition that until recently was thought to be an affliction of adults alone.

Attention deficit/hyperactivity disorder (ADHD) rates are exploding too. A Mayo Clinic study concluded that kids between 5 and 19 have at least a 7.5% chance of being diagnosed with ADHD. Other children are receiving diagnoses and pills for everything from obsessive-compulsive disorder (OCD) and social-anxiety disorder to post-traumatic stress disorder (PTSD), pathological impulsiveness to phobias and more.

OVER-PRESCRIBED?

Young Americans are taking drugs to fight depression, ADHD, bipolar disorder and a host of behavioral ills

Has the world—and American society in particular—simply become a more destabilizing place in which to raise children? Probably so. But other factors are at work, including sharp-eyed parents and doctors with a rising awareness of childhood mental illness and what can be done for it. Also feeding the trend for more diagnoses is the arrival of

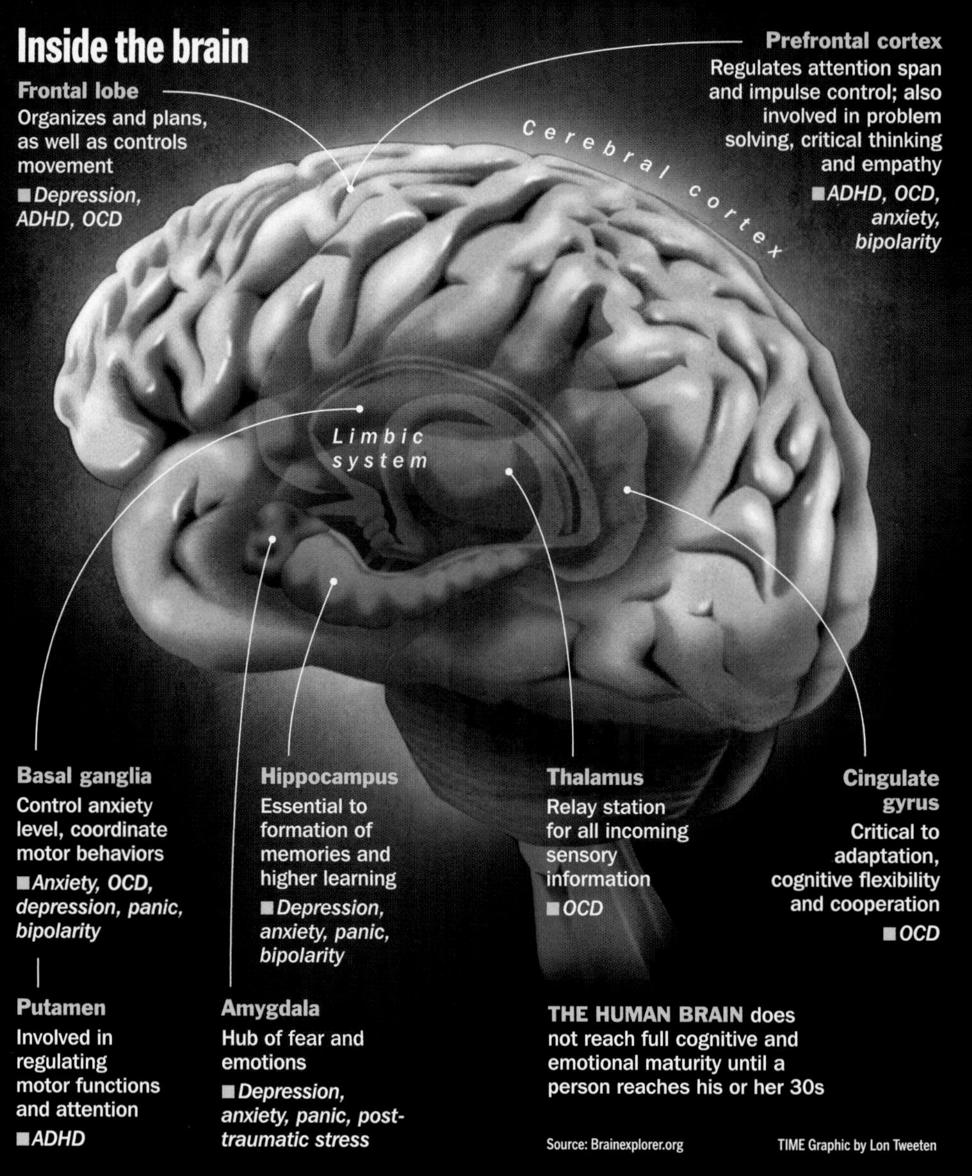
Inside the brain
Frontal lobe
Organizes and plans, as well as controls movement
■ Depression, ADHD, OCD
Prefrontal cortex
Regulates attention span and impulse control; also involved in problem solving, critical thinking and empathy
■ ADHD, OCD, anxiety, bipolarity
Cerebral cortex
Limbic system
Basal ganglia
Control anxiety level, coordinate motor behaviors
■ Anxiety, OCD, depression, panic, bipolarity
Putamen
Involved in regulating motor functions and attention
■ ADHD
Hippocampus
Essential to formation of memories and higher learning
■ Depression, anxiety, panic, bipolarity
Amygdala
Hub of fear and emotions
■ Depression, anxiety, panic, post-traumatic stress
Thalamus
Relay station for all incoming sensory information
■ OCD
Cingulate gyrus
Critical to adaptation, cognitive flexibility and cooperation
■ OCD
THE HUMAN BRAIN does not reach full cognitive and emotional maturity until a person reaches his or her 30s
Source: Brainexplorer.org
TIME Graphic by Lon Tweeten

whole new classes of psychotropic drugs with fewer side effects and greater efficacy than earlier medications, particularly the selective serotonin reuptake inhibitors (SSRIs) used to treat depression. One study found that the use of antidepressants among children and teens tripled between 1987 and 1996, and the numbers are increasing.

Nobody, not even the drug companies, argues that pills alone are the ideal answer to mental illness. Most experts believe that drugs are most effective when combined with talk therapy or other counseling. Nonetheless, there are now dozens of medications available for troubled kids, from the relatively familiar Ritalin (for ADHD) to Zoloft and Celexa (for depression) to less familiar ones like Seroquel and Depakote (for bipolar disorder), and more are being developed all the time.

While a few of the newest meds were developed or approved specifically for kids, the majority have been okayed for adults only. These are then used "off label" for younger and younger patients at children's-size doses. The practice is common and perfectly legal but potentially risky, because children and teens may metabolize medications differently than do adults.

WHEN PILLS DO WORK

Every time the use of antidepressants jumps 1%, suicide rates of kids age 10 to 19 fall, one study reported

Within the medical community—to say nothing of the families of the troubled kids—concern is growing about just what psychotropic drugs can do to still developing brains. Few people deny that the pills help—ask the untold numbers who have climbed out of depressive pits or shaken off bipolar fits thanks to modern pharmacology. But few deny either that in America's quick-fix culture, if you give us a feel-good answer to a complicated problem, we'll use it with little thought of long-term consequences.

➤Why Medicate? In one sense, we are using today's medicated teens as guinea pigs, for the mood-altering drugs they take are so new that no long-term tests have been performed on them. But when a child is suffering or suicidal, is it fair to deny him the prescription pad in conjunction with therapy? Is it even safe? Untreated depression has a lifetime suicide rate of 15%—with more deaths caused by related behaviors like self-medicating with alcohol and drugs. Severe and untreated childhood ADHD has been linked, according to some studies, to higher rates of substance abuse, dropping out of school and having trouble with the law.

Dr. Mark Olfson of the New York State Psychiatric Institute reported in a 2003 study that every time the use of antidepressants jumps 1%, suicide rates among kids 10 to 19 decrease, although only slightly. But that doesn't include the nonsuicidal depressed kids whose misery is eased by the same pills.

➤Are We Disrupting Development? For kids with less severe problems

APPROVED FOR TEENS?

A check indicates a drug has been tested and approved for teen use

Adderal	✓	Zoloft	No
Concerta	✓	Paxil	No
Strattera	✓	Effexor	No
Ritalin	✓	Depakote	No
Prozac	✓	Zyprexa	No
		Lithium	No

—children who are somber but not depressed, antsy but not clinically hyperactive—the pros and cons of using drugs are less obvious.

What concerns some doctors is that if you medicate a child's developing brain, you may be burning the village to save it. What does any kind of psychopharmacological meddling do, not just to brain chemistry but also to the acquisition of emotional skills—when, for example, antianxiety drugs are prescribed for a child who has not yet acquired the experience of managing stress without the meds? And what about side effects, from weight gain to jitteriness to flattened personality—all the things you don't want in the social crucible of grade school and, worse, high school.

Adding to the worries is a growing body of knowledge showing just how incompletely formed a child's brain truly is; it doesn't assume its mature form until age 30 or so (*see* Brain). That's a lot of time for drugs to muck around with cerebral clay.

For that reason, it may not always be worth pulling the pharmacological rip cord, particularly when symptoms are relatively mild. Child psychologists point out that nonpharmaceutical treatments can often reduce or eliminate the need for drugs. Anxiety disorders such as phobias can respond well to behavioral therapy—in which patients are gently exposed to graduated levels of the very things they fear until the brain habituates to the escalating risk.

Depression too may respond to new, streamlined therapy techniques, especially cognitive therapy, a treatment aimed at helping patients reframe their view of the world so that setbacks and losses are put in less catastrophic perspective. Sadly, medical insurance pays more readily for pills than for these other treatments for adults and children.

➤Hasty Prescriptions? Like adults taking mind meds, children often get their drugs not from a specialist in psychiatry and psychopharmacology but from any M.D. with the power of the prescription pad. Usually this means the pediatrician or family doctor, who isn't likely to have the time or training necessary for the extensive evaluations needed before drugs can be properly prescribed—much less the required follow-up visits. Part of the reason for all the hurry-up drugging, say psychiatrists, is managed care companies, which, already disinclined to pay for longer, more costly talk therapy, are equally reluctant to foot the bill to make sure patients on pills are well monitored.

Reacting to the controversy, the FDA in March of 2004 asked researchers at Columbia University to review the available data on the use of SSRIs in children and teens, aiming to issue a final ruling on the subject by the end of 2004.

For the present, though, the heaviest lifting will, as always, be left to the family. Perhaps the most powerful medicine a suffering child needs is the educated instincts of a well-informed parent—one who has taken the time to study all the pharmaceutical and nonpharmaceutical options and pick the right ones. There will always be dangers associated with taking too many drugs—and also dangers from taking too few.

■ Resources

FDA ADVISORY, ANTIDEPRESSANTS: *www.fda.gov/cder/drug/antidepressants*

Ivory Tower Blues

A shadow has fallen on America's colleges. A growing number of students arrive on campus suffering from depression and other emotional disorders—some diagnosed, some hidden. A rapid-fire trio of student suicides at New York University in the fall of 2003 focused attention on the problem. Two students leaped to their deaths from the inner balcony of the campus library, below; a third threw herself from the sixth-floor window of an off-campus apartment.

Behind these deaths lurks an array of grim statistics that show how prevalent mental disorders have become on campus. Data from a 2001 survey of college mental-health counselors, when compared with past findings, revealed that the percentage of students treated at college counseling centers who have had psychological problems diagnosed and are taking psychotropic drugs increased from 7% in 1992 to 18% in 2001. The survey also found that during the previous five years, 85% of North American student counseling centers reported an increase in students with "severe psychological problems."

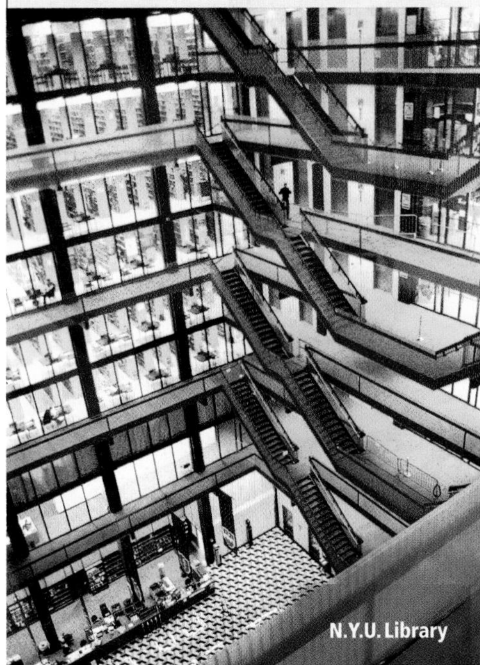

N.Y.U. Library

Despite concerns about their long-term effects, mood-altering drugs may be helping in the crisis. As the rate of their use on campus has gone up, overall reported college suicide rates, despite the cluster at N.Y.U., have fallen noticeably, from a total of 122 in 2000 to 80 in 2001. ■

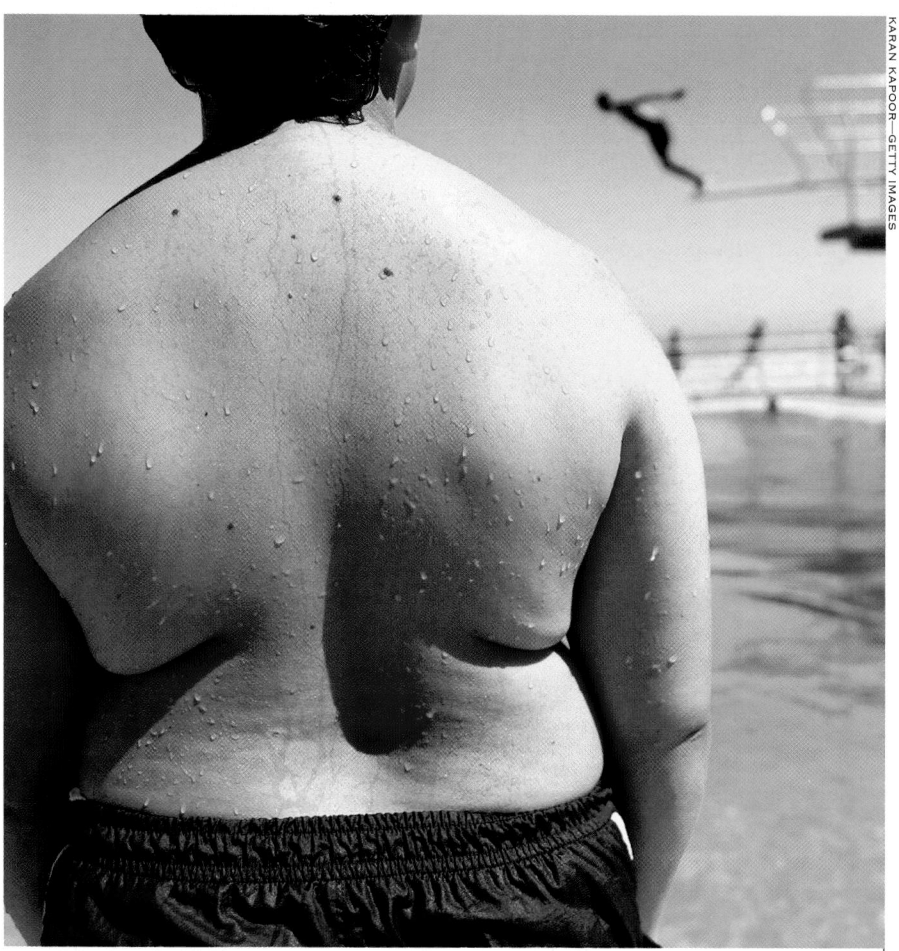

KARAN KAPOOR—GETTY IMAGES

Diabetes

The ailment that affects the way our bodies process sugar is surging in America. Yet some simple lifestyle changes can make a huge difference in warding off diabetes

Metabolic Syndrome Doctors have a new term for the symptoms that may lead to diabetes: metabolic syndrome. The signs to watch for: high blood pressure; resistance to insulin; high levels of triglycerides; low levels of HDL, the "good" cholesterol

The U.S. is under siege, beset by a raging epidemic of diabetes. Some 18 million Americans suffer from one form or another of the disease, with 1.3 million new cases diagnosed in 2002—up from 878,000 in 1997. The most common form of the ailment, Type 2 diabetes, is a chronic metabolic disorder that used to be called adult onset diabetes but was renamed in part because so many children were developing it, a fact of grave concern to health officials. Not only are these kids likely to face a lifetime of problems—including higher risks of blindness, heart disease and stroke—they are also a warning sign that something in our way of life has gone terribly wrong.

Yet scientists in just the past decade have learned that the most devastating complications of diabetes—and in some cases the disease itself—are almost entirely preventable. There are better techniques for monitoring diabetes and more effective drugs for treating it, and a major study published last year shows that by making only modest changes in diet and exercise, people at high risk of Type 2 diabetes can stave off the disease for at least three years and perhaps a lot longer.

A GRIM HARVEST

More than 200,000 Americans with diabetes will die from its complications in the year 2004

It's a puzzle. Never have physicians known so much about Type 2 diabetes and how to control it, yet the number of cases is expected to rise at an alarming rate. Epidemiologists predict that by 2025 the incidence in the U.S. will have doubled. Hardest hit will be certain ethnic groups—including African Americans and Native Americans, Hispanics and Asians—that for complicated reasons are more prone to the disorder.

Lots of doctors will tell you that the reason for the explosion is obvious: Americans are eating too much and exercising too little. There is no question that excessive weight increases your risk of becoming diabetic. But that explains only part of the problem. Diabetes has a strong genetic component, and scientists are beginning to suspect that certain evolutionary factors, as well as your mother's metabolic or nutritional status during pregnancy, may predispose you to develop it.

A complex picture is emerging that is changing the way we think about what was already a complex disease. It turns out that patients are not as helpless against its ravages as was once thought, especially if they are warned at the disease's very earliest stages. Changes in lifestyle and diet can, in the vast majority of cases, make a big difference. The future for anyone with diabetes has never been brighter, provided he or she has access to the right treatments. But the failure to act has never been more broadly devastating. In 2004 more than 200,000 Americans with diabetes will die from its complications.

➤**What Is Diabetes?** To understand the latest insights into the disease, it helps to know a little more about two key molecules—glucose and insulin—and the roles they play in the conditions doctors call Type 1 and Type 2 diabetes. We'll start with glucose, the sugar molecule that is a major source of fuel for the body. You can get your glucose levels tested at a doctor's office or at home with a device called a glucometer. What you're looking for is a reading measured in milligrams of glucose per deciliter of blood (or, on some glucometers, in millimoles per liter). Anyone whose glucose level before breakfast—the fasting level—is 126 mg/dL (7 mmol/L) or higher is considered diabetic. A normal fasting level runs anywhere from 65 mg/dL to just under 100 mg/dL (3.6 mmol/L to 5.6 mmol/L).

ADDING TO THE RISK

For reasons that are not yet clear, diabetes greatly increases your chance of suffering a heart attack or stroke

Insulin is a hormone made by specialized cells in the pancreas, whose job is to push glucose out of the blood into various cells in the body. Whenever the amount of glucose in the blood starts to rise, which happens just about whenever you eat, the pancreas pumps out more insulin to keep sugar levels stable. Here's where the difference between Type 1 and Type 2 is clearest. Type 1 diabetics have high glucose levels because their pancreas can no longer make insulin. By definition, Type 1 diabetics must eventually take insulin shots to get their diabetes under control. Type 2 diabetics can still make their own insulin, but their bodies don't respond as well to it—a situation called insulin resistance.

Any scientist who can figure out why Type 2 diabetics are insulin resistant will probably be a candidate for a Nobel Prize. It's not a simple consequence of being overweight. Many obese people are not insulin resistant, and not everyone who is insulin resistant is overweight. Researchers at the Salk Institute in La Jolla, Calif., believe that at least part of the answer lies not in the pancreas but in the liver. In a 2004 study of mice, they identified a protein that tells the liver to favor the metabolism of fat over that of glucose. The result is a buildup of glucose levels in the blood, a hallmark of insulin resistance.

➤The Sugar Blues What's so bad about being insulin resistant and having too much glucose in your blood? For reasons that researchers are still trying to figure out, having diabetes greatly increases your risk of suffering a heart attack or a stroke. A man with diabetes appears to have the same risk of cardiovascular problems as a nondiabetic who has had a heart attack. A woman who develops diabetes loses the cardioprotective benefits of being female. And kids with Type 2 diabetes are more likely to develop heart disease in their 20s and 30s.

The condition also damages small blood vessels throughout the body—especially in the eyes and kidneys. As many as 24,000 diabetics in the U.S. become blind each year; more than 100,000 require dialysis or kidney transplantation; and 82,000 need to have a toe, foot or leg amputated. Diabetics are twice as likely as nondiabetics to suffer from depression.

It doesn't have to be this way. Back in 1993 doctors proved that Type 1 diabetics could greatly reduce their risk of complications by intensively managing their

DIABETES SELF-TEST

Whether you have diabetes or one of its precursor conditions—prediabetes or metabolic syndrome—there's a lot you can do to safeguard your health. But it's tough to get the right treatment if you don't know there's a problem

Do You Have Prediabetes?

A person with prediabetes has slightly higher than normal glucose levels and is considered prediabetic if:

1	Your fasting glucose is at least 100 mg/dL but less than 125 mg/dL	☐
2	Your glucose-tolerance test is at least 140 mg/dL but less than 200mg/dL	☐

Do You Have Diabetes?

Your body can't control the amount of sugar in your blood, resulting in a fasting glucose of 126 mg/dL or higher. You should get tested if you notice any of these warning signs:

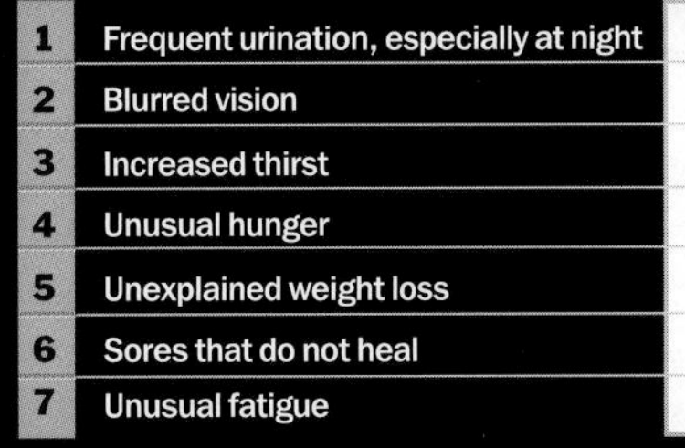

1	Frequent urination, especially at night	☐
2	Blurred vision	☐
3	Increased thirst	☐
4	Unusual hunger	☐
5	Unexplained weight loss	☐
6	Sores that do not heal	☐
7	Unusual fatigue	☐

Do You Have Metabolic Syndrome?

If three or more of the following are true, you have the syndrome and are at risk for heart disease or diabetes:

1	Your waist measures more than 40 in. (in men) or 35 in. (in women)	☐
2	Your fasting triglyceride level is 150 mg/dL or higher	☐
3	The level of HDL cholesterol in your blood is less than 40 mg/dL (if you're a man) or 50 mg/dL (if you're a woman)	☐
4	Your blood pressure is 130/85 mm Hg or higher	☐
5	Your fasting glucose measures 110 mg/dL or higher	☐

Blood glucose levels

In milligrams per deciliter of blood (mg/dl)

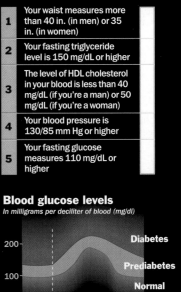

Sources: Dr. Frank Vinicor; Dr. David Nathan

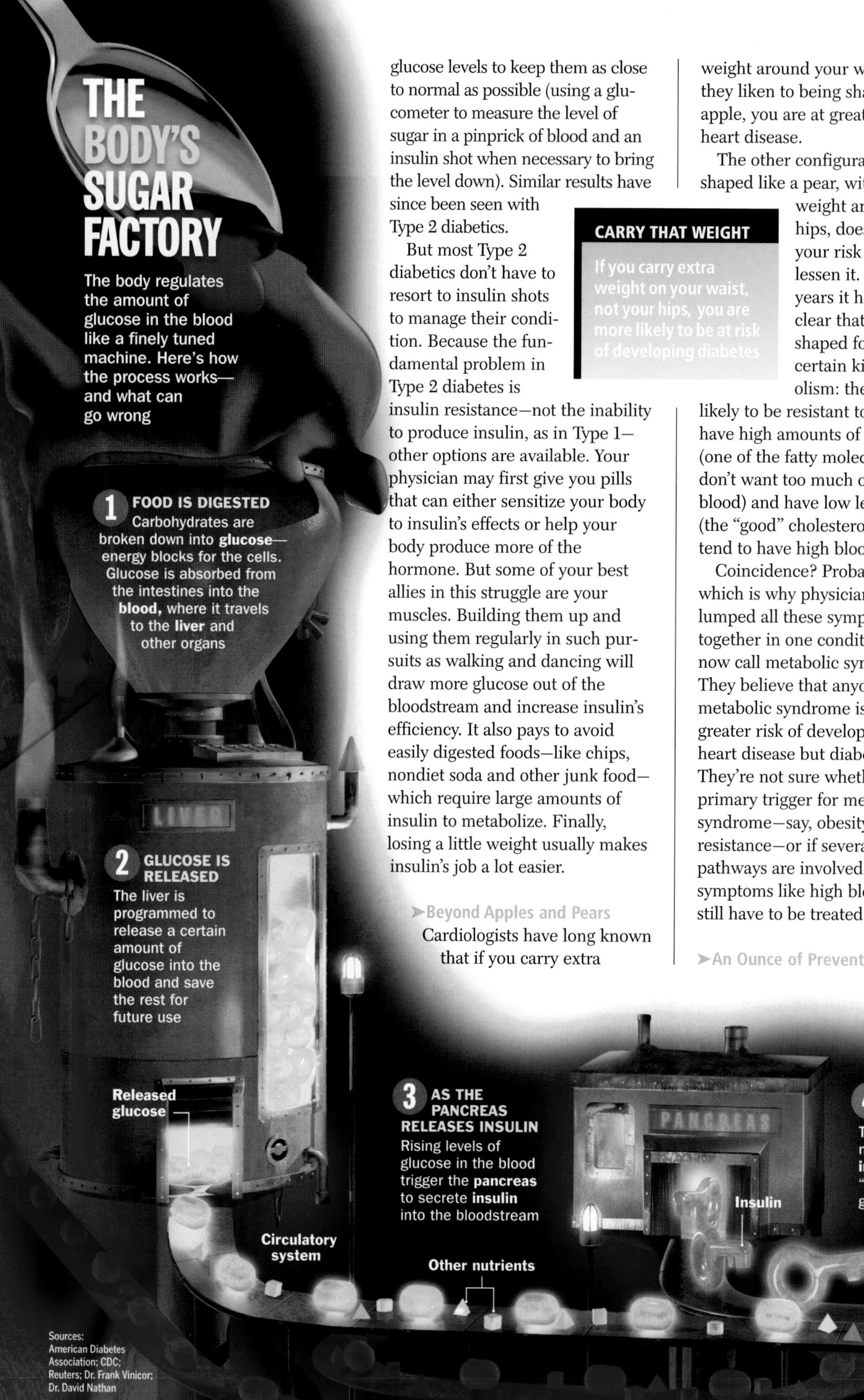

glucose levels to keep them as close to normal as possible (using a glucometer to measure the level of sugar in a pinprick of blood and an insulin shot when necessary to bring the level down). Similar results have since been seen with Type 2 diabetics.

THE BODY'S SUGAR FACTORY
The body regulates the amount of glucose in the blood like a finely tuned machine. Here's how the process works—and what can go wrong
1 FOOD IS DIGESTED Carbohydrates are broken down into glucose—energy blocks for the cells. Glucose is absorbed from the intestines into the blood, where it travels to the liver and other organs
LIVER
2 GLUCOSE IS RELEASED The liver is programmed to release a certain amount of glucose into the blood and save the rest for future use
Released glucose
Circulatory system
3 AS THE PANCREAS RELEASES INSULIN Rising levels of glucose in the blood trigger the pancreas to secrete insulin into the bloodstream
PANCREAS
Insulin
Other nutrients
4 AND CELLS RECEIVE ENER
The insulin "key" must fit into the cell' insulin-receptor "lock" for glucose to get inside the cells
Sources: American Diabetes Association; CDC; Reuters; Dr. Frank Vinicor; Dr. David Nathan

But most Type 2 diabetics don't have to resort to insulin shots to manage their condition. Because the fundamental problem in Type 2 diabetes is insulin resistance—not the inability to produce insulin, as in Type 1—other options are available. Your physician may first give you pills that can either sensitize your body to insulin's effects or help your body produce more of the hormone. But some of your best allies in this struggle are your muscles. Building them up and using them regularly in such pursuits as walking and dancing will draw more glucose out of the bloodstream and increase insulin's efficiency. It also pays to avoid easily digested foods—like chips, nondiet soda and other junk food—which require large amounts of insulin to metabolize. Finally, losing a little weight usually makes insulin's job a lot easier.

CARRY THAT WEIGHT

If you carry extra weight on your waist, not your hips, you are more likely to be at risk of developing diabetes

➤Beyond Apples and Pears Cardiologists have long known that if you carry extra weight around your waist, which they liken to being shaped like an apple, you are at greater risk of heart disease.

The other configuration, being shaped like a pear, with excess weight around the hips, doesn't eliminate your risk but seems to lessen it. Over the years it has become clear that apple-shaped folks have a certain kind of metabolism: they are more likely to be resistant to insulin, have high amounts of triglycerides (one of the fatty molecules you don't want too much of in your blood) and have low levels of HDL (the "good" cholesterol). They also tend to have high blood pressure.

Coincidence? Probably not, which is why physicians have lumped all these symptoms together in one condition that they now call metabolic syndrome. They believe that anyone with metabolic syndrome is at much greater risk of developing not just heart disease but diabetes as well. They're not sure whether there is a primary trigger for metabolic syndrome—say, obesity or insulin resistance—or if several biological pathways are involved. Individual symptoms like high blood pressure still have to be treated separately.

➤An Ounce of Prevention Advances

in diabetes research over the past few years have been swift and wide ranging. Scientists are beginning to identify the genetic and environmental factors that predispose some people to insulin resistance and increase their risk of diabetes. Researchers are looking beyond glucose levels to gauge patients' health and progress, and they have identified other pathways that may play a role in triggering diabetes.

Every new insight into Type 2 diabetes, from its biochemistry to its metabolic roots, makes clear that it can be avoided—and that the earlier you intervene the better.

The real question is whether we as a society are up to the challenge. "Our health-care system is currently set up to deliver care for acute disease," says Ann Albright, chief of the California Diabetes Prevention and Control Program. "It's get in, get your shot, and away you go."

NO TIME FOR EXCUSES

Every new insight into Type 2 diabetes tells us that it can be avoided, and the earlier you intervene, the better

Diabetes, however, is a chronic disorder that demands constant attention. You have to change your eating habits and incorporate physical exercise into each day's activities. You need to monitor your glucose levels several times a day to see how well you're doing. These prevention measures pay off in the long run in fewer heart attacks, strokes, amputations and cases of blindness and kidney failure. But very few insurance programs focus on them—or pay for health professionals who can teach folks how best to fit them into their lives. Comprehensive prevention programs aren't cheap, but the cost of doing nothing is far greater.

There are ways to keep costs down. It doesn't take a physician to teach a patient the principles of better nutrition or how to use a glucometer. Nurses, nutritionists, diabetes educators and other non-M.D.s can play a key role. "You can't give everybody the same diet to solve the problem," says Albright, a registered dietitian. "People obviously eat the foods they've grown up with. So you have to try to help them get as much of those things that they like into their eating plan but also make the changes that will help lower the fat or moderate the carbohydrates."

Resources

NIH DIABETES CENTER: *www.nlm.nih.gov/medlineplus/diabetes*
NIH HOTLINE: *800-860-8747*
CDC INQUIRY LINE: *877-232-3244*

Measuring Glucose

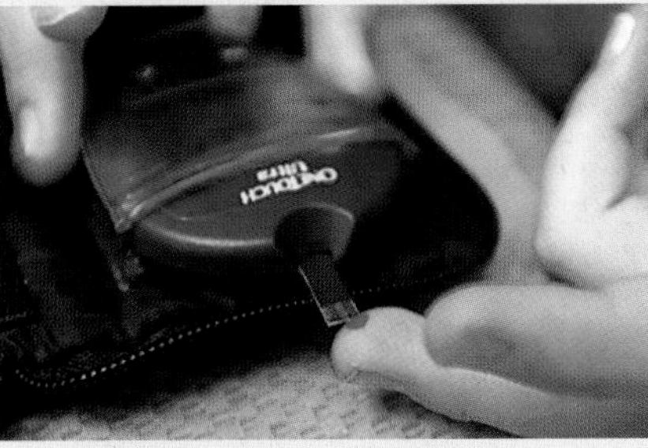

Once you've been given a diagnosis of diabetes, it's important to keep track of your blood-glucose levels. This can be done in one of several ways:

- **Finger Stick** The most common way to keep track of blood-sugar levels—pricking the finger for blood before meals and bed—has become more convenient and less painful than it used to be. Automatic lances, above, make the drawing of blood easier, and computerized devices can record readings automatically.
- **A1C** Also known as the glycatede hemoglobin test, A1C is a blood test that provides a record of your glucose levels over two to three months. Glucose in the blood attaches to hemoglobin, and because red blood cells circulate in the body for several months, levels of glycated hemoglobin are a good indicator for average blood-glucose levels over time.
- **Urine** When the body can't make enough insulin and blood sugar levels get too high, it begins to break down fat, forming ketones. These compounds spill out into the urine, signaling too little insulin at work.

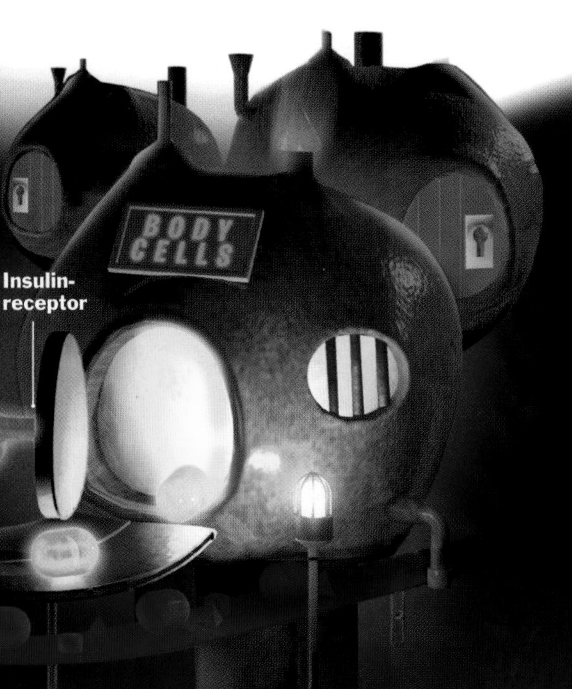

DIABETES: WHAT GOES WRONG

In Type 2 diabetes, faulty insulin-receptors prevent the key from opening the cell. At other times the insulin does not work properly or the pancreas does not produce enough of it. Either way, glucose cannot enter the cells and builds up in the blood. Eventually, this can damage small capillaries

At risk:

HEART High blood pressure, high cholesterol, blood-clotting problems and heart failure

EYES Retinopathy, cataracts and glaucoma

NERVOUS SYSTEM Strokes, impotence and foot ulcers leading to amputations

KIDNEYS Kidney disease

BODY CELLS

TIME Graphic by Lon Tweeten; text by Kristina Dell

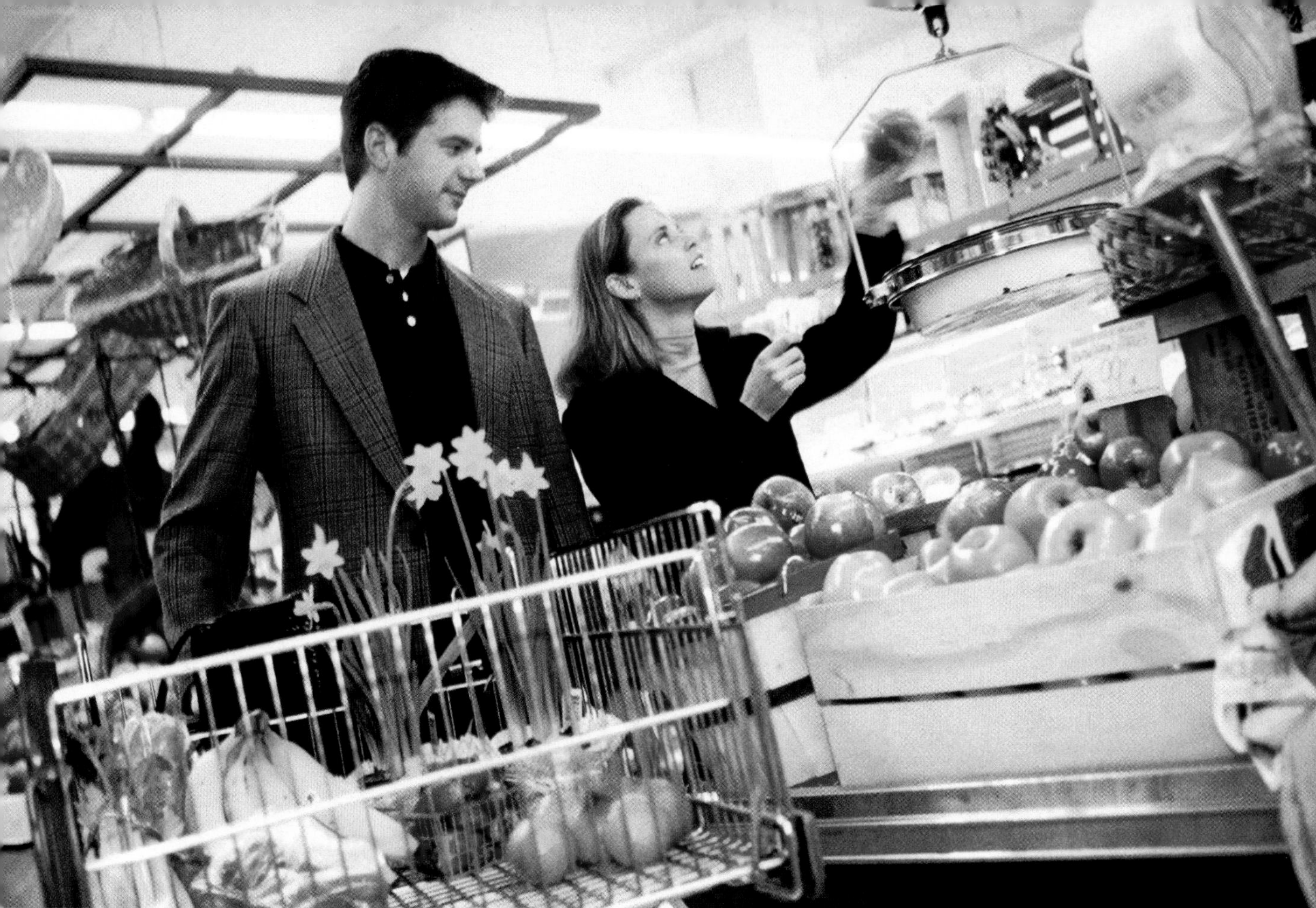

Diet and Nutrition

So many Americans embraced the low-carb diet craze in 2004 that we treat that subject in a separate entry, under Carbohydrates. Here, we treat other news of nutrition

Where to Begin? Here's a suggestion: eat lots of fruits and vegetables, favor whole grains over highly processed cereals and make red meat an occasional treat rather than the centerpiece of most meals. And spud lovers: bid adieu to all those toppings

It's 6:45 p.m. After a bruising day at the office and a hair-raising commute on the freeway, you are standing in the kitchen about to prepare a healthy, satisfying dinner for your spouse, your two school-age children and yourself. As usual, all they want to know is, "What's for dinner?" and "When do we eat?" You dump a box of thin spaghetti into a pot of boiling water, zap 3 cups of green beans in the microwave, pop a loaf of frozen garlic bread into the toaster oven and pour a medium-size jar of marinara sauce into a saucepan to simmer. While all that's bubbling, you chop up half a head of iceberg lettuce and a couple of tomatoes for the salad, which you'll sprinkle with a light dressing. Dessert will be two scoops of frozen yogurt per person and a plate of assorted low-fat cookies for the family to share.

Sounds pretty healthy, right? Wrong. While this meal may be better than what most Americans eat for dinner, it's enough food for a family twice the size of most. In addition, it contains some nutritional traps that in the best-case scenario will make you fat and in the worst will increase your chances of developing diabetes, heart disease and certain types of cancer. Think you know the pitfalls? Read on. You may be surprised.

THE VEGGIE RAINBOW

Pick vegetables across the spectrum: the brighter their hue, the more likely they are to be good for you

Here are a few of the problems:

- Most light salad dressings are too heavy on sugar and salt and too light on nutrition. A better choice is a simple oil-and-vinegar dressing, which—although packed with calories—contains lots of heart-healthy monounsaturated fatty acids and no saturated fat.
- You're serving your family too many highly processed foods. The latest research shows that such foods won't keep them satisfied for very long and may make them hungrier in the long run.
- Having different kinds of cookies to choose from makes it more likely that your family will eat more cookies than they should. The fewer our choices, the less we eat.
- Your portion sizes are far too generous. According to the U.S. Food Guide Pyramid, you're giving each member of your family 4 servings of spaghetti, 112 servings of marinara sauce and 2 servings of frozen yogurt. The

What You Need to Know About . . .

FRUITS & VEGETABLES

The news isn't that fruits and vegetables are good for you. It's that they are so good for you they could save your life

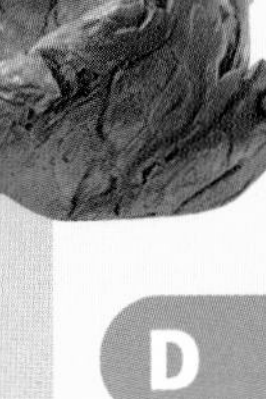

TOP VEGGIES

Average amount Americans eat each year:

Iceberg lettuce
25 lbs. per person

Tomatoes
92 lbs per person (80% in a processed form, such as catsup or pasta sauce)

French fries
51 lbs. per person

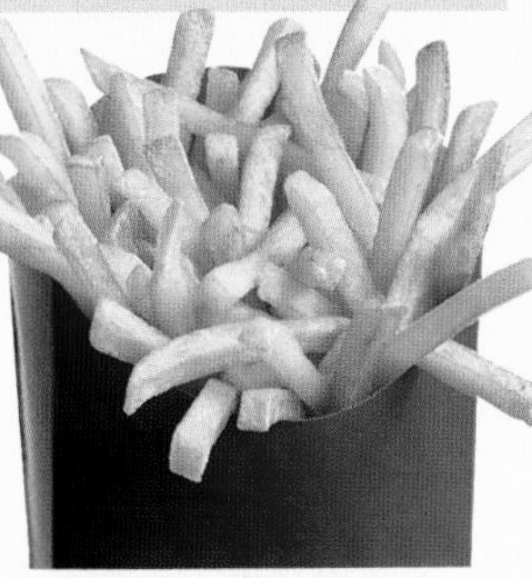

BOTANICAL BOUNTY

The latest scientific research has shown—and the evidence continues to mount—that the plant kingdom is filled with gifts that can help fight off the ravages of chronic disease. A large group of compounds called **phytochemicals** (*see below*), found in plants ranging from garlic to cabbage to tea leaves, have been shown to help fight disease by preventing the cellular damage caused by chemicals called free radicals. A diet rich in fiber also has been shown to help reduce the risk of heart disease, stroke, high blood pressure, obesity, diabetes and cancer. Fiber and phytochemicals are a one-two punch that should be reason enough to eat your peas and broccoli.

DEFINITION

FIBER

Soluble fiber, which dissolves and becomes gummy in water, slows digestion, promoting a sense of fullness. Found in apples, citrus fruits and carrots

Insoluble fiber, also known as roughage, speeds the passage of food through the intestines. Found in wheat bran, veggies and whole grains

SO, WHY DON'T WE EAT OUR VEGGIES?

The trick is not to force yourself to eat stuff you hate but rather to find ways

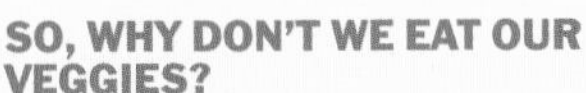

to turn the plant kingdom into dishes you enjoy. Don't want to face a plate of okra or Brussels sprouts? You don't have to. Aim for variety, and put your energy into getting— on a daily basis—as many different vegetables as you can into salads, soups, stews, sides, salsas and pasta sauces. **Fresh is best,** but frozen is fine, and even canned will often do (although mind the added sodium).

AN APPLE A DAY

Fruit is a natural energy source, and there's nothing wrong with eating an apple a day. But why stop there? As always, variety is key, and there's a whole world of fruit to be savored and enjoyed. Look for new ways to **add fruit to your daily routine.** Begin your day with a fruit smoothie or throw a handful of banana slices and mixed berries on your cereal. Add peaches, pears or melons to your lunch, and make fresh or dried fruit a sweet, satisfying snack. Try fish and meat with tropical-fruit salsa. Be adventurous. Find out—finally—what a loquat or a persimmon tastes like.

SPUD TROUBLE

Americans love their potatoes—but too much for their own good. We eat 140 lbs. per capita yearly. And while an **unadorned** potato is low in fat and a good source of nutrients, it is also primarily a carbohydrate that is almost immediately turned into sugar in the body. Besides, who eats plain potatoes? We love to dress them up—mashed with butter or gravy, baked with sour cream, deep-fried, scalloped or au gratin. Putting the humble potato at the center of every meal might have been a necessity a century ago. It isn't now. You don't have to stop eating potatoes—just don't eat them to the exclusion of other vegetables.

THE JUICE TRAP

Starting each day with a glass of juice is a healthy morning ritual. But we need to remember that the juice has more calories—sometimes even added sugar—and **less fiber than the fruit.**

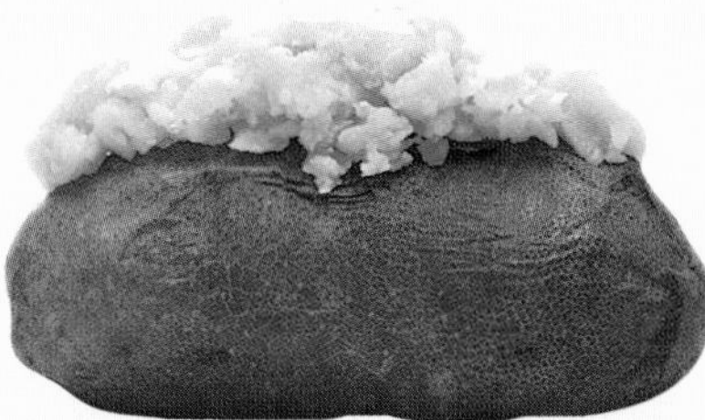

Phytochemicals

You may have seen these compounds touted as supplements. Flavonoids grow naturally in citrus fruits, onions, apples and grapes. Researchers think flavonoids may protect against cancer. Indoles, another kind of phytochemical, are found in cruciferous vegetables (such as broccoli and Brussels sprouts) and may offer protection against a host of chronicdiseases. Other phytochemicals:

CAROTENOIDS

Beta-carotenes, the best-known carotenoids, give color to carrots and other orange, red and yellow produce and are converted to vitamin A in our bodies. Lutein and zeaxanthin (from green vegetables) and lycopene (from tomatoes) may protect against coronary-artery disease, cataracts, macular degeneration and cancer. All the more reason to eat colorful meals

ISOFLAVINS

Plant estrogens—soy foods are a particularly rich source—seem to have some of the same effects as estrogen. Benefits may include:

- **Lower blood-lipid levels**
- **Decreased risk of hormone-related cancers of the breast, ovaries, endometrium and prostate**
- **Relief from menopausal symptoms**

AND ...

Don't like tofu? Soybeans—when roasted—make a good snack. Or try cooking green soybeans (edamame) like lima beans. Soy milk also makes a delicious milk shake

What You Need to Know About . . .

MEAT, FISH & EGGS

Forget fad diets for a minute—even if they do work—and find out how to eat smarter at the top of the food chain. Hint: watch your portion size

BRAIN FOOD

Meat has been a precious food commodity and a great source of **complete protein,** vitamins and other nutrients since prehistoric times. In fact, many anthropologists think meat may have played a key role in the evolution of our species. And although vegetarianism has become increasingly popular in recent years, meat of some variety is still at the center of the American plate.

PUMPING IRON AND THE B VITAMINS

Red meat in particular is a rich source of iron, which plays an important part in **building muscles** and healthy blood. Studies of vegetarians have discovered that they risk becoming iron deficient, which can lead to anemia. The B vitamins found in ample quantities in meat are critical for proper energy production.

OVERPROTEINED

Our ancient ancestors hunted for their meat and expended a lot of energy chasing it down. Today our animal protein is raised on feedlots and in cages and delivered in great abundance nearly to our door. We eat roughly twice as much protein as we need, according to some estimates, risking injury to our kidneys and livers. Many cuts of meat—red meat in particular—are high in the saturated fats that have been linked to heart disease. Some studies suggest that eating meat may predispose us to cancer.

TAME YOUR INNER CARNIVORE

Go ahead, enjoy your bacon cheeseburger. But make it a once- or twice-a-month extravaganza. **Go lean** if you can, but above all, go easy. Remember that meat doesn't have to be an all-or-nothing proposition. Many dishes, such as stir fries and salads, can incorporate small quantities of meat but still satisfy. A pasta sauce can be 25% meat and 75% vegetables. Dr. David Katz of Yale suggests eating lean beef, pork or lamb once or twice a week, chicken or turkey once or twice a week, and fish and other seafood three to four times a week. For most meat eaters, the harder goal will be to bring their portion sizes down to earth. The USDA considers 3 oz. of meat to be one serving. When was the last time you ordered a 3-oz. hamburger or rib-eye steak? Most steak houses serve portions large enough to fulfill your

Burgers: Save for special occasions

whole meal contains 1,500 calories per person, or 80% of the daily requirement for a sedentary office worker.

■ Let's not even get started on whether the tomatoes should be cooked or raw, how much salt and trans fats there are in the garlic bread, or how many calories are packed into that marinara sauce.

It just goes to show that it's hard to eat healthy even when we try. We've all heard that fruits and vegetables are good for us, that restaurant portions are too big, that we should exercise more. But even a casual glance at public-health statistics suggests that Americans don't know how to put that information into practice. Two out of three Americans are overweight or obese. The incidence of Type 2 diabetes among children is climbing. And any gains we've made against heart disease by quitting smoking may be ... up in smoke.

➤A Glut of Information? Alarmed by the worsening trends, health experts have unleashed a flood of nutritional advice for consumers—much of it contradictory. One expert says red meat is bad. Another diet maven says bacon keeps you trim. Someone says skip the potatoes, and someone else says eat the skin. And let's face it, controversy sells. Diet books and magazine articles try to grab our attention by telling us everything we thought we knew was wrong. (It's not.)

EAT RIGHT, LIVE LONG

As much as 80% of heart disease and 90% of diabetes can be tied to unhealthy eating and lifestyle habits

Even the government-approved labels on our food can lead us astray. Serving sizes bear no relationship to the helpings we usually eat. Low-fat products are not necessarily low in calories. And now the Food and Drug Administration says we should be on the lookout for trans fats—a lesser-known type of fat that is every bit as bad for the heart as saturated fat—although we won't learn which products are the worst offenders until 2006.

Meanwhile, the food pyramid, which serves as the basis for all meals prepared in the federal school-lunch program, is about to be changed. The next revision, however, won't be out until 2005. Not that we necessarily mind the data smog: being perplexed can ease our conscience. As long as we can point to a general state of nutritional confusion, we don't have to take responsibility for our ever expanding waistlines.

The truth is that nutritionists have a fairly good idea about what constitutes a healthy diet as

red-meat rations for a couple of months.

FRUITS OF THE SEA

For a low-fat alternative to red meat, it's hard to beat seafood. Fish and shellfish with high levels of **omega-3 fatty acids** have been shown to lower the risk of heart disease and may reduce men's risk of prostate cancer.

STINKERS IN THE BAIT BUCKET

Seafood, however, is not perfect. Among the problems it presents:

- Fish, particularly oily fish, can concentrate **toxins** in their flesh. The heavy metal mercury is a particular concern. Among fish with the highest levels of mercury: swordfish, shark, tilefish and king mackerel.
- More bad news: salmon (both farmed and, to a lesser extent, caught) can contain worrisome levels of PCBs.
- Freshwater anglers are advised that their catch can contain various toxins, depending on the waters they come from. In some cases , the Environmental Protection Agency advises anglers to limit their intake to one fish a week. And some species from particularly polluted waters should never be eaten under any circumstances.

GUIDELINES

The jury is still out on some of these recommendations, but to play it safe, **children and pregnant or nursing women** should eat no more than 12 oz. of fish a week and completely avoid swordfish, shark, mackerel and tilefish. (The rest of us can eat these once or twice a month.) It's uncertain whether tuna is a concern for children and pregnant women, but the FDA gives it safe marks for the rest of us.

GO FISH

The news is not all cautionary. You can catch—and eat—your limit with shellfish, flounder, cod, tilapia and a host of other catches-of-the-day. And don't forget the **small fry:** herring and sardines are high in omega-3s and low in toxins.

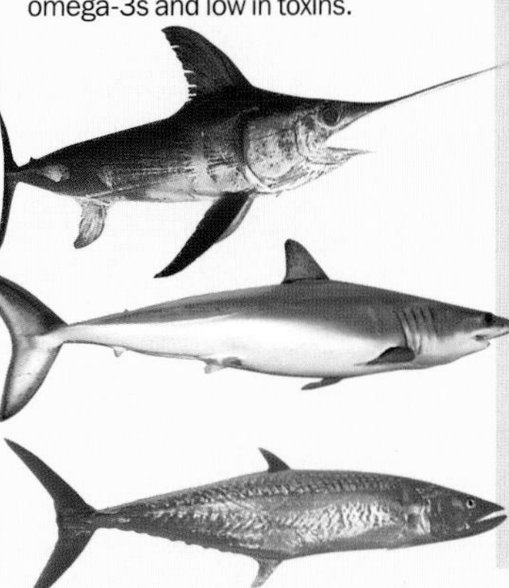

SIRLOIN TIPS

Fat grams per portion size

	8-oz.	3-oz.
Prime rib	83	31
Lamb chop	66	25
Sirloin steak	59	22
Pork chop	20	8
Roasted chicken breast (no skin)	8	3
Broiled fish	2	trace

Source: *Encyclopedia of Foods* (Academic Press)

Meat Rack

Annual pounds per capita consumed in the U.S.

	1950-59	2000
Total meats	**138**	**195**
Beef	53	64
Pork	45	48
Veal/Lamb	9	2
Chicken	16	53
Turkey	4	14
Fish/shellfish	**11**	**15**
Eggs (Number)	**374**	**250**

Source: USDA Economic Research Service

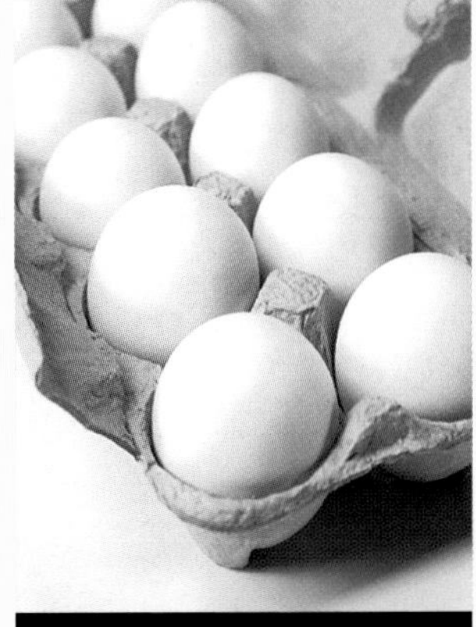

INCREDIBLE, EDIBLE?

Yes, it's safe to go back to the henhouse. Eggs are a complete protein and loaded with nutrients and vitamins A, B_{12}, folic acid and riboflavin—probably the best bargain in the grocery store. But this doesn't mean you should start each day with a mountain of scrambled eggs. Eggs have twice the cholesterol of beef, so three or four a week are plenty.

well as plenty of solid evidence to back that up. As a rule, they tell us, we should eat lots of fruits and vegetables, favor whole grains over highly processed cereals and make red meat an occasional treat rather than the daily centerpiece of our evening meal. And we shouldn't eat any more than our body needs.

Small Changes, Big Rewards The problem is that no matter how much we think we know about what goes into a healthy meal, we often misjudge the results. Some vegetable dishes, it turns out, are healthier than others, some grain products are less processed than others, some fish are safer than others. You may think you are eating right, but by making subtle changes in what you eat and how you eat it, you could start eating considerably healthier.

The rewards are worth the effort. Studies show that as much as 80% of heart disease and 90% of diabetes can be tied to unhealthy eating and lifestyle habits. Doctors have proved that a diet emphasizing fruits and vegetables as well as small amounts of nuts and dairy products can lower blood pressure and "bad" cholesterol as effectively as many medications. Evidence is growing that adding fiber to your diet and avoiding highly refined foods can help prevent or delay the onset of Type 2 diabetes.

You don't have to sacrifice flavor. You don't have to go hungry. You do need to put in some effort—much of it in the kitchen—and accept that there really is no free lunch. But with a little planning and a better understanding of some of the basic food traps, we can all eat better and smarter.

Pomegranate: It's time you got acquainted

Begin by Eating Less "Everything In Moderation" is a great motto—until you realize that *moderation* means different things to different people. Better to nail down some specifics and measure them using a tough-to-fudge yardstick—the much dreaded but ultimately very helpful concept of the calorie.

At its heart, the rule for losing weight is simple: eat fewer calories than you burn. As anyone who has ever tried to shed a couple of pounds knows all too well, that's often harder than it sounds. Eat too little, and your body ratchets down its metabolism so that it doesn't need as much energy and you regain weight more easily.

Nutrition Facts
Serving Size 1 cup (228g)
Servings Per Container 2

Amount Per Serving	
Calories 260	Calories from Fat 120
	% Daily Value*
Total Fat 13g	**20%**
Saturated Fat 5g	**25%**
Trans Fat 2g	
	10%
	28%
	10%
Dietary Fiber 0g	**0%**
Sugars 5g	
Protein 5g	

Vitamin A 4% • Vitamin C 2%
Calcium 15% • Iron 4%

*Percent Daily Values are based on a 2,000 calorie diet. Your Daily Values may be higher or lower depending on your calorie needs:

	Calories:	2,000	2,500
Total Fat	Less than	65g	80g
Sat Fat	Less than	20g	25g
Cholesterol	Less than	300mg	300mg
Sodium	Less than	2,400mg	2,400mg
Total Carbohydrate		300g	375g
Dietary Fiber		25g	30g

Calories per gram:
Fat 9 • Carbohydrate 4 • Protein 4

Fats: Now there are two villains, saturated fats and trans fats

One way to counteract that is to boost your level of physical activity to increase the number of calories you burn. But when it comes to weight control, exercise—though necessary—can take you only so far.

Think about it, and you'll understand why. Food is so plentiful and so readily available that you're always going to be able to eat more than you can sweat off. The average American consumes 530 calories more per day now than he or she did in 1970. That's roughly what you'd get from eating 2½ cups of cooked pasta. You would have to walk an extra two hours a day to burn that off.

That doesn't mean you should forget about exercising—the benefits to your heart, bones and peace of mind are just too great. It does mean you have to pay more attention to the "calories in" side of the equation. Even if you're happy when you step on the scales, you can't eat the way you did when you were a teenager. As you grow older, your body needs fewer calories to keep going. Certain exercises—like yoga and weight training—help counteract the trend because they build muscle, which burns more calories than fat. But to avoid gaining weight, you will have to eat less.

What You Need to Know About . . .

NUTS, BEANS & OILS

Nuts and beans are packed with protein, vitamins and minerals. And if you choose wisely, even oils can be good for you

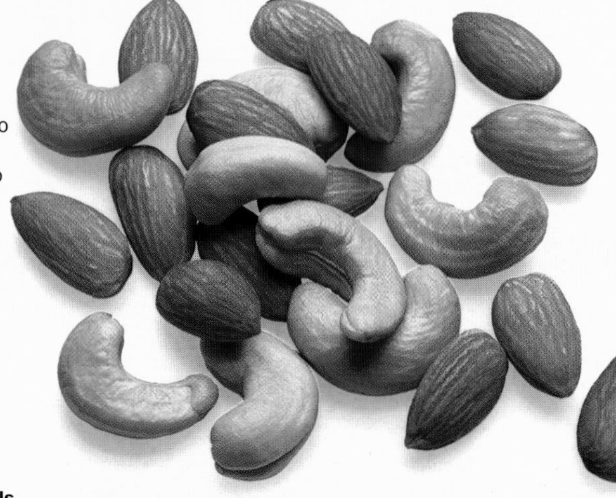

MAGIC FOODS

In other cultures, nuts, seeds and beans make up a major part of the diet, supplying all sorts of **key nutrients** that are hard to replace. If Americans could incorporate more of them into meals, much as we have embraced olive oil to replace less healthy sources of fat, our collective health would improve, and our average waistline would shrink. Here's why:

SEAL OF APPROVAL

Although we tend to think of them as snack foods, nuts and seeds are actually terrific sources of protein, **healthy oils** and other nutrients, especially vitamin E. For that reason, the American Heart Association has allowed packages of nuts to carry the qualified health claim that they "may reduce the risk of heart disease."

RESTRAINING ORDER

But, yes, you can have too much of a good thing. For all their benefits, nuts and seeds are high-calorie foods because of the oils they contain. Beyond that, they often come **heavily dosed with salt,** sugar or both. Tossing back bagfuls of salted, sugared beer nuts while watching the ball game on TV is not the same as going to the gym.

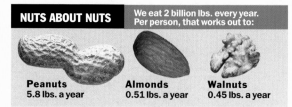

NUTS ABOUT NUTS — **We eat 2 billion lbs. every year. Per person, that works out to:**

Peanuts	Almonds	Walnuts
5.8 lbs. a year	0.51 lbs. a year	0.45 lbs. a year

WARNING

We usually know when we eat animal or butterfat. But we often don't know when we are consuming palm and coconut oils, used to fry chips and frequently found in margarine, chocolates, whipped cream and toppings, even nondairy creamers.

SOMETIMES YOU FEEL LIKE A NUT

As a healthier alternative to chips or pretzels, try reaching for almonds, walnuts, pecans or plain old goobers. But, again, use moderation. Once you start eating nuts, it's hard to stop. **Think handfuls, not bowlfuls.** Eat like a bird: add seeds such as sunflower, pumpkin and sesame to your diet in trail mix, granola, muffins, bread and occasionally even cookies.

FOLLOW THE PATH OF THE BEAN

No restraint is necessary with kidney beans, lentils, chickpeas and their brother beans. They're low in fat and calories and packed with fiber, protein and minerals—and they fill you up to boot. There's a big, beautiful world of legumes, and they play an important role in many ethnic cuisines. Use them dried, fresh, canned or frozen in soups, stews, chilies, curries, pilafs and falafel.

BATTLE OF THE FOOD PYRAMIDS

The USDA's Food Guide

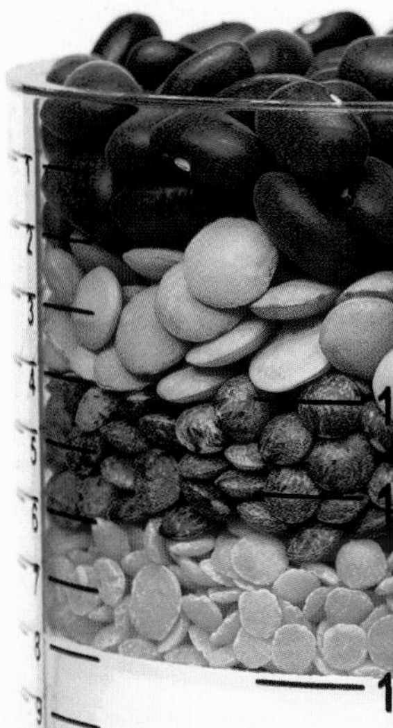

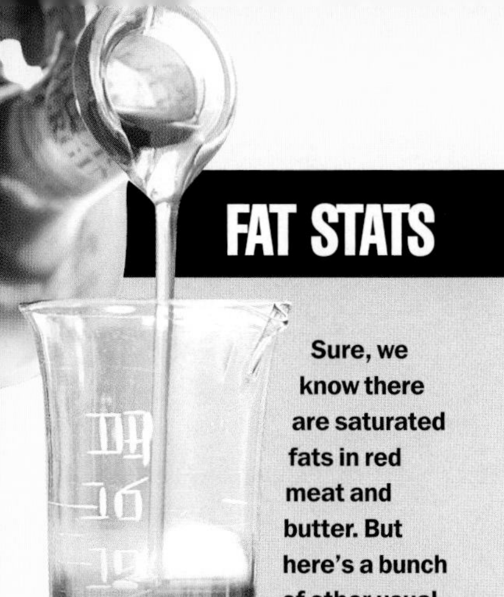

FAT STATS

Sure, we know there are saturated fats in red meat and butter. But here's a bunch of other usual suspects, showing what percentage of total fat is saturated

Coconut oil	**92%**
Butterfat	**64%**
Beef fat	**52%**
Palm oil	**51%**
Lard	**41%**
Chicken fat	**31%**
Peanut oil	**18%**
Soybean oil	**15%**
Olive oil	**14%**
Corn oil	**13%**
Sunflower oil	**9%**
Safflower oil	**9%**
Canola oil	**6%**

Recommended daily grams of total fat/saturated fat

53/17	73/24	93/31
Women and older adults	Men, active women, teen girls, children	Active men and teen boys

Pyramid has turned into a battleground over **how much fat is good for you.** On one side are those like Dr. Dean Ornish of the University of California, San Francisco, who want you to slash fat intake to 10% of daily calories. On the other is Harvard's Dr. Walter Willett, who favors the Mediterranean diet, which permits as much as 40% of calories to come from fat as long as they are from a healthy source of fat, like olive oil.

LESSER OF TWO EVILS? When all fat became bad, anything nonfat became good. Unfortunately, "low-fat" or "fat-free" products are often high in sugar, making them caloric catastrophes.

➤Secrets of Portion Control So, what are some smart ways of cutting back? Start by fooling both your eyes and your stomach. As you reduce the amount of food you eat, use smaller plates to keep your meals from looking skimpy. Begin a couple of meals each week with an apple or a cup of soup. Either will help curb your appetite.

Watch out for the portion-size trap. For reasons known only to bureaucrats, the portion sizes provided in the U.S. government's food pyramid can differ dramatically from those indicated on a product's food label. (One set of figures is regulated by the Department of Agriculture, and the other, which appears on product labels, is regulated by the Food and Drug Administration.) A single serving of pasta is ½ cup (cooked) according to the USDA, 1 cup according to the FDA, and at least 2 cups according to most families.

Eat a variety of fruits and vegetables, but limit your choices of everything else, particularly snacks. Giving folks a wide choice of foods in a single meal, scientists have shown, encourages them to eat more. "It works for every species ever tested—humans, rats, fish, cats," says Susan Roberts, professor of nutrition at Tufts University in Boston. If there are two types of cookies on a plate, the temptation is to eat one of each.

Eventually, you will have to become familiar with the calorie count of your foods. Just a couple of days of measuring or weighing what you eat and calculating the calories you consume can be a real eye opener. You don't have to do this for the rest of your life, just long enough to get a feel for it. Many nutritionists recommend eating healthy frozen dinners, whose calorie counts are printed on the package, as a good way to make the transition to smaller-portion sizes. How many calories you should eat in a day depends on whether you want to lose or maintain weight. The American Heart Association's rule of thumb is to multiply your weight in pounds by 13 (15 if you're active). If you want to lose weight, subtract 250 calories.

➤All Fats Are Not Created Equal For more than 30 years, most researchers agreed that the healthiest diets were those low in percentage of calories attributable to fat. Now they realize that just as there are good and bad types of cholesterol, there are good and bad types of fat. The good fats—found in foods like fish, olive oil, avocados and walnuts—actually improve cholesterol levels in the blood and significantly reduce the risk that the heart will suddenly stop.

As for the bad fats, there are now two villains instead of just one. Saturated fats—typically found in red meat, butter and ice cream—are still champion artery cloggers. But trans fats—found primarily in processed foods, such as margarines and many commercially baked or fried foods but also in whole milk—may be even worse.

Good fats do more than help protect the heart. They also seem to delay hunger pangs. "People on these high-starch, low-fat diets are often hungry soon after they eat. They would be more satisfied eating nuts or a salad with a full-fat dressing," says Dr. Walter Willett, chairman of the department of nutrition at the Harvard School of Public Health and author of *Eat, Drink and Be Healthy* (Fireside; 2001). "And longer-term studies are showing that people tend to be able to control their weight better over the long run on a moderate or higher-fat diet than on a low-fat diet."

Fats have more flavor—just remember that there's a smart way to include fat in your diet and lots of unhealthy ones. Good fats contain double the calories (9 calories per gram) of either proteins or carbohydrates (4 calories per gram). So there's little room for error. If

What You Need to Know About . . .

GRAINS & CEREALS

They are the staff of life, but that doesn't mean our daily bread should be Krispy Kremes or Cinnabons

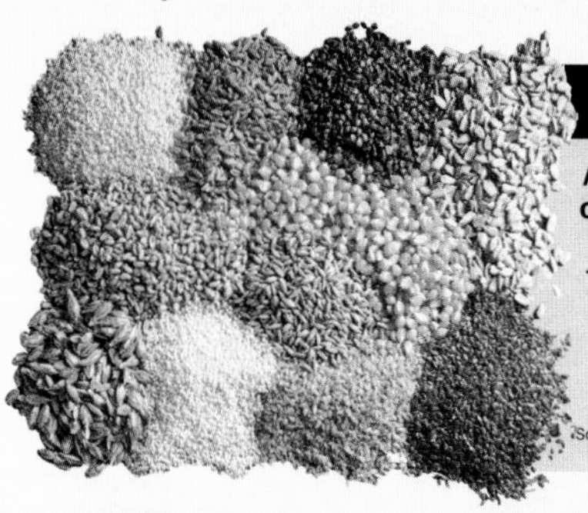

GRAIN GLUT

Annual lbs. per capita consumed in the U.S.

	1950-59	2000
Total grains	155	200
Wheat	126	146
Corn	15	28
Rice	5	20

Source: USDA Economic Research Service

CEREAL SOLUTION

You should replace as many refined carbs as you can with whole grains such as **brown or wild rice,** bulgur, barley and whole-grain flours. A seven-grain dinner roll isn't as scary as it sounds. And if you don't relish a side dish of buckwheat groats, add some to soups and salads. If you don't like whole-wheat pasta (and who does?), eat your favorite but less of it.

BRAIN FOOD

Thousands of years ago, our forebears learned how to **domesticate staples** such as rice, wheat and millet (as well as such less well known grains as amaranth and quinoa), which led in turn to cities, civilization and telemarketing. Packed with complex carbohydrates and essential vitamins such as B and E, grains still account for most of the calories consumed in the world.

PHYSICS LESSON

But the more we grind, mill, refine and strip grains of their constituent parts, such as **bran,** the fiber-rich outer layer, the more quickly our bodies are able to digest them—and the sooner we're hungry again. In ascending order of processing:

- **Whole Grain** Only outer husk removed
- **Cracked or steel cut** Grains are cut into pieces
- **Flaked or rolled** Kernels are flattened by rollers
- **Flour** Whole or polished grains ground into a powder

BEYOND RICE AND PASTA

- **Amaranth** More protein than most grains
- **Wild rice** A marsh grass, native to North America
- **Millet** Ancient grain used as birdseed in the U.S.

you eat nuts, you're going to have to eat less of something else.

What about the Mediterranean diet? you ask. Researchers have long been fascinated by the traditional Greek and Italian diets of the 1960s, which contained as much as 40% fat but didn't trigger a lot of heart attacks. Don't assume that what worked for Greeks and Italians 40 years ago will work for you. After all, they typically ate a pound of fruit a day (equal to four medium apples) and little red meat, and many of them got lots of exercise tilling fields and tending livestock.

Moreover, you can go overboard trying to avoid trans fats. Yes, there is a small amount of trans fat in whole milk, but whole milk is what most pediatricians recommend for children from the age of 1 to 2. Their brains need all kinds of fats to develop properly. After they reach age 2, you've got to be on the lookout for saturated fats as well.

Finally, no matter how much McDonald's reduces the amount of trans fat in its French fries, they are never, alas, going to be a health food. Which brings us to . . .

➤**The Potato Factor** It's not that spuds are so bad; it's that they're misunderstood—not to mention deep-fried and drowned in sour cream and cheese. America's much beloved tuber definitely has a dual personality. A good source of potassium (particularly if you eat the skin) and a great thickener for soups, the potato still doesn't have all the benefits bestowed by more colorful produce like broccoli, Brussels sprouts and green beans.

Make sure the vegetables you eat are as colorful as possible—in order to get a wide variety of nutrients and those ever important antioxidants. Using spinach instead of iceberg lettuce in a salad, for example, will double the dietary fiber consumed, more than quadruple the calcium and potassium, more than triple the folate and provide seven times as much vitamin C. If you don't like spinach, try a more nutritious lettuce like romaine or Boston. Your goal should be to eat at least five ½-cup servings of fruits and vegetables a day—and preferably more. (Nine is divine, according to the latest nutritional research.)

Don't assume that fresh is the only game in town. Because frozen fruits and vegetables are chilled immediately after being picked, they often contain more nutrients than produce that has been sitting on the shelf for a few days.

➤**Sirloin, Salmon or Beans?** Protein from any number of sources can be part of a healthy diet. But figuring out just how much or how little of each to include can be tricky. We've known for some time that most Americans need to cut back on their consumption of red meat because of its high saturated-fat content. But now some health experts are raising the possibility that eating too much fish—long a staple of heart-healthy diets—may expose folks to dangerous levels of mercury and other poisons. That's still being debated. A study published in August 2003 suggests that most of the mercury found in fish is of a form that is not particularly toxic to humans. So if your choice is between the third helping of swordfish that week and a Big Mac, go for the swordfish.

Overall, how much protein do you need? Given the popularity of high-protein diets, you may be surprised to learn that there hasn't been much research on the long-term health benefits and risks of eating lots of protein, although there is concern that too much protein can lead to kidney and liver problems. Scientists have calculated the minimum amount needed to keep your muscles from breaking down—just under 70 grams, or about 2½ oz., a day for someone who weighs 150 lbs. (Food is so plentiful that Americans rarely develop protein deficiencies.) Whether high levels of protein are linked to an increased risk of developing cancer or heart disease remains unclear.

What is known is that too much protein of any kind can leach calcium out of your body and that eating lots of animal protein usually means you're increasing your intake of saturated fat as well. "I don't believe any nutritionist would argue that 30% protein isn't a reasonable upper limit for long-term safety," says Roberts at Tufts. But what is safe and what is ideal are two different matters. Current federal guidelines suggest that adults should get as little as 10% to 15% of their daily calories from protein.

Ice cream: a now-and-then treat

If you're like most people, what interests you about high-protein diets is the possibility that they might make it easier to slim down. Preliminary evidence suggests this may be the case over the short run, but in many ways, that is almost beside the point. "People forget they should be eating a nutritious, healthy diet for other reasons," says Barbara Rolls, professor of nutrition at Pennsylvania State University. "They go on these kooky weight-management fad diets, and they lose all sight of bone and cardiovascular health."

So remember, a little protein goes a long way. Your muscles will not fall apart if you don't eat protein at every meal. Stick with leaner cuts of meat, and give preference to beans, fish, chicken or pork over red meat.

The basic rules for eating smarter couldn't be simpler. Watch your total intake of calories. Burn off as many calories as you take in. And be choosy about the foods you eat—not just for a couple of weeks or months but for the rest of your life. "It takes work," says Dr. John Swartzberg, who chairs the editorial board of the U.C. Berkeley *Wellness Letter.* "We live in a fast-food world." The sooner we accept that that is not the healthiest of environments for us, the better off we'll be.

So, what's for dinner?

Resources

FDA FOOD LABEL INFORMATION: *www.cfsan.fda.gov/~dms/foodlab-*

NIH DIET WEBSITE: *www.health.nih.gov/search.asp/29m.n*

What You Need to Know About . . .

DAIRY & SNACKS

Craving for snacks and desserts is the bane of most dieters. But you can indulge yourself without fattening up your calorie count

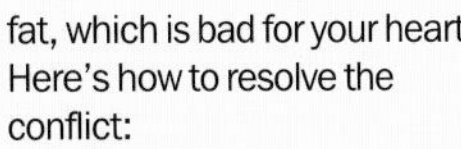

GOOD NEWS, BAD NEWS

Milk, cheese and other dairy products are terrific sources of protein and calcium—the latter a crucial **building block of bones and teeth.** That's why kids especially but adults too should eat plenty. Yet dairy foods are also full of saturated fat, which is bad for your heart. Here's how to resolve the conflict:

COMFORT-FOOD FOLLIES

A nightly bowl of Häagen-Dazs may help smooth out the day's frustrations, but it also gives you 12 grams of saturated fat, 330 calories and 85 mg of cholesterol in a 4 oz. serving. You can satisfy your craving almost as well with low-fat frozen yogurt. The dairy case is also packed with low- and nonfat milk, yogurt and cheeses. Aim for two to three servings a day, says the USDA, and remember that serving sizes may be a lot smaller than you think.

SNACK SMARTER

The way many of us pig out between meals, you would think snacks were a vital food group that included such high-calorie staples as potato chips, cheese curls, buttered popcorn, cookies and soda. **No wonder we're obese.** But between-meal cravings can be tamed without loading up on the fat and processed sugar that most of these foods contain. Fruits and vegetables are far less fattening, and as a bonus they are actually good for you. Even nuts are fine in moderate portions.

SECRET FORMULA

The basic ingredients in a lot of sweet snacks are **sugar, trans fats and refined starch,** all fattening and low in nutrition—but also so cheap that it costs almost nothing to double the size of a product. You may think that getting 12 more oz. for only half the price is a real steal, but it sure is no dietary bargain.

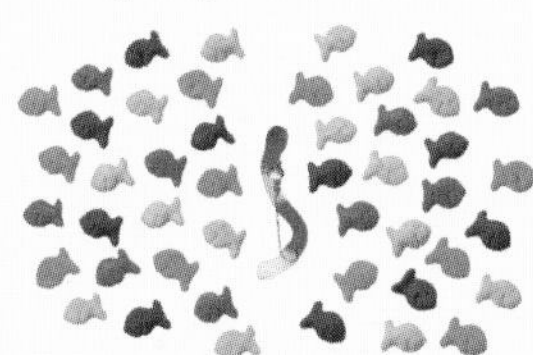

E

Ecstasy

The "hug drug" is still fueling raves, and more scientists and parents are asking: How dangerous is it?

a.k.a. Other street nicknames for the synthetic psychoactive substance: Adam, XTC, hug, X, beans and the love drug

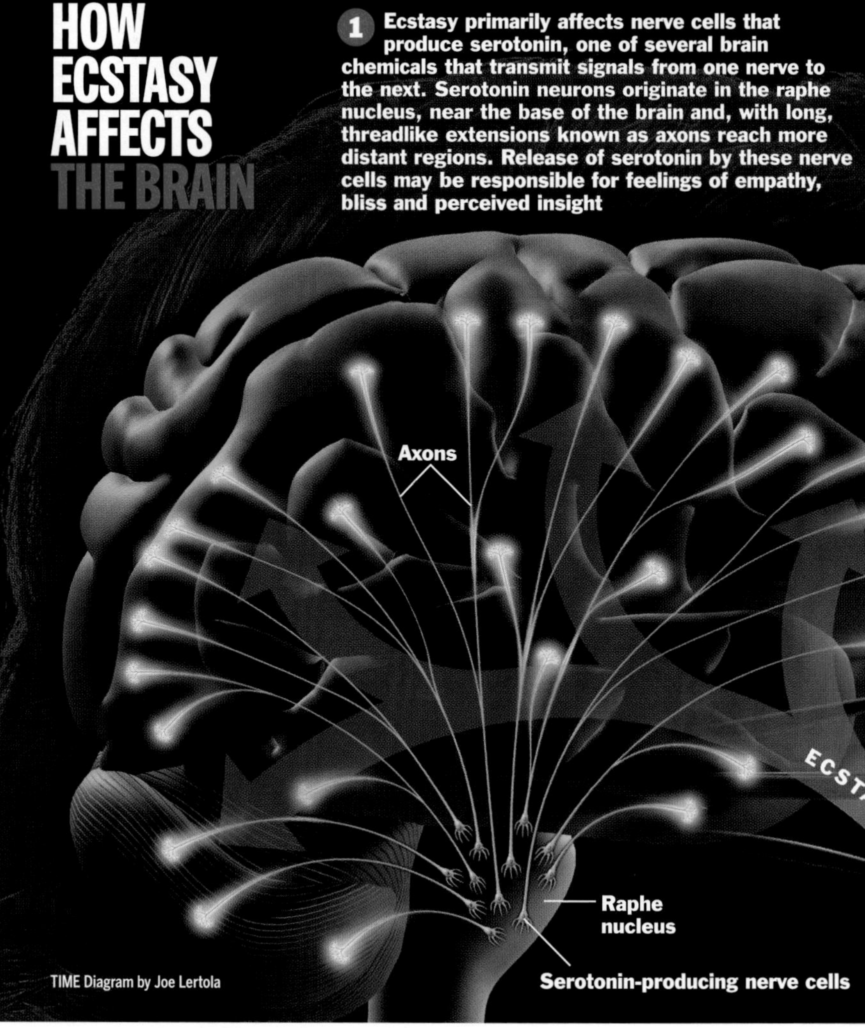

HOW ECSTASY AFFECTS THE BRAIN
1 Ecstasy primarily affects nerve cells that produce serotonin, one of several brain chemicals that transmit signals from one nerve to the next. Serotonin neurons originate in the raphe nucleus, near the base of the brain and, with long, threadlike extensions known as axons reach more distant regions. Release of serotonin by these nerve cells may be responsible for feelings of empathy, bliss and perceived insight
Axons
Raphe nucleus
Serotonin-producing nerve cells

TIME Diagram by Joe Lertola

On the street or at the all-night dance parties that made it famous, it's called ecstasy, "e" or the love drug, and as a pure designer drug not found in nature, it's unlike pretty much every other illicit drug. Ecstasy pills are made of a compound called methylenedioxymethamphetamine, or MDMA. It's an old drug: Germany issued the patent for it in 1914 to the E. Merck company; the U.S. Army studied it in the 1950s and it enjoyed a following among avant-garde psychotherapists in the early 1980s, when it was still legal. As it spread to club culture, it acquired its catchy name—and came under the scrutiny of the U.S. Food and Drug Administration, which declared it illegal in 1985.

Use of the drug is spreading, particularly among high school and college-age kids, who claim it has few negative effects; they rave that the drug heightens their senses, gives them energy, makes them feel loving toward all. Federal drug-abuse officials strongly disagree; they insist ecstasy use involves a number of both long-term and short-term dangers.

NOT FOUND IN NATURE

A "designer drug," ecstasy is unlike most commonly abused drugs: fabricated in a lab, it is not based on an organic substance like poppies or pot

After MDMA enters the bloodstream, it aims with laser-like precision at the brain cells that release serotonin, a chemical that is the body's primary regulator of mood. MDMA causes these cells to disgorge their contents and flood the brain with serotonin.

But forcibly catapulting the brain's serotonin levels can be risky. Of course, millions of Americans manipulate serotonin when they take Prozac (*see* Depression). But ecstasy actually shoves serotonin out of its storage sites, according to Dr. John Morgan, a professor of pharmacology at the City University of New York. In contrast, Prozac merely prevents the serotonin that's already been naturally secreted from being taken back up into our brain cells.

Normally, serotonin levels are exquisitely maintained, which is crucial because the chemical helps manage not only the brain's mood but also the body's temperature. In fact, overheating is the worst short-term danger posed by MDMA. Flooding the system with serotonin, particularly when users take several pills over the course of one night, can short-circuit the body's ability to control its temperature.

Dancing in close quarters doesn't help, and because some novice users don't know to drink water, their temperatures can climb as high as 110°. At such extremes, the blood starts to coagulate. In the past two decades, dozens of users

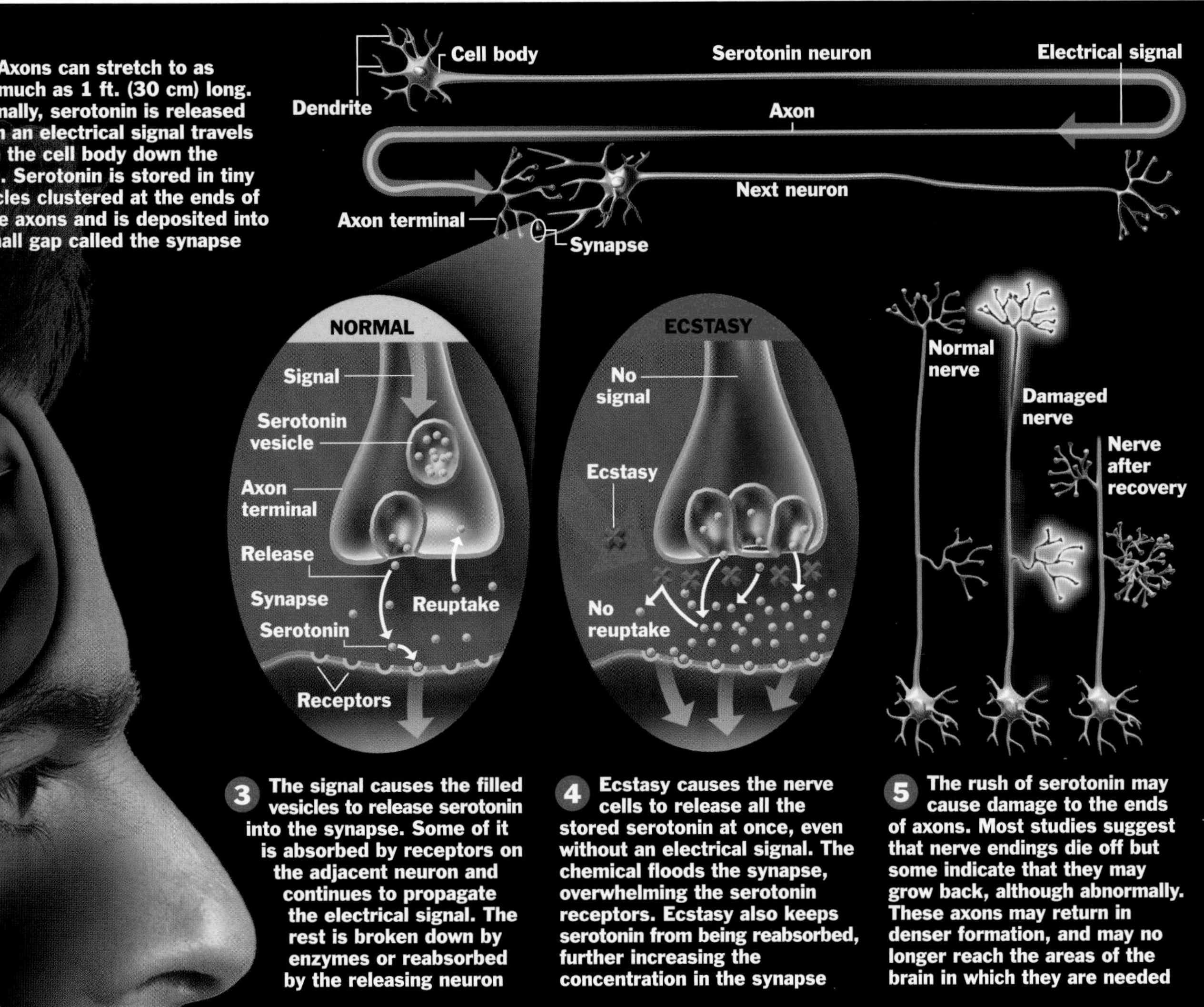
Axons can stretch to as
much as 1 ft. (30 cm) long.
mally, serotonin is released
n an electrical signal travels
the cell body down the
. Serotonin is stored in tiny
cles clustered at the ends of
e axons and is deposited into
all gap called the synapse
Cell body
Serotonin neuron
Electrical signal
Dendrite
Axon
Next neuron
Axon terminal
Synapse
NORMAL
Signal
Serotonin vesicle
Axon terminal
Release
Synapse
Serotonin
Reuptake
Receptors
ECSTASY
No signal
Ecstasy
No reuptake
Normal nerve
Damaged nerve
Nerve after recovery
3 The signal causes the filled vesicles to release serotonin into the synapse. Some of it is absorbed by receptors on the adjacent neuron and continues to propagate the electrical signal. The rest is broken down by enzymes or reabsorbed by the releasing neuron
4 Ecstasy causes the nerve cells to release all the stored serotonin at once, even without an electrical signal. The chemical floods the synapse, overwhelming the serotonin receptors. Ecstasy also keeps serotonin from being reabsorbed, further increasing the concentration in the synapse
5 The rush of serotonin may cause damage to the ends of axons. Most studies suggest that nerve endings die off but some indicate that they may grow back, although abnormally. These axons may return in denser formation, and may no longer reach the areas of the brain in which they are needed

of ecstasy around the world have died in this manner.

There are long-term dangers associated with the use of ecstasy as well. By forcing serotonin out, MDMA resculpts the brain cells that release the chemical. The changes to these cells could be permanent. Johns Hopkins neurotoxicologist George Ricaurte has shown that serotonin levels are significantly lower in animals that have been given about the same amount of MDMA as you would find in just one ecstasy pill.

There's no doubt concerning one of ecstasy's after-effects: a depressive hangover, a down day that users sometimes call Terrible Tuesdays. Another downside: because users feel empathetic, ecstasy can lower sexual inhibitions. Men generally cannot get erections when high on ecstasy, but they are often ferociously randy when its effects begin to fade. One Columbia University psychiatrist found that men in New York City who use the drug were 2.8 times as likely to have unprotected sex as nonusers.

Another problem: most people who end up in the emergency room after taking ecstasy are almost certainly not taking MDMA but adulterated versions masquerading under its name. One pro-ecstasy organization found that as much of as 20% of the so-called ecstasy sold at raves contains something other than MDMA. The most common adulterants in such pills are aspirin, caffeine and other over-the-counter substances. Perhaps the worst stand-in is DXM (dextromethorphan), a cheap cough suppressant that can cause hallucinations in the 130-mg dose usually found in fake "e." Because DXM inhibits sweating, it easily causes heatstroke.

Finally, did we mention ecstasy is illegal?

RAVING FAKES

A major concern surrounding ecstasy is that many users are not taking the real thing: fake ecstasy, cut with other, more harmful, substances, can circulate at raves

Resources

NATIONAL INSTITUTE ON DRUG ABUSE: *www.nida.nih.gov/drugpages/mdma.html*

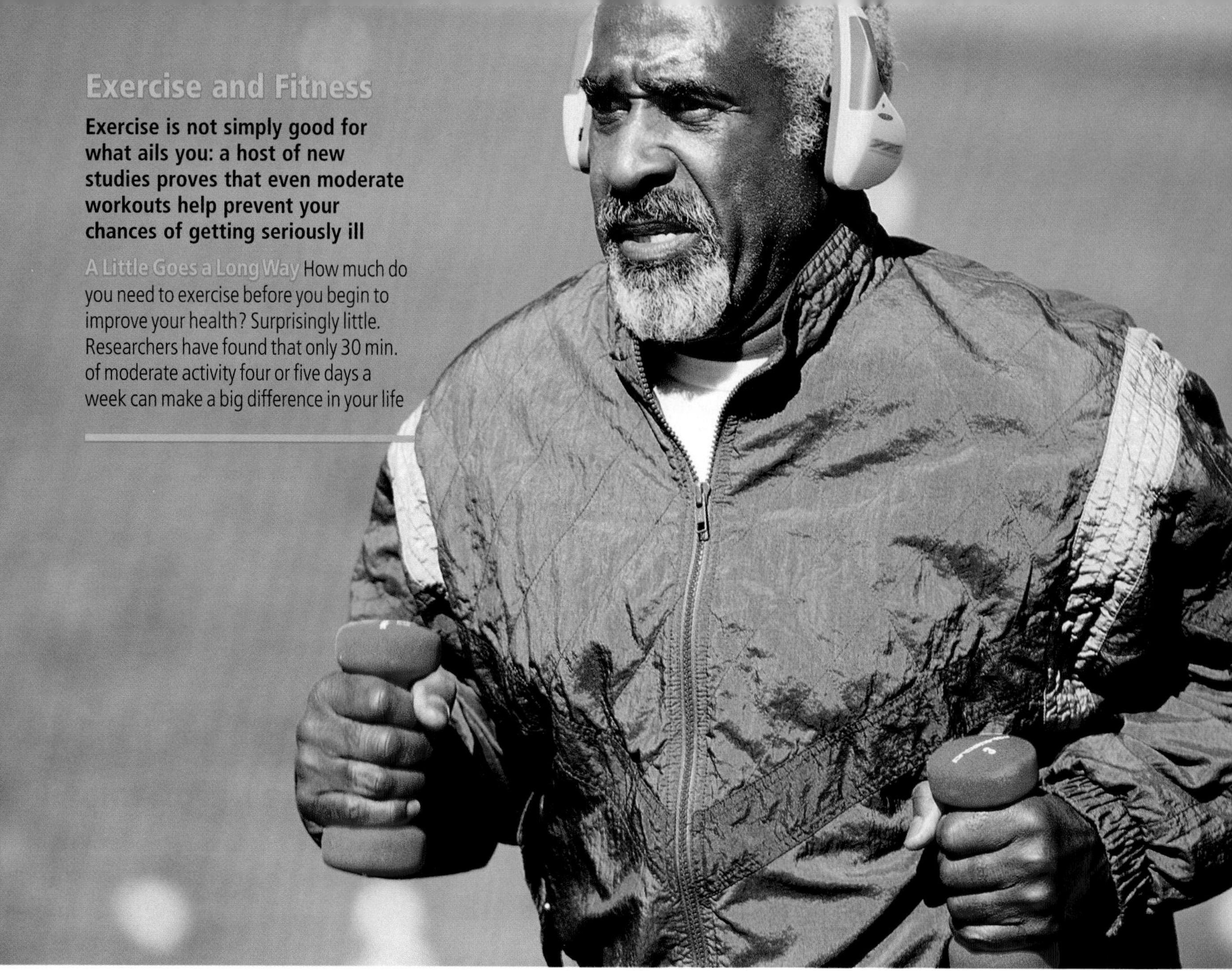

Exercise and Fitness

Exercise is not simply good for what ails you: a host of new studies proves that even moderate workouts help prevent your chances of getting seriously ill

A Little Goes a Long Way How much do you need to exercise before you begin to improve your health? Surprisingly little. Researchers have found that only 30 min. of moderate activity four or five days a week can make a big difference in your life

When it comes to exercise, there's plenty of good news to print for the fit. The latest research shows that even a little bit of regular physical activity holds surprising benefits for just about every cross section of the population: women; seniors; the young; and people concerned about arthritis, breast cancer, heart disease, stroke, diabetes, colon cancer, osteoporosis, depression, and Alzheimer's—to name only a few of the problems that getting up off the couch can help head off. The only dark cloud on the exercise horizon is that not enough people are taking advantage of one of the closest things to a magic bullet that modern health care has to offer: according to government data, only 1 in 4 U.S. adults satisfies the minimum recommendation of 30 minutes of moderate activity most days of the week.

PREVENTION ENGINE

If you don't exercise regularly, your risk of contracting a serious ailment may increase as much as 20% to 50%

Of course, there's a flip side to these discouraging words: for those who choose to pass on the benefits that exercise offers, the risk of most of the ailments listed above can increase 20% and 50%, as does the overall likelihood of premature death.

➤Getting Started The hardest part about starting a new exercise routine is just that: starting. But two new studies should help get into your sweats. In the first, researchers put 184 sedentary, overweight women on diets of 1,200 to 1,500 calories a day and exercise plans of varying intensity that ranged in duration from 30 to 60 minutes a day. The scientists expected that more exercise would yield greater benefits, and it did. But to their surprise, the benefits to those who spent more of their day exercising were only marginal.

Even 30 minutes a day of moderate exercise, such as walking, led to a weight loss of 14 lbs. over a year. Women who worked out vigorously for an hour a day lost only 6 lbs. more. The second study showed that women who exercised moderately for 75 to 150 minutes a week were 18% less likely than inactive women to develop breast cancer. The more the women exercised, the more their risk declined, but once again the incremental difference was small. Conclusion: you don't have to run a marathon; you just have to get moving.

➤Good News for Women Although it has been long accepted that exercise plays a role in reducing the risk of invasive breast cancer, new research has shed light on its potential for lowering a woman's chances of developing breast carcinoma in situ (BCIS), a precursor that may help indicate invasive breast cancer. One study found that women who did even minimal exercise were 35% less likely to develop BCIS than women who did no exercise at all. Separate research concluded that post-menopausal women may be able to lower their risk of breast cancer by using a routine of moderate exercise (45 minutes, five days a week) to lower their levels of estrogen, which has been linked to the development of breast cancer.

NEVER TOO OLD

Hit the gyms! Adults 55 and over have become the fastest-growing segment of the fitness industry in America

➤Sweating Seniors Doctors once warned older adults against vigorous exercise. Now many promote the benefits of physical activity as prevention against age-related decline. Dr. Laurel Coleman, a geriatrician in Augusta, Maine, gives her patients written prescriptions for weekly weight-training sessions. "Some of them say, 'Oh, come on, you're kidding!' because they don't picture themselves lifting weights," she says. "So we start off doing biceps curls with cans of soup, or leg extensions with tiny ankle weights."

After age 40, adults lose a quarter to a third of a pound of muscle a year and gain that much body fat, a condition known as sarcopenia. "You get that typical, pudgy 'old-person look,'" says Miriam Nelson, director of Tufts University's Center for Physical Activity and Nutrition, "and eventually you become so weak, you can't walk up stairs or get out of a chair without help."

But as seniors have grown more conscious of the benefits of exercise, adults 55 and older have become the fastest-growing segment of the fitness industry, with health-club memberships for this age group up more than 350% since 1987, according to one study. Why? "Exercise for older adults is not something considered vaguely deviant anymore," says Harvey Lauer, president of the firm that compiled the data. "Women are allowed to sweat, and men don't have to be highly trained athletes to enter a gym. It's a big switch."

Slow but steady is the best approach for exercise neophytes, says Bess H. Marcus, director of physical-activity research at Brown University's Center for Behavioral and Preventive Medicine. "You don't take a sedentary person and say, 'O.K., go to the gym every day, or go run five miles.' You help them set realistic short-term goals so they are successful." A user-friendly class at a Y, community center or health club can ease a first-timer into a routine, she says.

➤Exercise and Stroke A rigorous 11-year study that precisely gauged the fitness of elderly test subjects by measuring maximum oxygen consumption of the heart and lungs during strenuous activity (instead of using written questionnaires, which are not always reliable) found that those who ranked in the lowest of

Get In the Swim

Exercise has long been a widely prescribed treatment for osteoarthritis. Now new research has shown that hydrotherapy (exercise that takes place while a patient is immersed in water) may yield the same benefits as other aerobic exercises like walking and running, while going much easier on the joints of people whose knees and hips are sensitive to higher-impact forms of exercise, like jogging or walking on a treadmill.

In one recent study, test subjects who tried swimming and other forms of hydrotherapy for six weeks reported improvements in walking speed and distance similar to that found in a group who tried more traditional gym-based exercises—but the hydrotherapy group also reported a significant reduction in joint pain, which the test subjects who worked out performing land-based exercises in a gym did not exhibit.

Because swimming helps build balance, flexibility and muscle strength in the elderly, it is an excellent way to help defend against falls that can lead to hip injuries. However, swimming does not help build bone mass, and it is not a substitute for proper nutrition and body-building exercises like lifting weights.

Swimming uses all the major muscle groups, and its aerobic nature helps maintain proper heart and lung health. To double its benefits, seniors can swim and exercise with friends, for research shows social activities help fight senior blues. ■

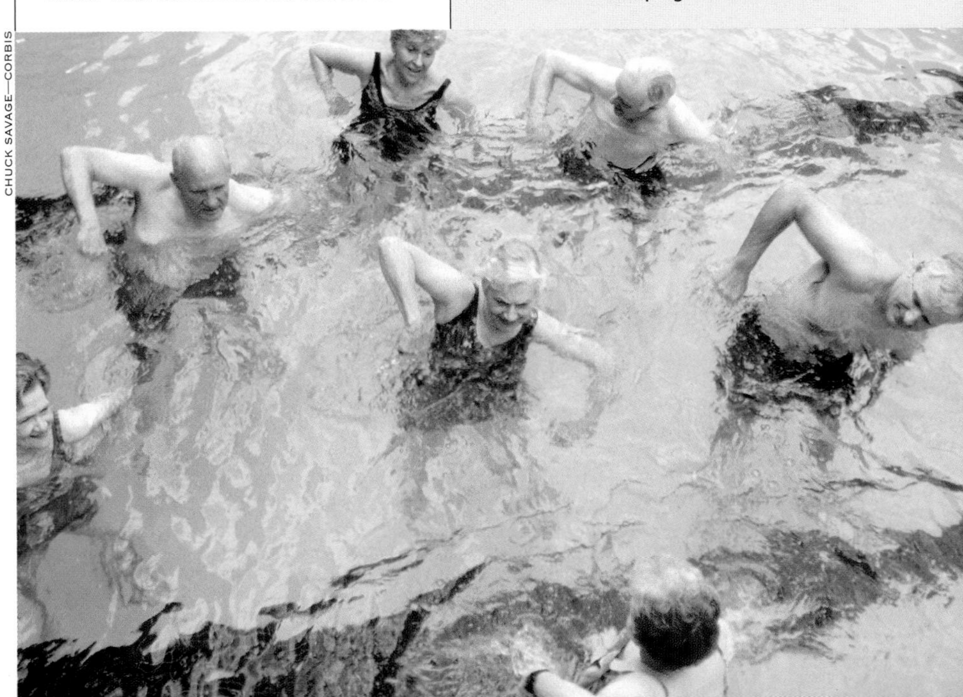
CHUCK SAVAGE—CORBIS

The Amish Example

Ever wonder why the Amish look so fit? In an experiment, 100 adults in an Amish farming community in southern Ontario wore pedometers (on trouser waistbands and apron strings, since the Amish don't wear belts) and logged their physical activity for a week. Not surprisingly, the Amish, who favor a 19th century lifestyle, were quite active. The men reported 10 hours of physically intense work (such as heavy lifting, shoveling or digging, shoeing horses and tossing straw bales) each week and averaged 18,425 steps a day, while women logged 3.5 hours of hard labor per week and walked an average of 14,196 steps a day. (The rest of us walk an average of fewer than 3,000 steps per day.) When it came to moderate physical activity (like gardening, feeding farm animals and doing laundry), men put in 53 hours each week, women 42. All told, the Amish engaged in six times as much physical activity as did their "modern" counterparts.

The bottom line? Only 4% of the Amish men were obese, vs. 31% of non-Amish men. And this despite a 3,600-calorie-a-day diet that includes potatoes, gravy, pies and cakes. As one of the Amish (who made an exception to their ban on electronic devices for the pedometers, with the proviso that they be taken away at the study's end) said of their flabbier non-Amish neighbors, "Maybe they have it a little too easy." ■

four categories of physical fitness had three times the stroke risk of those in the highest category. This means that lack of exercise may be comparable to such risk factors as high blood pressure, high blood cholesterol and obesity in predicting the chances of a stroke.

STEP LIVELY

Some tout the benefits of walking 10,000 steps a day. But that's probably far more than you need to stay fit

➤The Walking Cure Walking has been much touted of late as a pretty-close-to-ideal exercise. But how many steps should you rack up? The figure you see most often is 10,000 a day. That's a nice, round number, based on Japanese research. But like so many one-size-fits-all solutions, those 10,000 steps may not all be necessary. In fact, if all you want is to stop gaining weight, you may need only 2,000 steps more than your normal routine—provided you also pay attention to what you eat.

At least that is the contention of James Hill, an obesity researcher at the University of Colorado in Denver. The average American office worker takes about 5,000 steps a day, Hill says. Trying to double that right away may be too much too fast. He calculates that taking an extra 2,000 steps while eating 100 fewer calories a day is enough to keep most people from gaining the pound or two a year that comes with middle age. But Hill concedes that 10,000 steps may be necessary to control Type 2 diabetes or to lose weight and keep it off.

Ready to strap on a pedometer (a little pagerlike device that attaches to your belt and counts the number of steps you take) and give it a try? A good model will set you back anywhere from \$10 to \$25. The brand used most often in research is the Digi-Walker by Yamax, but you don't need all the fancy mileage and calorie-counter features. A no-frills pedometer is quite accurate if worn for walking, and you will get the best results if you keep the pedometer in line with what would be the crease line on a pair of trousers.

➤Heavy Petting Two new studies showed that dog owners who regularly walk their pets reap significant benefits from this accidental exercise. In the first study, more than half of a group of new dog owners lost some weight, averaging a reduction of 3 lbs. over six months—at a time when the average weight of Americans is growing at about the same rate. The second study compared overweight people who owned dogs with similar test subjects who didn't, and found that even dog owners who don't lose weight are deriving health benefits from walking their pets.

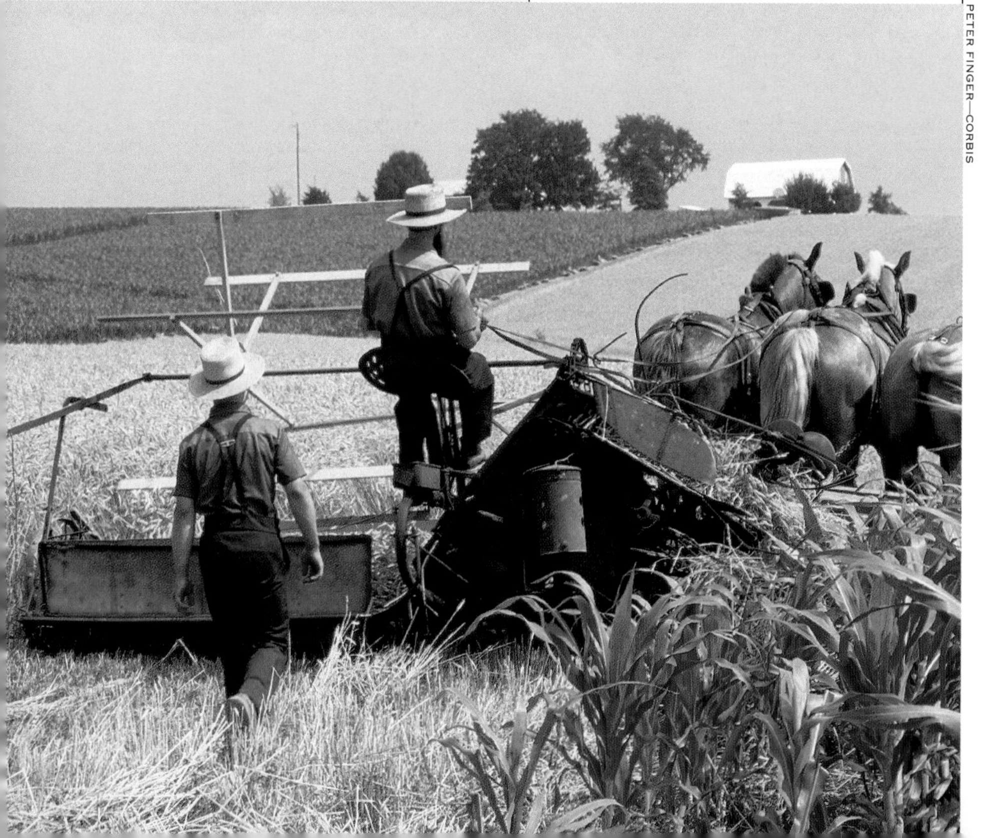

PETER FINGER—CORBIS

■ Resources

NIH WEBSITE ON EXERCISE FOR SENIORS: *www.nihseniorhealth.gov/exercise/benefitsofexercise/01*

FOR KIDS: *www.nlm.nih.gov/medlineplus/exerciseforchildren*

PRESIDENT'S COUNCIL ON FITNESS: *www.fitness.gov*

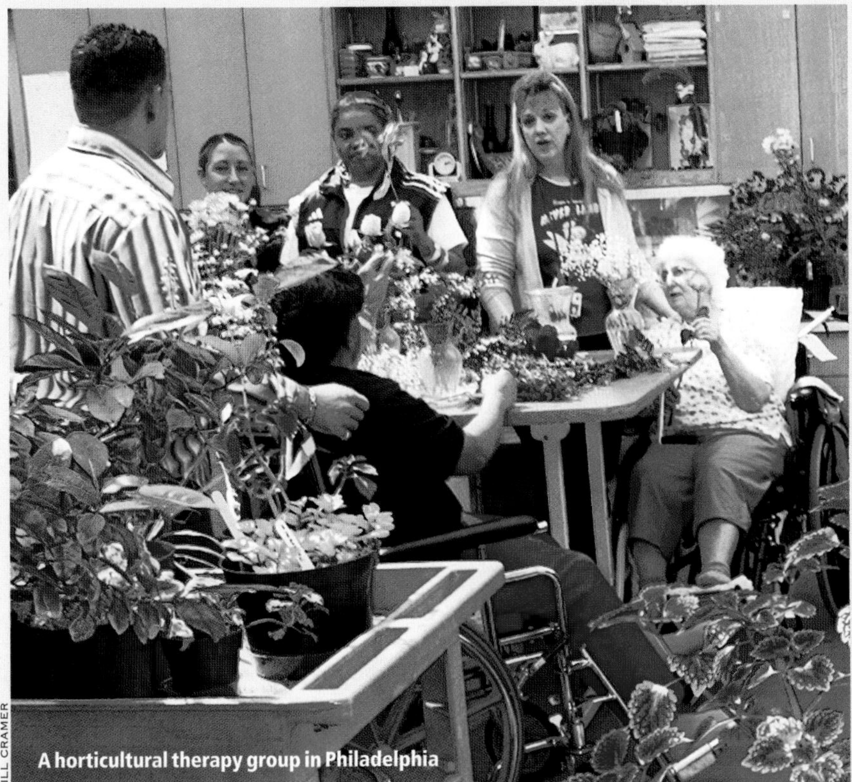

BILL CRAMER

A horticultural therapy group in Philadelphia

Stop and smell the roses has always been sound advice—but who knew it was also a medical prescription? A growing number of researchers and therapists have found that working with plants can enhance your physical and mental health, giving the green-thumb crowd yet another reason to play in the dirt.

Studies have shown that regular yard work can lower stress levels and provide a workout that compares with other exercise regimes. It's also an effective weapon in battling osteoporosis. Researchers at the University of Arkansas found that women over 50 who engaged in regular home gardening had higher bone-density readings than those who performed activities more typically thought of as exercise, including jogging, cycling, swimming, walking and aerobics.

Just looking at a garden can be good for you. In a study published in the *Journals of Environmental Psychology*, Terry Hartig and colleagues at the University of California at Irvine split 112 stressed-out young adults into two groups. One group spent time in a room with an arboreal view and then took a walk in a nature preserve. The second group sat in a windowless room and then strolled through an urban setting. The group exposed to greenery had decreased blood pressure and elevated mood, some in just a few minutes. Studies by Texas A&M University's Roger Ulrich have found that surgical patients in hospital rooms with landscape views recover faster than those without.

Such benefits provide the basis for horticultural therapy (HT), a field with deep historical roots that is blossoming anew in light of these findings. Ancient writings show that the Egyptians thought gardening activities to be beneficial, says Nancy Easterling, president of the 700-member American Horticultural Therapy Association. In the modern era veterans' organizations used gardening as physical and emotional therapy for soldiers returning from World Wars I and II. But only since the 1970s has horticultural therapy emerged as a distinct discipline used in hospitals, rehabilitation centers and even prisons. Many public gardens, arboretums and conservatories are also developing HT programs.

At the North Carolina Botanical Garden in Chapel Hill, Easterling oversees HT programs for adult day care, at-risk teens, adults with developmental disabilities and patients with Alzheimer's. HT is also a valuable tool for treating depression and substance abuse. "It's about using plants as the tool to reach therapeutic goals," says Easterling, who began her career as a clinical social worker but became frustrated when "words were not enough to reach some patients." By using plants, she says, you "create a connection with the natural world. Learning that you can take care of a living thing—and it responds—can be very powerful."

Gardening is also an excellent tool for physical rehabilitation because it uses large and small muscles and fine and gross motor skills. Linda Ciccantelli, who founded the HT program at Magee Rehabilitation Hospital in Philadelphia, works in the hospital's lush rooftop greenhouse with patients who have suffered spinal-cord and head injuries as well as stokes. "When people have a devastating illness, you try to tap into something they want to do," she says. "I have seen standing tolerances improve while people are planting. When you are in the flow of an activity, you aren't as aware of your pain. Gardening helps our patients focus on their ability, not their disability."

Like any other activity, gardening has its hazards as well. Health experts advise wearing sunscreen, keeping a water bottle on hand to stay hydrated and exercising caution when attempting any heavy lifting. ■

STOCKBYTE

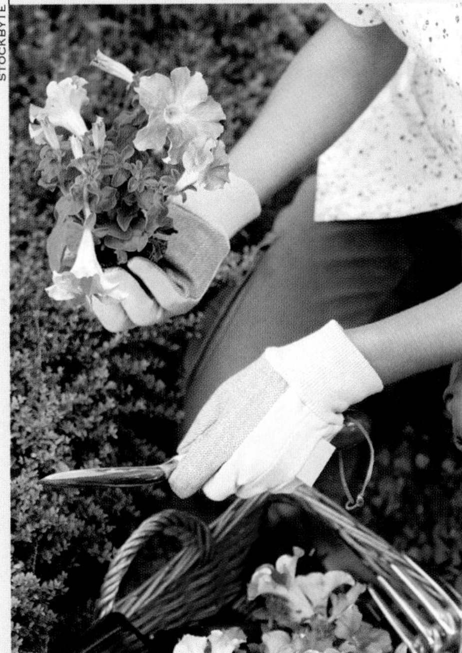

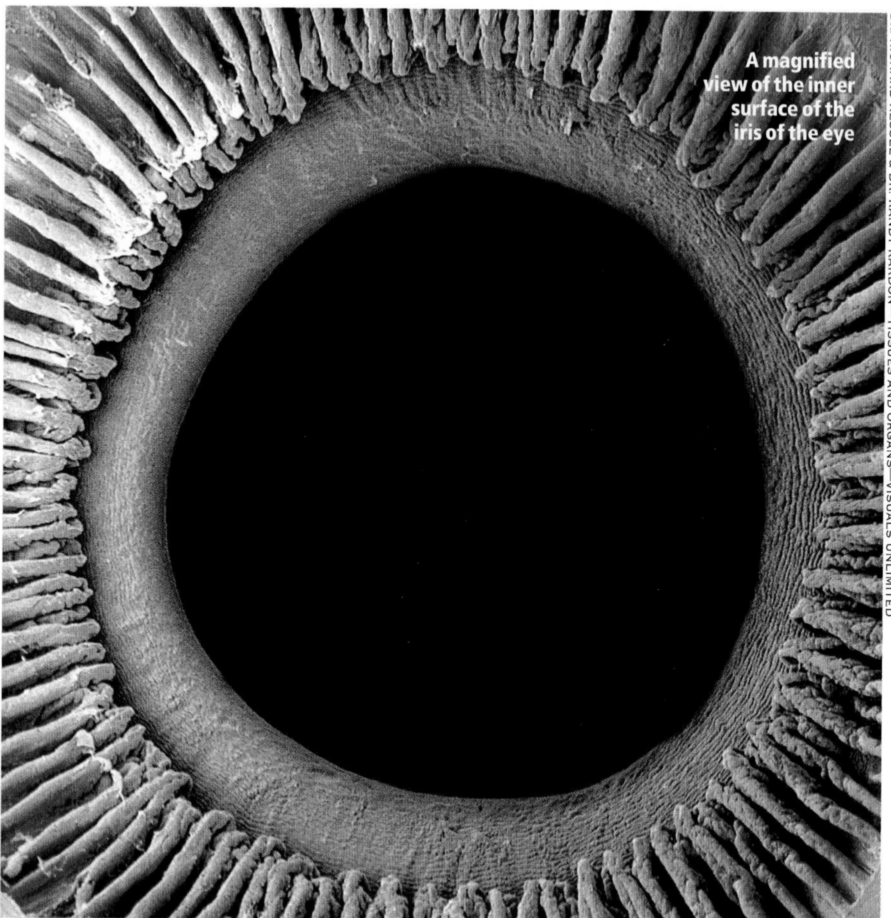

A magnified view of the inner surface of the iris of the eye

DR. RICHARD KESSEL & DR. RANDY KARDON—TISSUES AND ORGANS—VISUALS UNLIMITED

Eyesight

As baby boomers age, research into preserving the health of our eyes is booming. We're finding aid in one surprising place, the cholesterol-lowering medications called statins

Definition Age-related macular degeneration (AMD) takes two forms. In the more common "dry" AMD, lesions appear on the macula, the region of the retina responsible for seeing. In "wet" AMD, abnormal blood vessels cover the macula, obscuring vision

A 2004 National Eye Institute study predicted that, as baby boomers age, the number of blind Americans over 40 will rise from 3.3 million to 5.5 million by 2020, chiefly due to ailments like age-related macular degeneration (AMD) and glaucoma, which are preventable, or at least manageable, if detected early and treated properly. And there are intriguing new treatments on the horizon.

➤Statins and AMD Statins are cholesterol-lowering medications whose health-enhancing powers are just being explored. The latest word: statins may help reduce damage from the most common cause of irreversible blindness among older adults, AMD. About 85% to 90% of patients with AMD have the dry form, rather than the more serious, wet form. A 2004 study of more than 300 people with dry AMD showed that those who were taking statins were half as likely to develop wet AMD. Taking aspirin—with or without a statin—worked almost as well.

It isn't yet clear why statins and aspirin work against AMD: the leading hyptothesis focuses on their ability to dampen inflammatory processes in the body. Before doctors begin using these drugs to treat AMD, they consider their side effects. Statins, though remarkably safe, can trigger severe muscle and joint pain, while long-term use of aspirin increases one's risk of internal bleeding.

➤Prevention How can aging Americans prevent AMD? At the top of the list is quitting smoking. Eating lots of fruits and vegetables and wearing sunglasses that block harmful ultraviolet rays may also help. A 2001 study showed that a high-dose regimen of vitamins (including C, E and beta-carotene) plus zinc was moderately successful for intermediate cases of AMD. Most important of all are regular visits to an eye doctor, who can monitor the risk of AMD, as well as cataracts and glaucoma.

YOU SEE WHAT YOU EAT

People on high-fat diets are 2.9 times as likely to develop AMD as those whose diet is rich in fish and nuts

➤ViewPoint CK Even those lucky enough to have perfect vision for their first 40 years will almost inevitably develop presbyopia, a loss of elasticity in the lens that makes it hard to focus on close objects, like a magazine. But it may be possible to avoid reading glasses now that the FDA has approved ViewPoint CK (conductive keratoplasty) as a treatment. CK uses radio waves to tighten small areas of collagen, creating a constrictive band, like a belt, that increases the curvature of the cornea and brings near vision back into focus.

■ Resources

FDA WEBSITE, VIEWPOINT CK: *www.fda.gov/cdrh/pdf/P010018S005*

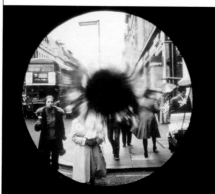

ARGENTUM—PHOTO RESEARCHERS

Simulation of the view of a person afflicted with macular degeneration

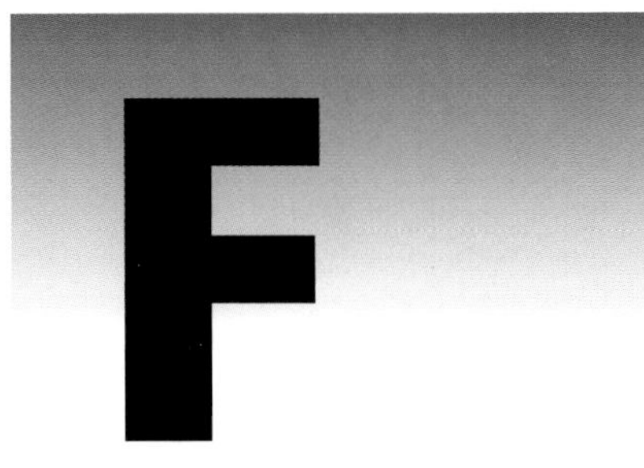

Fertility

A new study questions our view of female fertility, suggesting women may generate eggs for decades

What Next? If proved, the theory could usher in dramatic advances in treating infertility and dealing with menopause

The standard story on female fertility has always tested the limits of logic. A few months before the birth of a girl, textbooks say, her ovaries contain about 1 million egg cells each—all she will ever have. Those numbers decrease as eggs deteriorate or get washed out of the body during menstruation. When a woman is about 50, they're essentially gone, signaling the hormonal changes known as menopause.

Men, by contrast, churn out new sperm all the time. Insects make new eggs too, well into maturity. But a 2004 study discovered that mice, at least, have specialized stem cells in their ovaries that make new eggs throughout the animals' lives. The research suggests the same might be true for humans, and the implications are vast.

The researchers found that the egg cells in adult-mouse ovaries are constantly dying off—but at a remarkable rate of up to 1,200 a day, or about a third of the total. Simple arithmetic suggested that the eggs were being replenished.

In one experiment, researchers transplanted normal ovarian tissue into mice genetically engineered to carry a jellyfish gene that glows a faint fluorescent green. If the mice really did have egg-producing stem cells, they reasoned, some should migrate into the new tissue to generate new, green eggs—while the follicles that enveloped them, coming from normal tissue, would be white. Result: green eggs (no ham)—and strong evidence for the new theory.

The finding will have to be confirmed by others before it's fully accepted. But even if the cells exist, it will be a while before anyone benefits from the research. Scientists will have to figure out how to purify ovarian stem cells, then transfer them into depleted ovaries to see if they can restart egg production—first in mice, then, if possible, in humans.

And the potential uses? You might extract the cells and freeze them, and if a woman got cancer, you could reintroduce them after chemotherapy shut down her ovaries. Or you might freeze some of the vigorous stem cells in a young woman so she would have a reserve as her own supply aged and weakened. Or, if you could keep existing stem cells viable longer, you might stave off the discomforts of menopause by staving off menopause itself. Now that's a hot flash.

■ **Resources**

WEBSITE: *ww.newscientist.com/news/news.jsp?id=ns99996104*

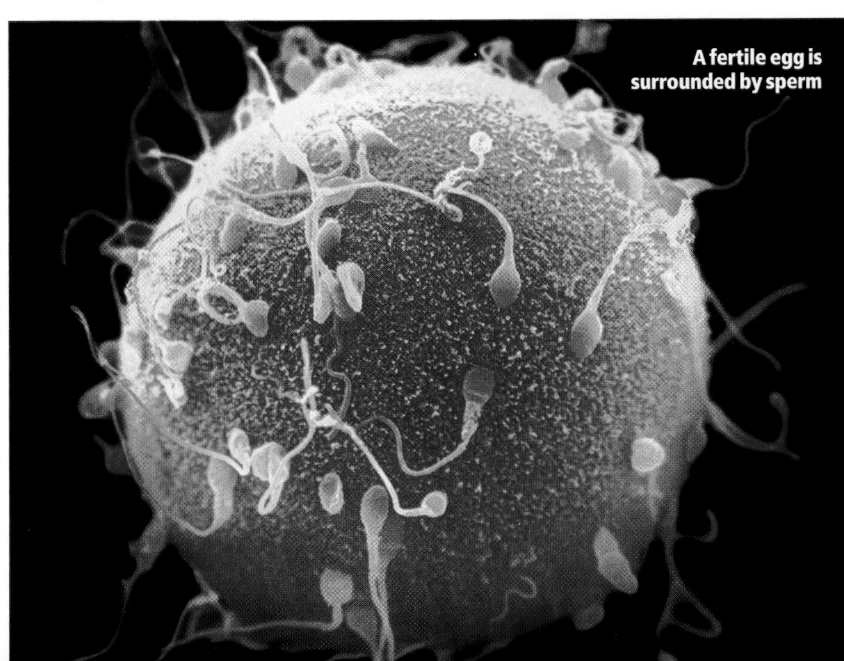

A fertile egg is surrounded by sperm

DAVID M. PHILLIPS—PHOTO RESEARCHERS

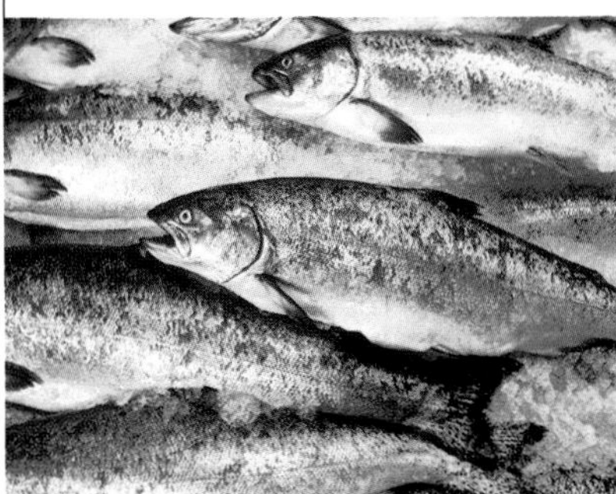

RANDY FARIS—CORBIS

Food Safety

How safe is salmon? Though we know it's great for your heart, fears of contamination increase

Take Care To be safe, try to find wild salmon, not the farm-raised kind

Salmon steaks are great sources of heart-healthy omega-3 fatty acids. But according to the Environmental Working Group (EWG), salmon can also contain dangerous doses of cancer-causing polychlorinated biphenyls (PCBs), especially if the fish comes from your local grocery store. EWG found that store-bought salmon, most of which is farmed, contained 16 times the PCB levels of salmon caught in the wild. The EPA considers these levels a health hazard: if they were found in wild salmon, the agency would suggest eating the fish only once a month. The FDA, the agency responsible for fish sold in stores, says these PCB levels are safe—for now.

■ **Resources**

FDA MERCURY AND FISH WEBSITE: *www.fda.gov/oc/opacom/hottopics/mercury/backgrounder*

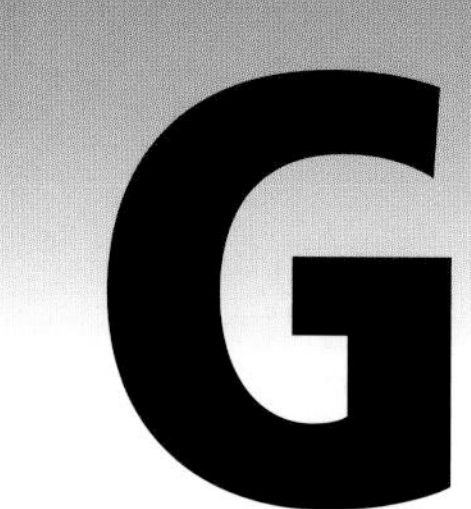

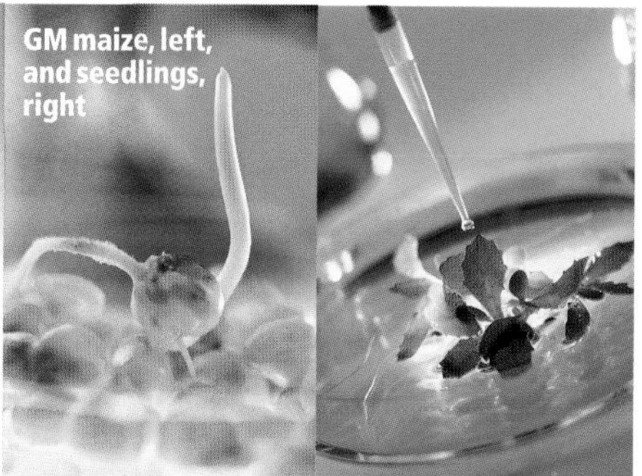

GM maize, left, and seedlings, right

Genetically Modified Food

The battle over GM foods goes on: activists in Vermont and Hawaii are seeking state bans against them

On the Horizon Taking a stand amid the fury, the FDA said it would issue new rules to regulate the use of GM foods in 2005

The controversy surrounding the genetic modification of food and animals continues to rage. While U.S. farmers have embraced new versions of old crops like corn, soybeans and cotton—genetically modified to boost yield or thrive with less help from pesticides or fertilizers—the rest of the world has shunned "Frankenfoods." The European Union has been especially skeptical, enacting a five-year ban on new genetically modified products that was partially lifted only in the summer of 2003, when new regulations (including tighter labeling requirements) went into effect.

Many Americans share these reservations. In January 2004 the National Academy of Sciences issued a report detailing the challenges in keeping GM plants and animals contained and enumerating the dangers of their accidental release into the environment. Among them: weeds and parasitic insects could acquire the same resistance that has been built into the genes of high-tech crops; powerful drugs cultivated in the body fluids of GM livestock could end up inside cold cuts and dairy products. The report urged stricter "bioconfinement" measures.

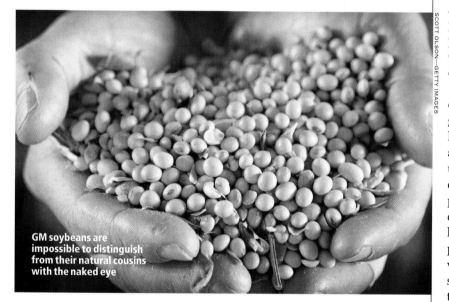

GM soybeans are impossible to distinguish from their natural cousins with the naked eye

SCOTT OLSON—GETTY IMAGES

Resources

HUMAN GENOME PROJECT SITE: *www.ornl.gov/sci/techresources/Human_Genome/elsi/gmfood*

Genetics

The latest advances in genetic research offer tantalizing hints to the answers of medical questions both large and small, from bad hair to very good food

Bad-Hair DNA? Researchers have located a gene in mice (called Frizzled 6) that seems to be a marker for unruly hair patterns. Scientists are trying to determine whether a virtually identical human gene has the same effect

Every cell in your body contains a copy of your entire genetic makeup—some 50,000 known genes and gene variants. But to make those data useful to scientists who are trying to identify genetic markers for cancer and develop drugs that target specific genes, a tool was needed to isolate each gene and make it easily identifiable. The new GeneChip from California-based Affymetrix does just that. While previous chips each contained a portion of the human genome, the GeneChip is the first to contain an entire genome.

Another team of researchers has engineered a new way to insert a gene from worms into mice and help them produce omega-3 fatty acids, the heart-healthy chemicals usually found in salmon and other oily fish that most mammals cannot produce on their own. If this discovery can be extended to the livestock we eat, it is theoretically possible that cattle and chickens with designer DNA will someday supply T-bone steaks and omelets that your cardiologist will nag you to eat more frequently.

Resources

GENECHIP: *wwww.affymetrix.com/index.affx*

TEK IMAGE—PHOTO RESEARCHERS

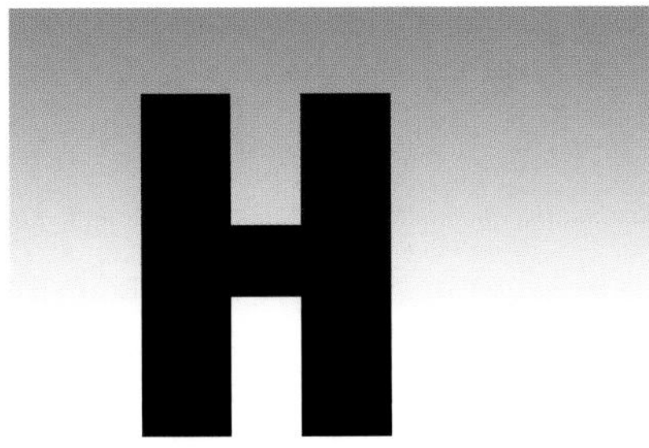

Hair and Baldness

Speaking out on a condition long deemed off-limits, more and more women are confronting baldness

Hair Raising The most drastic remedy is also the most effective: hair transplants for women are booming, doctors report

More than 30 million U.S. women experience androgenetic alopecia, or hereditary hair loss. For years, most of them suffered in silence,

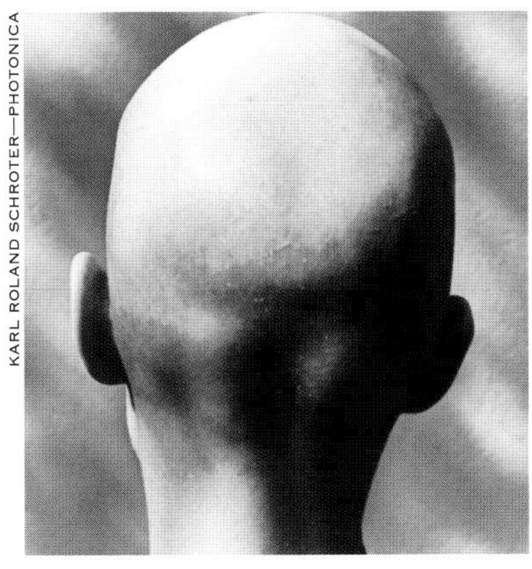
KARL ROLAND SCHROTER—PHOTONICA

fretting about thinning hair but saying nothing. Suddenly, it seems, they are speaking up. Television ads tout cures for the problem, and the topic is getting more airtime as sufferers become more comfortable confronting this condition, which can be triggered by causes as diverse as menopause, giving birth, undergoing a hysterectomy, eating disorders or depression.

Many medications can also be culprits, including high-blood-pressure drugs, antidepressants and cholesterol-lowering remedies. (Also suspect: frequent permanents and overuse of hair dyes.) The closest thing to a miracle cure for hair loss in women is minoxidil, best known by the brand name Rogaine. A majority of women with genetic hair loss show hair growth within four months of using it. Rogaine is applied topically, and its use must be continued to sustain the results.

Headaches

Good news for those who battle headache pains: acupuncture and an epilepsy drug may help

Needle Aid As Western scientists learn how acupuncture affects the brain, they are growing more comfortable with testing it against a variety of ailments

Two recent studies offer hope for those who suffer from migraine headaches. In the first, people who experience at least three migraines a month were given the epilepsy drug topiramate (Topamax). Compared with a control group given a placebo, the topiramate test subjects experienced a greater reduction in the frequency of their migraine attacks, and this reduction became more pronounced as the dosage of the drug was increased. One caveat: the drug's side effects include nausea and fatigue.

In a second study, which looked at both migraine sufferers and patients with chronic but less severe headaches, treatment with acupuncture (along with traditional headache medications) was found to be more than twice as effective as treatment with headache medicine alone. The apparent benefits often lasted for months after the treatment ended and were most dramatic in those with the most severe headaches.

CHARING CROSS HOSPITAL—PHOTO RESEARCHERS

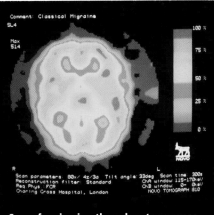

Scan of a migraine; the red spots are areas of most pain

■ **Resources**

NIH WEBSITE: *wwww.nlm.nih.gov/medlineplus/headache*

Hearing

Cochlear implants, miracle workers for many, turn out to have unexpected side effects

All Ears The National Campaign for Hearing Health's goal of testing all newborns for hearing problems, the most common form of birth defect, is nearing success: 85% of all babies are now being tested for hearing

It's a dark cloud wrapped inside a silver lining. The cochlear implant is a technological miracle that has restored hearing to thousands of children with severe to profound hearing loss. But according to a study conducted by the FDA and the CDC, children who receive implants are more than 30 times as likely to develop bacterial meningitis infections, which are lethal in some 10% of cases.

NOW HEAR THIS

Cochlear implants have helped thousands of kids hear better, but they also may lead to bacterial infections

This certainly doesn't mean parents should give up on implants. The risk of infection is still tiny. The study advises that all children getting implants have the shots (pneumococcal and Hib) that protect against meningitis. Also, parents should watch for warning signs of infection, such as a high fever and a stiff neck.

■ **Resources**

NIDCD WEBSITE: *www.nidcd.nih.gov/health/hearing/coch.asp*

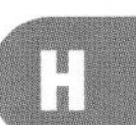

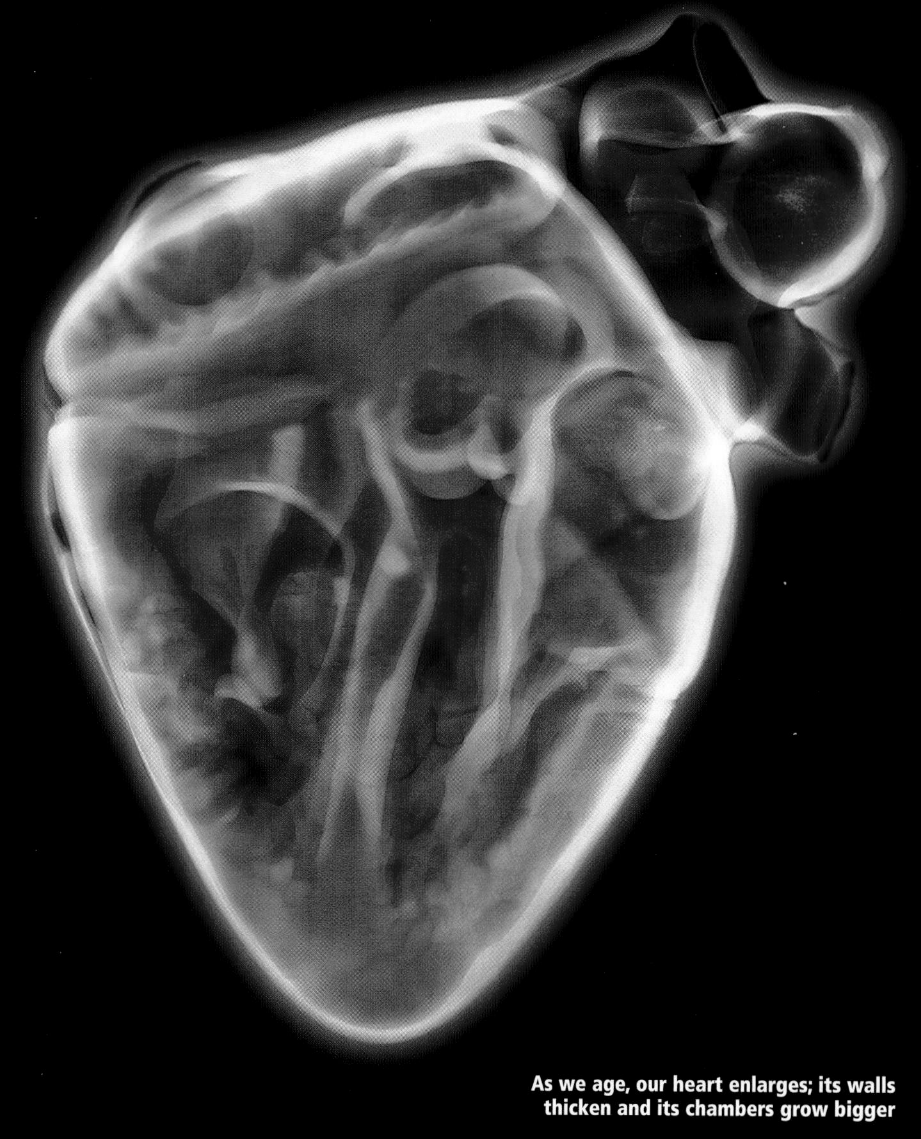
As we age, our heart enlarges; its walls thicken and its chambers grow bigger

DAVID ARKY—CORBIS

Heart Disease

More Americans die from heart disease than from any other ailment. But new treatments, new drugs and a new artificial heart may help reduce the killer's toll

Pumping Station A new treatment, enhanced external counterpulsation, or EECP, is helping patients overcome chest pain (angina). Now we're finding the benefits may last for years, suggesting that it is helping ailing hearts regain their vigor

Heart disease is the No. 1 killer of Americans: 1.5 million of us die from it each year, while 1.1 million Americans have heart attacks every 12 months, and about 5 million suffer from some form of heart failure. Outside the U.S., the news is, if anything, worse. In developing countries—where exercise is rare, obesity is increasingly rampant, and few people are trying to quit smoking—rates of heart disease are skyrocketing. In Russia, for example, 576 of every 100,000 men between ages 35 and 59 die each year from some form of cardiovascular disease, compared with 116 American men from the same age group.

INSOMNIA WARNING

For men, chest pain is often an indicator for heart ailments; for women, sleeping problems are a tip-off

➤Risk Factors Doctors have long accepted the mystifying conventional wisdom that 50% of all heart disease patients do not exhibit any of the four major risk factors known to predict heart disease: smoking, diabetes, high cholesterol and high blood pressure. The problem, according to a new investigation into the source of this widely held belief, is that it just isn't true. It's an old wives' tale.

Two new studies, in fact, prove just the opposite, documenting that as many of 90% of all heart disease patients fall into one or more of these risk groups, and any patient who ranks in all four categories is virtually ensured of developing heart disease.

■ **Risk: Metabolic Syndrome** A new risk factor is the combination of health problems like high blood pressure and high blood triglyceride and sugar levels that doctors call "metabolic syndrome." Though most common in heavy people, this condition, also an indicator for diabetes, occurs in people of all weights. For those with heart disease, a new study shows, metabolic syndrome may double the risk of complications or death, regardless of the patient's weight.

■ **Risk: CRP** One risk factor that may not be as bad as previously thought is the level of C-reactive protein (CRP) in an individualt's blood. This sign of inflamed arteries had been linked by previous studies to a doubled risk of heart attack. But new research indicates that while CRP does put a patient at increased risk of heart attack, the heightened danger is more in the range of 50%. Even so, the CDC and the American Heart Association are still considering whether to recommend CRP testing for millions of Americans judged to be at moderate risk of heart disease.

■ **Risk: Depression** One's mental state is also emerging as a major risk factor, both for heart disease and for death after heart surgery. Multiple new studies have shown that depression can double a man's lifetime risk of heart disease and triple his chances of dying in the first 12 months after a heart attack. For both men and women, depression can double the risk of dying in the years following bypass surgery.

➤Risk: A Female View For women, sleeping problems may be a cardiac warning sign. Although heart disease is as threatening to women as it is to men, it doesn't strike them the same way. While men often complain of chest pain during a heart attack, for example, many women experience no chest pain whatsoever. What they do experience is sleeping problems. A new survey of female heart-attack survivors shows that 70% reported unusual fatigue a month before their attack, and 48% said they had been having trouble sleeping. At least 1 in 3 also experienced indigestion, anxiety or shortness of breath.

MIND AND BODY

A number of new studies demonstrate that there is a clear link between depression and risk of heart attack

And finally, some good news for women with heart disease: new research shows that in the past decade, heart-attack death rates have fallen sharply among women with diabetes—evidence that significant progress is being made in the treatment of this major risk group.

➤Treatment: Angioplasty and Stents A study of heart-attack patients in Denmark suggests that emergency angioplasties (the unclotting of heart artieries by an internal balloon) work so much better than anticlotting drugs that the wait for a patient to reach a hospital where the procedure can be performed is often worthwhile. The study followed 1,129 patients. Of those treated with drugs, 14% died or had a second heart attack or a disabling stroke. The figure was lower—8%—for those given an angioplasty rather than drugs within two hours of the attack.

But angioplasties are not without risks. Doctors have long known that patients who undergo the procedure in combination with stenting (the placing of a metallic scaffold inside the blood vessel to keep it open) face a high risk of restenosis, or reblockage. Now research indicates that a stent that gradually releases an anti-inflammatory drug can prevent restenosis, reducing the rate of this problem from 30% to 5%.

As the technology has advanced, some stents inserted years ago have collapsed within heart patients' arteries. A new design, called the Cypher stent, is designed to be inserted in old stents. This configuration was approved by the FDA in 2003 and is now so common that nearly 1 of out every 1,500 Americans has one of them inserted in his or her chest. The use of stents has become so widespread, in fact, that it has led to a decline in bypass operations, which carry a higher risk and involve a much longer recovery period.

➤Treatment: Surgery Coronary artery bypass surgery once entailed rerouting circulation through a heart-lung pumping device, which sometimes resulted in lasting harm to brain cells. A more modern version of the procedure can be done without this pump, reducing the risk of brain damage. The surgery, however, is more complicated. A new study shows that three months after surgery, patients who underwent off-pump surgery run a reduced risk of restenosis, compared with those who opted for the traditional procedure.

➤Technology: Defibrillators An American Heart Association study indicates that installing defibrillators (which use electric current to "shock" an ailing heart back into the correct proper rhythm) in public places, where bystanders

A Helping Heart

For more than 30 years, scientists have been building artificial human hearts for people who are beyond help from a pacemaker or defibrillator, but the FDA has never given its full blessing to any of them. That may soon change. In March, 2004, a panel of experts recommended that the FDA approve the CardioWest Total Artificial Heart for use as a stop-gap, fully implantable replacement heart that can keep a patient alive until a transplant can be found. That's lifesaving news for the 3,500 Americans who were waiting for a heart donor in 2003 (only some 2,000 human hearts become available through donation each year).

Sixteen-year-old Arizona resident Alex Rowe ,whose heart had atrophied from muscular dystrophy, received a CardioWest artificial heart in October 2003 as part of an FDA-approved clinical trial. The artificial unit kept Rowe (who may be the world's youngest artificial heart recipient) alive until December, when he received a donated human heart. He is now back in high school.

The National Institutes of Health have underwritten a $5 million grant to Jarvik Incorporated, a leading designer of artificial hearts, to begin development of an artificial heart the size of an AA battery for young children, and an even tinier unit for infants. Tests of the prototype on animals should begin by 2005. ■

SYNCARDIA SYSTEMS

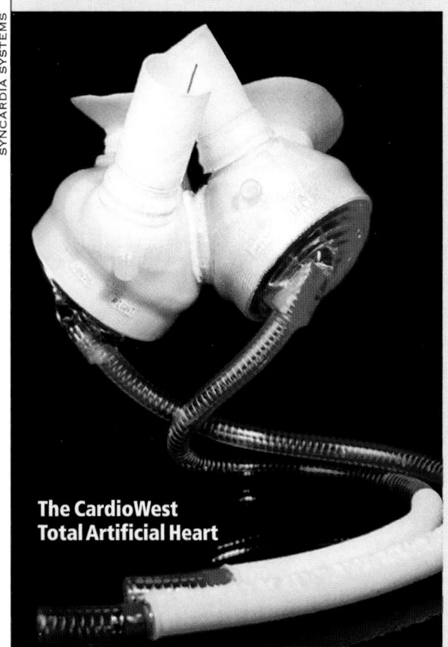

The CardioWest Total Artificial Heart

H

can use them without waiting for emergency help, could save as many lives as the most effective emergency system. Indeed, a recent National Institutes of Health test of so-called public-access defibrillators (PADs) found that twice as many lives were saved in locations where they were available.

A variation of the device, the Automated External Defibrillator, which features a robotic voice designed to instruct an untrained user in the machine's operation, can further magnify this advantage. But a third study has found that defibrillators offer a limited (but still significant) benefit when there is no one trained in their operation available at the time of a heart emergency.

The best news on this front: as of April 2004, every large passenger jet in the U.S. fleet is required by the FAA to have a defibrillator aboard: having a heart attack at 30,000 ft. may thus be better than having one in your home.

Implanted defibrillators, which are surgically inserted into the chest of a patient with heart failure, are also saving lives. A new study found that patients with implanted defibrillators were one-third less likely to die from disturbances in the heart's rhythm than those who were being treated with medication alone. But they're expensive, costing about $25,000. A second study shows that dual-chamber pacemaker defibrillators (which synchronize the two halves of a diseased heart while also shocking a heart that needs it back into beating) can cut the risk of death for some heart failure patients up to 50%.

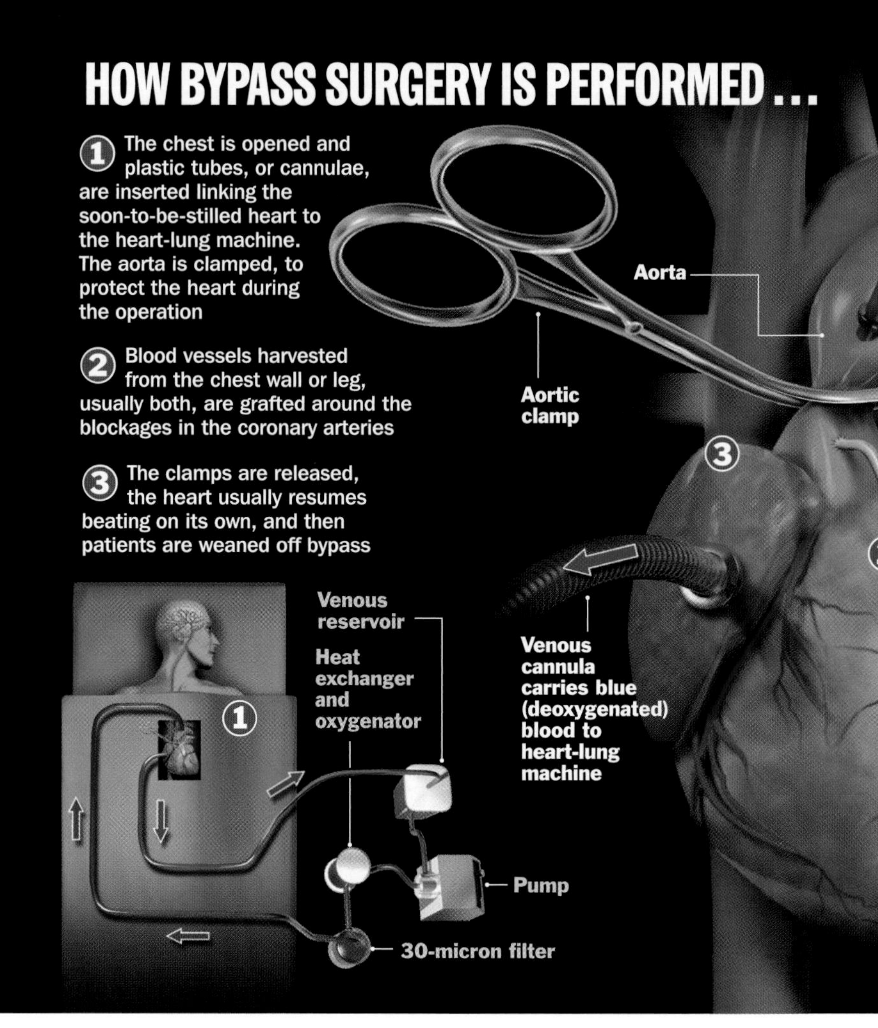

HOW BYPASS SURGERY IS PERFORMED . . .
① The chest is opened and plastic tubes, or cannulae, are inserted linking the soon-to-be-stilled heart to the heart-lung machine. The aorta is clamped, to protect the heart during the operation
② Blood vessels harvested from the chest wall or leg, usually both, are grafted around the blockages in the coronary arteries
③ The clamps are released, the heart usually resumes beating on its own, and then patients are weaned off bypass
Aorta
Aortic clamp
Venous reservoir
Heat exchanger and oxygenator
Venous cannula carries blue (deoxygenated) blood to heart-lung machine
Pump
30-micron filter

A PUBLIC LIFESAVER

Placing defibrillators in public locations has proved to halve the number of deaths from heart attack

➤Prevention: The Drug Frontier

As researchers seek to reduce the root causes of heart disease, a new study found that infusing patients with an experimental drug, ApoA-1 Milano, can reduce the fatty arterial plaque that triggers most heart attacks an average of 4.2%—about 10 times better than statins, the most effective drugs now on the market. The new drug works in the almost unbelievably short period of just five weeks.

Although this first study was too too small to be definitive, the news has the cardiology world holding its breath. The discovery is tied to a rare type of HDL (or "good") cholesterol known as ApoA-1 Milano that is evidently much more protective than ordinary HDL. In the 1990s, researchers began testing a synthetic version of this variant HDL on rabbits and mice and found that ApoA-1 Milano could not only reverse plaque buildup but also stabilize and reduce inflammation of the remaining plaque.

If these initial results hold up in larger trials, they could be revolutionary. Statin drugs, which lower the "bad" LDL cholesterol that causes plaque in the first place, reduce the risk of dying from heart disease 30% or so, but ApoA-1 Milano might even halve the risk.

Nevertheless, there's plenty of work ahead before ApoA-1 Milano is certified as an effective treatment for heart disease. For one thing, it may be logical to assume that reducing plaque always lowers the risk of heart disease, but this remains unproved. Another question mark: nobody really knows how ApoA-1 Milano does what it appears to do. Some believe the

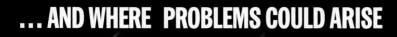

cannula
s red
genated)
from
ung
ne

s

ed

... AND WHERE PROBLEMS COULD ARISE

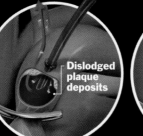

Dislodged plaque deposits

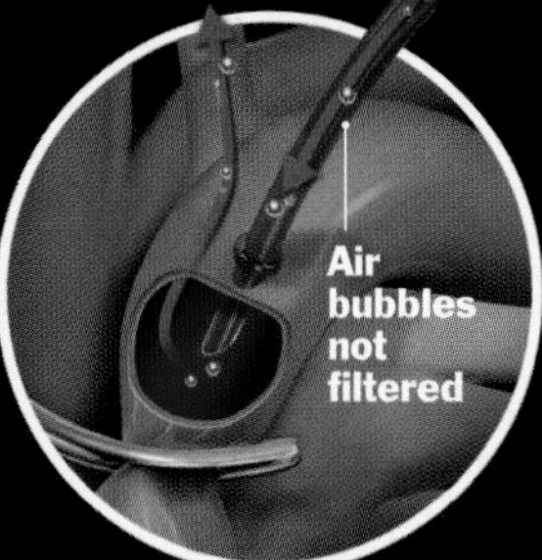

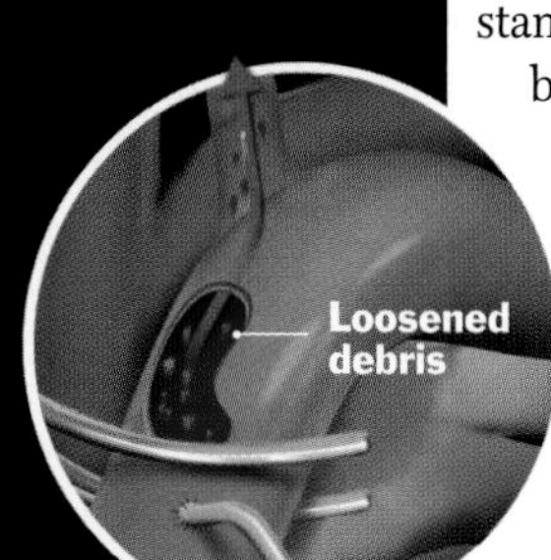

AORTIC CANNULA
Insertion of the cannula into the aorta may dislodge fatty deposits into the bloodstream

HEART-LUNG MACHINE
Filter systems may not remove all air bubbles introduced during oxygenation

CROSS CLAMP
Clamping and unclamping the aorta may unleash microscopic showers of debris

DECLINING TEST SCORES

Percentage of 261 patients whose mental acuity diminished after bypass surgery

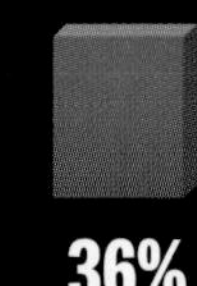

53%	36%	24%	42%
At discharge	After six weeks	After six months	After five years

Source: *New England Journal of Medicine*, New York-Presbyterian/Weill Cornell

TIME Graphic by Ed Gabel

synthetic HDL works by a "dump truck" mechanism, binding to cholesterol molecules in plaque and carting them off to the liver (this is no more than a theory). But even if ApoA-1 Milano turns out to be too good to be true, it's the opening salvo in an entirely new strategy for fighting heart disease. After two decades of focusing on lowering "bad" LDL, doctors are now looking at raising "good" HDL.

Another piece of good news: the same research team that tested ApoA-1 Milano also published test results showing that high doses of the statin Lipitor not only slow down the accumulation of arterial plaque but also seem to stop it. Other new studies confirm this, indicating that high-dosage regimens of several statins can reduce the risk of a heart attack even more than we had believed previously .

Separate research documents that the blood pressure drug perindopril (Aceon) lowers the risk of major heart problems and death for people with relatively mild heart disease, while other research indicates that carvedilol (Coreg), a combination of alpha- and beta-blockers, appears to enhance chances of survival in heart failure patients more than the standard treatment of a beta-blocker taken alone.

Elsewhere on the drug front, two studies have shown that clopidogrel (Plavix) may be more beneficial than aspirin, both in preventing heart attacks in patients with chest pain and in warding off a second heart attack.

➤Treatment: New Strategies

Patients with heart disease usually receive one or more of four traditional treatments: aspirin (to reduce inflammation), statins (to lower cholesterol), beta-blockers (to control adrenaline) and ACE inhibitors (to keep blood pressure low). But a new study indicates that treating a patient with all four of these therapies can lower the risk of a heart attack as much as 90%.

Meanwhile, an American Heart Association study concluded that inducing hypothermia (a rapid lowering of body temperature) in patients who have been resuscitated after cardiac arrest increases their chances for survival.

➤Treatment: Angina and Chest Pain

The latest in off-beat therapies: strapping oversize blood-pressure cuffs to a patient's legs and

H

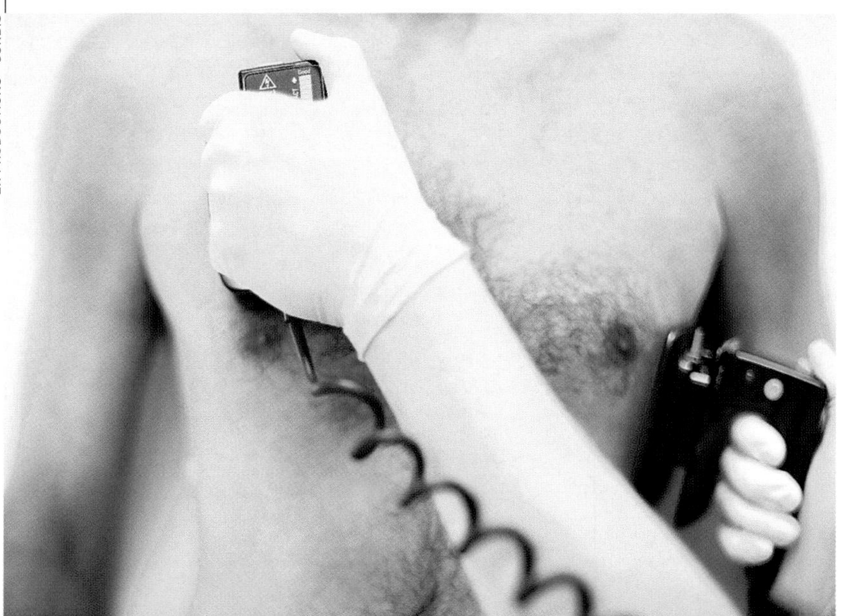

ER PRODUCTIONS—CORBIS

buttocks and pulsing them in synch with the heartbeat. The idea behind this wacky-sounding treatment, known as enhanced external counterpulsation (EECP), is to decrease the demand on an ailing heart by helping it push blood through the body. Perhaps the oddest thing about EECP is that it works amazingly well in reducing angina (chest pain) in many patients.

First approved by the FDA in 1995, EECP is most often used in folks with stable angina—the kind that often lasts five minutes or less, is brought on by physical exertion and is usually relieved by drugs like nitroglycerin. (Unstable angina tends to be severe, occurs suddenly or unexpectedly, often while a person is at rest, and requires immediate attention.) Stable angina isn't always easily controlled with medications, and some people just aren't good candidates for angioplasty or surgery. That's where EECP comes in.

Patients lie down during the procedure, which lasts an hour and is performed once a day, five times a week, for seven weeks. (The cost is about $6,000, compared with as much as $60,000 for bypass surgery.) The pneumatic cuffs are timed to inflate in progression when the heart reaches its resting phase between beats. As each cuff inflates, it squeezes blood out of the legs and back to the heart. The most common side effect of the process is chafing of the skin, which can be prevented by wearing elastic clothing. Those patients who have very high blood pressure, valve disease, phlebitis (inflammation of a vein) or are pregnant should not undergo EECP, doctors caution.

Intriguingly, recent studies suggest that the heart responds to the extra flow of blood created by EECP by growing tiny blood vessels to better nourish it. That may be why the procedure's benefits often last several years. EECP may also be useful in other hard-to-treat conditions, like congestive heart failure.

➤Lifestyle Choices Doctors have long emphasized the importance of a diet low in saturated fats for those seeking healthy hearts. But rather than simply concentrating on what not to eat, they now promote what to eat: new studies indicate that adding nutrients like soy, fiber and nuts to a diet low in saturated fats can significantly reduce cholesterol levels and thus contribute to a reduced risk of heart attack.

Drinking alcohol in moderation also appears to lessen the risk of heart disease (at least in men with high blood pressure), according to a new study that challenges the widespread belief among doctors that these patients should avoid alcohol. And a third study finds that among heart attack survivors age 60 and older, those who have a network of close relationships with friends and family are half as likely to suffer a second heart attack as those who don't have such a support network.

SEVEN STEPS TO A HEALTHIER HEART

- Quit smoking (if you're a nonsmoker, don't start)
- Adopt a healthy diet. Avoid foods high in saturated fat and salt
- Exercise. Perform 30 min. of aerobic exercise (the kind that raises your heart rate) at least four times a week
- Control your weight. If overweight, consult your doctor about a plan for losing weight
- If diabetic, learn to control your blood sugar
- If hypertense, learn to control your blood pressure
- Consult your doctor: Could aspirin help reduce your risk of a heart attack?

■ Resources

AMERICAN HEART ASSOCIATION: *www.americanheart.org*

DEPRESSION AND HEART DISEASE: *www.nimh.nih.gov/publicat/depheart.cfmm*

A Surprising Death

Sudden death is always shocking, but there was something particularly unsettling about the way popular TV actor John Ritter died in September 2003: quickly and without warning. He suffered what is known as an aortic dissection, a rare condition in which the major artery that carries blood from the heart to the rest of the body basically tears itself apart. More precisely, blood, which is propelled by the beating heart, gets between layers of the arterial wall and pushes them apart, moving down the blood vessel like a run racing down a nylon stocking.

As you might expect, if the tear occurs close to the heart, death can occur in minutes. Indeed, half of all patients who suffer this kind of aortic catastrophe die within 24 hours. "The key is to make the diagnosis," said Dr. Michael Deeb, a cardiac surgeon at the University of Michigan in Ann Arbor. The pain of aortic dissection is often mistaken for that of a heart attack. But if the dissection is detected in time and there's no damage to other organs in the body, surgeons can successfully replace the torn section of aorta with a synthetic graft.

Unfortunately, aortic dissections are impossible to predict. "You can't get screened for dissection," says Dr. Ann Bolger, a cardiologist at the University of California, San Francisco. "It's not there until it starts, and when it starts, it's almost over." ■

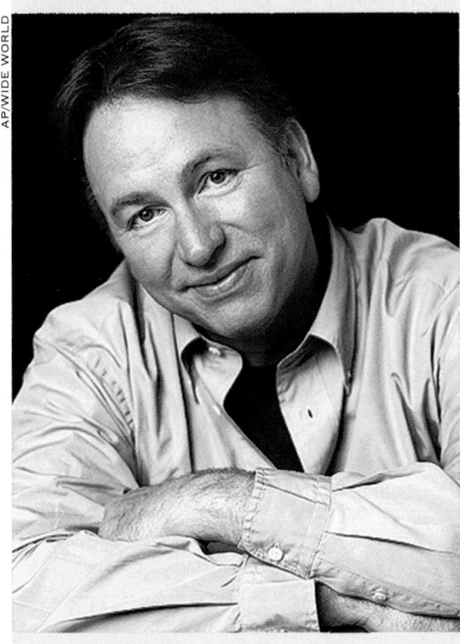

AP/WIDE WORLD

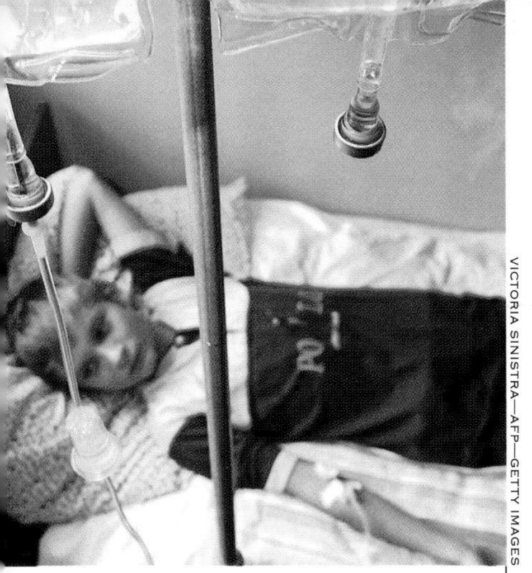

VICTORIA SINISTRA—AFP—GETTY IMAGES

Hepatitis

The largest outbreak of hepatitis in U.S. history trained a spotlight on the need for safer food preparation

Definition Hepatitis is a virus-borne, highly contagious disease that causes inflammation of the liver and can be fatal

The largest hepatitis A outbreak in U.S. history hit four states (Pennsylvania, Georgia, North Carolina and Tennessee) in November 2003, sickening more than 600 people and killing four. In the Pittsburgh area, hundreds of patrons of a Chi-Chi's restaurant got sick. An investigation by the FDA linked the outbreak to tainted green onions from Mexican farms, where FDA investigators found poor sanitary conditions and inadequate facilities for hand washing—two risk factors linked to hepatitis contamination. The farms were shut down.

➤**Drug Use** In another hepatitis-related development, a new study found that drug users who inject illegal drugs are 50 times more likely to develop hepatitis C than those who inhale them. The findings suggest that since most users of heroin, crack and cocaine begin by sniffing the substances, persuading them to avoid moving on to needles may be an effective strategy in fighting the spread of hepatitis C.

Resources

CDC HEPATITIS A WEBSITE: *www.cdc.gov/ncidod/diseases/hepatitis*

Hip Injuries

Two popular blood-pressure medications may also help seniors avoid debilitating hip fractures

On the Other Hand A widely-used group of drugs, the corticosteroids, may increase one's chances of sustaining a hip fracture

New research shows that two widely used categories of medications may significantly affect a senior's chances of suffering a hip fracture. The good news: thiazide diuretics, prescribed to help control blood pressure, are known to reduce calcium loss and may slow down the reduction of bone density associated with aging. A new, nine-year study that looked at more than 7,000 test subjects over age 55 found that those who took thiazide diuretics for more than a year were half as likely to suffer a hip fracture as those who didn't—but also found that such benefits disappeared within four months of discontinuing the medication.

The bad news: a second group of drugs, the corticosteroids widely prescribed to treat ailments such as rheumatoid arthritis and asthma, may actually increase one's chances of suffering a hip fracture. A study that looked at more than 39,000 seniors found that the likelihood of a such an injury was measurably greater among patients who had been prescribed a corticosteroid, and that the risk grew as the dosage or length of time on the medication increased.

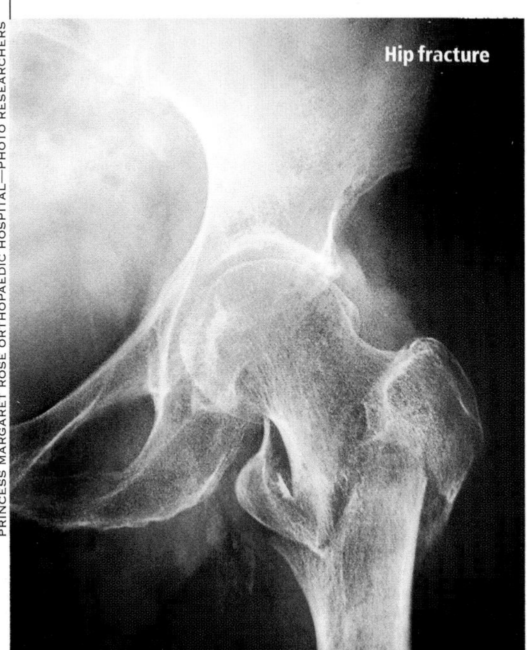

Hip fracture

PRINCESS MARGARET ROSE ORTHOPAEDIC HOSPITAL—PHOTO RESEARCHERS

Resources

NIH WEBSITE: *www.nlm.nih.gov/medlineplus/hipinjuriesand-disorders*

Hodgkin's Disease

A new study has found that aspirin may help prevent this uncommon form of lymphatic cancer

By the Numbers 7,000 Americans come down with Hodgkin's Disease each year

The millions of Americans who take aspirin each day to ward off heart disease and other ailments may also be reducing their risk of Hodgkin's, a study found. It concluded that regular aspirin users have a 40% lower long-term risk of developing Hodgkin's than those who don't use aspirin, but the authors caution that this disease is too rare (and the potentially harmful side effects of aspirin too common) to make aspirin therapy advisable as a prevention strategy.

Another new study determined that women whose Hodgkin's disease was treated with high doses of radiation may be up to eight times more likely to develop breast cancer, and that their increased risk may last as long as 25 years after radiation therapy. For this reason, the American Cancer Society advises that women whose Hodgkin's therapy included radiation ought to consider beginning yearly mammograms at age 30, rather than at the standard age, 40.

Resources

NIH WEBSITE: *www.nlm.nih.gov/medlineplus/hodgkinsdisease*

H

Hormone Replacement Therapy

Studies find another reason why HRT is rapidly falling out of favor

The Threat A major study has linked HRT to breast cancer, heart attack and stroke; now there's a new link to Alzheimer's

In more bad news for hormone-replacement therapy (HRT), the FDA in February 2004 asked makers of HRT pills (most of which contain the hormones progestin and estrogen) to add another warning to their labels: that HRT may raise the risk of dementia in older women. A watershed 2002 study had linked the drugs to increased risk of breast cancer, heart attack and stroke, leading experts to conclude that for many women the risks of long-term use outweigh the benefits. The FDA directive was based on 2003 data showing that women on Prempro, an HRT drug, doubled their risk of Alzheimer's.

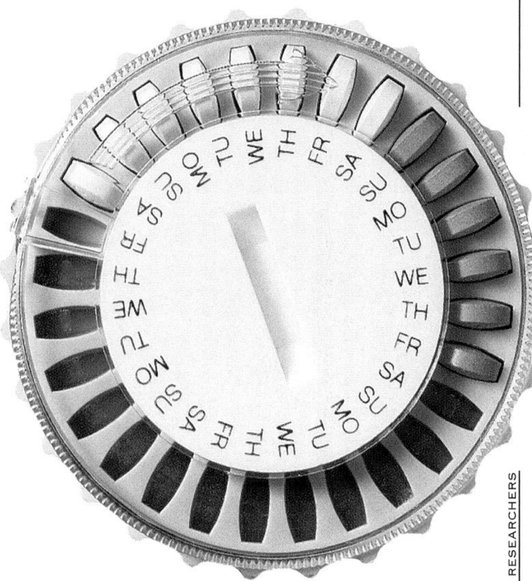
SHEILA TERRY-PHOTO RESEARCHERS

Maybe the most positive thing to be said about HRT at this point is that the debate over its benefits and risks isn't over quite yet. Some experts insist that the studies showing harmful side effects from HRT were conducted on female test subjects too old to derive any benefit from the therapy, and that tests that claimed increased risk for ovarian cancer were inconclusive. However, the central conclusion of recent studies is inescapable: most women should not take hormone replacement therapy for extended periods of time after menopause.

■ **Resources**

NIH HRT WEBSITE: *www.nlm.nih.gov/medlineplus/hormonereplacementtherapy*

Hypertension

Commonly known as high blood pressure, hypertension has long posed a threat to seniors, but now it's afflicting young Americans

The Percentages Reversing a three-decade decline, blood pressure is on the rise for all Americans. Experts estimate some 29% of all U.S. adults suffer from the ailment, up from 25% in 1988

The most alarming news about hypertension (a.k.a. high blood pressure) is that it's affecting growing numbers of American youth. A May 2004 report showed for the first time that blood pressure rates among children and teens across the U.S. have inched up over the past 15 years, a consequence of their growing girth. A separate study also suggests that teenagers who exhibit two of the three defining characteristics of a Type A personality, hostility and impatience, may also be at increased risk of high blood pressure later in life. (The third trait, a strong urge to achieve, appears to be less directly related to hypertension.)

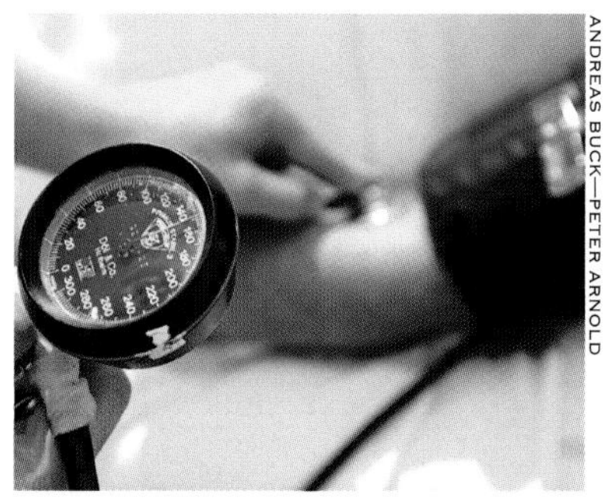
ANDREAS BUCK—PETER ARNOLD

A SENIOR CHALLENGE

Six of every 10 U.S. citizens over age 65 currently suffer from high blood pressure

The reported jump may seem inconsequential at first: up 1.4 points, to 106 mm Hg (millimeters of mercury), for systolic pressure and up 3.3 points, to 61.7 mm Hg, for diastolic. Indeed, that would not be a problem for an individual child. But these are averages for the entire U.S. population of young people, and that has doctors and health experts concerned.

High blood pressure has long been recognized as a significant risk factor for diseases like heart attack, stroke, heart failure and kidney failure. And the list keeps getting longer: a new study has added memory loss to the ailments linked to hypertension.

■ **Resources**

NIH HYPERTENSION WEBSITE: *www.nlm.nih.gov/medlineplus/highbloodpressure*

Teens and Coffee

Most doctors prefer to treat high blood pressure in younger patients with lifestyle changes first: getting them to lose weight, if necessary, and step up their physical activity. A new threat: preliminary evidence suggests that caffeine—found in soda, coffee and some candy—may boost blood pressure, particularly in African Americans.

A new study aims to gauge the effect on children and teenagers of a diet that has been shown to lower blood pressure in adults: it's long on fruits, vegetables, whole grains and low-fat dairy. Blood pressure can jump high enough among young people, however, that diuretics and beta-blockers (in child-size doses) may be needed to bring it under control.

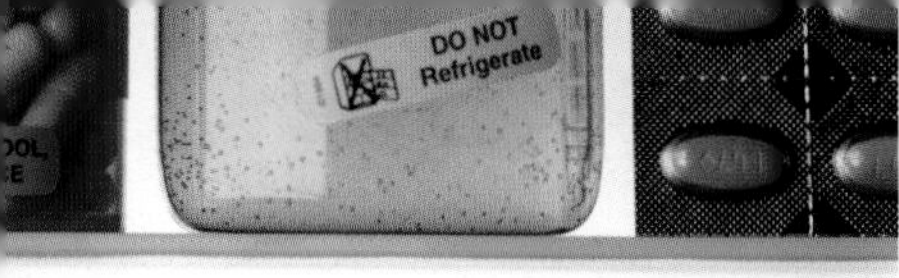

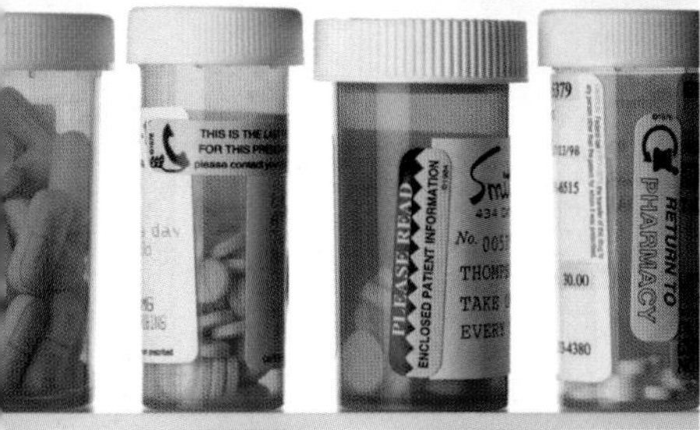

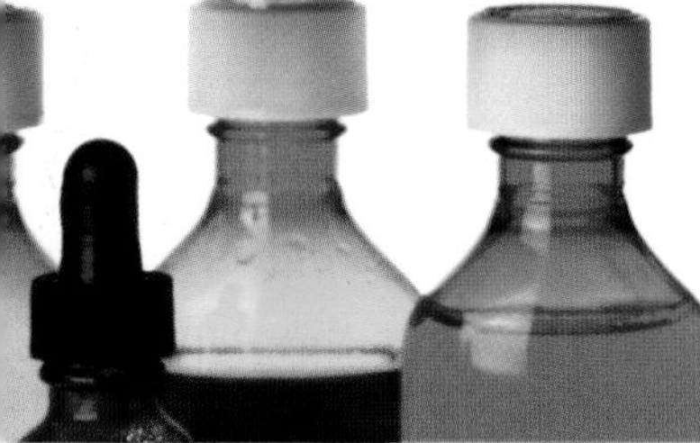

ED ECKSTEIN-PHOTOTAKE

Hypochondria

The Internet is a downloadable feast for hypochondriacs—so much so that doctors have a new term for such virtual patients: "cyberchondriacs"

The Bottom Line The key to treating hypochondria is teaching patients to counter its self-reinforcing spiral

For the tens of thousands who suffer from hypochondria, living in constant terror that they are dying of some awful disease (or two) is an everyday reality. Doctors can assure them that there's nothing wrong, but since no physician or test can offer a 100% guarantee that one doesn't have cancer or an ulcer, a hypochondriac always has fuel to feed his or her worst fears.

Hypochondriacs don't harm just themselves; they clog the whole health-care system. Although they account for only about 6% of doctor visits each year, these visits take up expensive time, costing the U.S. some $20 billion in wasted medical resources each year. The problem is getting worse, thanks to the proliferation of medical information on the Internet; doctors have tagged this phenomenon "cyberchondria."

Recent research suggests that hypochondriacs may actually represent three different groups whose problems look superficially similar. Those in the first have a variant of obsessive-compulsive disorder (OCD). Those in the second have a problem more like depression, often triggered by something that makes them feel guilty or by a loss, like the death of a close relative. The third group consists of people who somatize, which means they focus an inordinate amount of attention on their bodies. For them, a pain most people wouldn't even notice feels like a punch in the nose.

In all cases, though, the descent into hypochondria takes the form of a self-reinforcing spiral. You notice a symptom, decide it's unusual and begin to explore for more. Since we all have minor twinges from time to time, when you go looking for others, you find them. Even if doctors insist you're healthy, your symptoms prove to yourself that the docs are wrong.

The key to treatment is disrupting the cycle. One approach that has led to some success is cognitive behavioral therapy, in which patients are trained to force their attention away from the symptoms and counter panicky thoughts with self-reassurance, reminding themselves, for example, that stomach pain almost never means stomach cancer. Drug-based therapy is another promising approach. Research shows that roughly three-quarters of test subjects with hypochondria show significant improvement after medication with Prozac and other brain-regulating drugs.

CLOGGING THE SYSTEM

Hypochondriacs are responsible for some $20 billion in wasted medical resources in the U.S. each year

Resources

NIH HYPOCHONDRIA WEBSITE: *www.nlm.nih.gov/medlineplus/ency/article/001236*

THINK YOU'VE GOT A DEADLY DISEASE?

The standard self-test for hypochondria is called the Whiteley Index. To take it, circle the number that best fits the way you feel for each question, then add them all up. The higher the total, the more likely that you are a hypochondriac

1 = Not at all
2 = A little bit
3 = Moderately
4 = Quite a bit
5 = A great deal

1. Do you worry a lot about your health? **1 2 3 4 5**

2. Do you think there is something seriously wrong with your body? **1 2 3 4 5**

3. Is it hard for you to forget about yourself and think about all sorts of other things? **1 2 3 4 5**

4. If you feel ill and someone tells you that you are looking better, do you become annoyed? **1 2 3 4 5**

5. Do you find that you are often aware of various things happening in your body? **1 2 3 4 5**

6. Are you bothered by aches and pains? **1 2 3 4 5**

7. Are you afraid of illness? **1 2 3 4 5**

8. Do you worry about your health more than most people do? **1 2 3 4 5**

9. Do you get the feeling that people may not take your ailments seriously enough? **1 2 3 4 5**

10. Is it hard for you to believe your doctor when he or she tells you there is nothing for you to worry about? **1 2 3 4 5**

11. Do you often worry about the possibility that you have a serious illness? **1 2 3 4 5**

12. If a disease is brought to your attention (through the media or by a friend), do you worry about getting it yourself? **1 2 3 4 5**

13. Do you find that you are bothered by many different symptoms? **1 2 3 4 5**

14. Do you often have the symptoms of a very serious disease? **1 2 3 4 5**

There are no hard-and-fast cutoffs in the index, but people who score between 32 and 55 are generally considered to be hypochondriacs, whereas those who score between 14 and 28 are generally considered not to be. The numbers are only indications; people suffering from depression often score high. The best way to find out for certain is to consult a physician you trust.

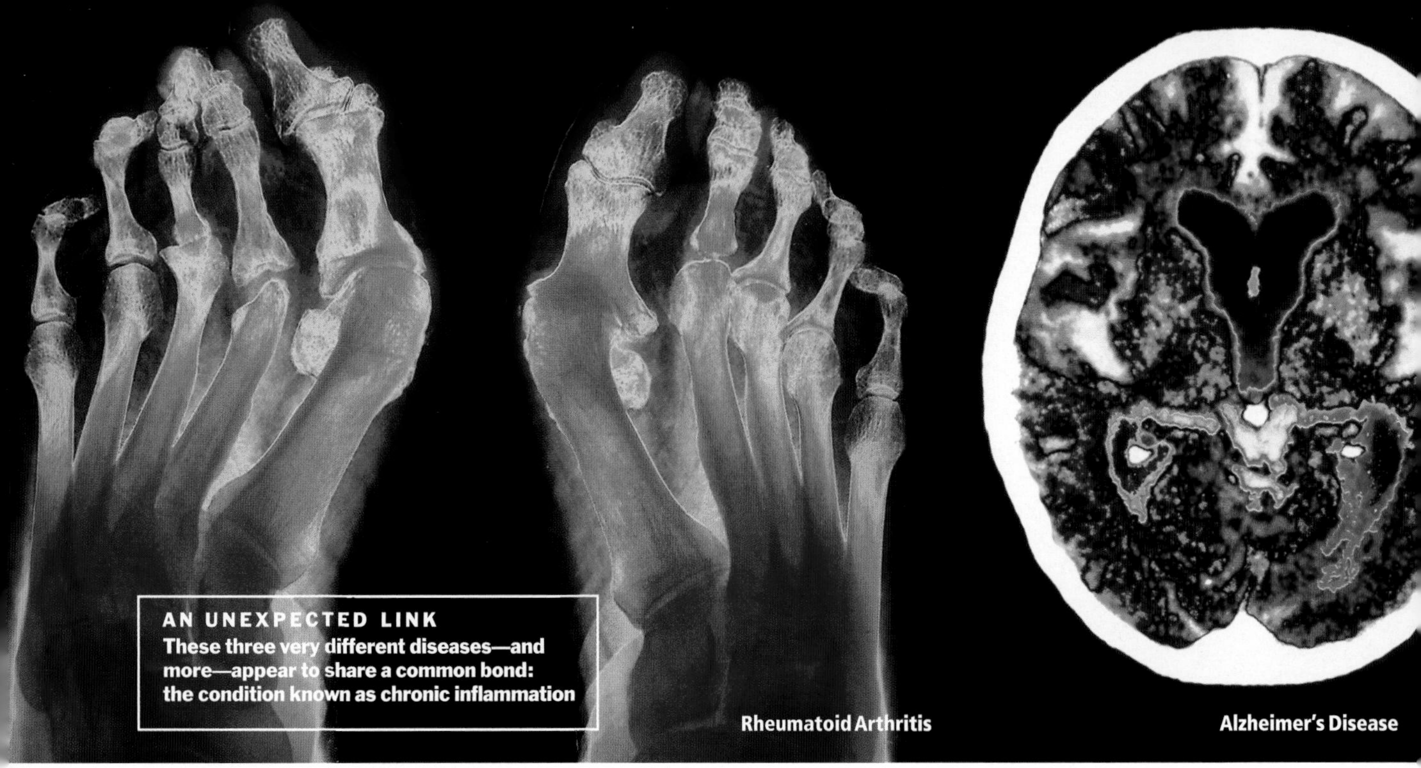

AN UNEXPECTED LINK
These three very different diseases—and more—appear to share a common bond: the condition known as chronic inflammation

Rheumatoid Arthritis

Alzheimer's Disease

Inflammation

Researchers are finding that heart disease, arthritis and Alzheimer's share a common link to the body's immunological defense system, via the process known as inflammation

The Crystal Ball Doctors are beginning to suspect that understanding the workings of inflammation may help us learn how to ward off a wide variety of illnesses before they take hold in our body, rather than treating their symptoms once they develop

What does a stubbed toe or a splinter in a finger have to do with your risk of developing Alzheimer's disease, suffering a heart attack or succumbing to colon cancer? More than you might think. As scientists delve deeper into the fundamental causes of those and other illnesses, they are starting to see connections to an immunological defense mechanism called inflammation—the same biological process that turns the tissue around a splinter red and causes swelling in an injured toe. If they are right—and the evidence is starting to look good—it could radically change doctors' concept of what makes us sick. It could also prove a bonanza to pharmaceutical companies looking for new ways to keep us well.

Most of the time, inflammation is a lifesaver that enables our bodies to fend off various disease-causing bacteria, viruses and parasites. The instant that any of these potentially deadly microbes slips into the body, inflammation marshals a defensive attack that lays waste to the invader and any tissue it may have infected. Then, just as quickly, the process subsides, and healing begins.

Once in a while, however, the whole feverish show doesn't shut down on cue. Sometimes the problem is a genetic predisposition; other times something like smoking or high blood pressure can keep the process going, and the inflammation becomes chronic rather than transitory. When that occurs, the hyper-active immune system turns on itself—like a child who can't resist picking a scab—with aftereffects that seem to underlie a wide variety of diseases.

OUT OF CONTROL

Inflammation is the body's natural healing process, but chronic inflammation opens the door to disease

Suddenly, inflammation has become one of the hottest areas of medical research. Hardly a week goes by without the publication of yet another study uncovering a new way that chronic inflammation does harm to the body. It destabilizes cholesterol deposits in the coronary arteries, leading to heart attacks and potentially even strokes. It chews up nerve cells in the brains of Alzheimer's victims. It may even foster the proliferation of abnormal cells and facilitate their transformation into cancer. In other words, chronic inflammation may be the engine that drives many of the most feared illnesses of middle and old age.

This concept is so intriguing because it suggests a new and possibly much simpler way of warding off disease. Instead of different treatments for, say, heart disease, Alzheimer's and colon cancer, there might be a single, inflammation-reducing remedy to prevent all three.

Chronic inflammation also fascinates scientists because it indicates

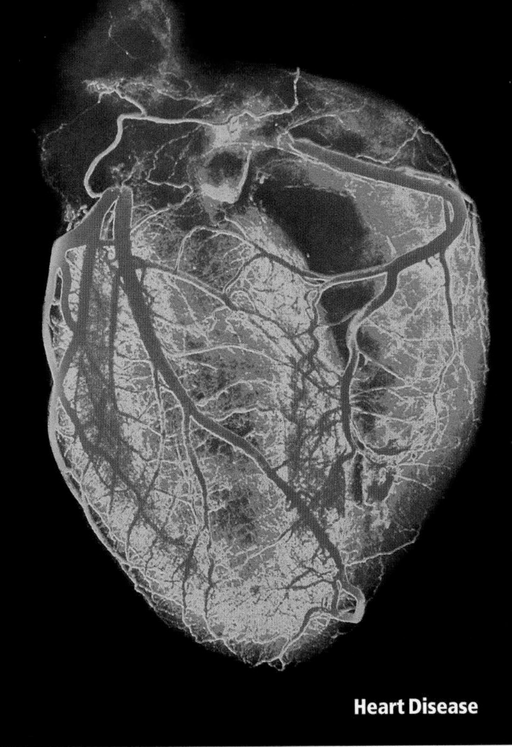
Heart Disease

that our bodies may have, from an evolutionary perspective, become victims of their own success. "We evolved as a species because of our ability to fight off microbial invaders," says Dr. Peter Libby, chief of cardiovascular medicine at Brigham and Women's Hospital in Boston. "The strategies our bodies used for survival were important in a time when we didn't have processing plants to purify our water, when we didn't have sewers to protect us."

But now that we are living longer, those same inflammatory strategies are more likely to slip beyond our control. Making matters worse, it appears that many of the attributes of a Western lifestyle—such as a diet high in sugars and saturated fats, accompanied by little or no exercise—also make it easier for inflammation to stay out of control.

At least that's the theory. For now, most of the evidence is circumstantial. (A few researchers think chronic inflammation can in some cases be good for you.) Doctors are testing the anti-inflammatory drugs already on pharmacy shelves to see if they have broader benefits. The findings are encouraging:

CELEBRATE CELEBREX

Celebrex, a drug used to treat arthritis, is turning out to prevent the intestinal polyps that can lead to cancer

■ In 2000 researchers found that patients who take Celebrex, a prescription drug originally designed to treat inflammation in arthritis, are less likely to develop intestinal polyps, abnormal growths that can become cancerous. Now there are dozens of clinical trials of Celebrex, investigating, among other things, whether it can also prevent breast cancer, delay memory loss or slow the progression of the devastating neurodegenerative disorder known as Lou Gehrig's disease.

■ As cardiologists gain more experience prescribing statins to lower cholesterol, they are finding that the drugs are more effective at preventing heart attacks than anyone expected. It turns out that statins don't just lower cholesterol levels; they also reduce inflammation. Now statins are being tested for their anti-inflammatory effects in cases of Alzheimer's disease and sickle-cell anemia.

■ DeCode Genetics, an Icelandic biotech firm, announced early in 2004 that it is launching a pilot

WHAT YOU CAN DO

The damaging effects of inflammation can be kept to a minimum with drugs, diet and even dental hygiene

DRUGS

■ Aspirin
A well-known inflammation fighter, aspirin can cool reactions raging in heart arteries and in the colon. Similar agents are also showing promise in controlling inflammation in the brains of Alzheimer's patients.

■ Statins Not only do statins lower cholesterol, but they also drive down levels of C-reactive protein as well as other inflammatory proteins.

■ Beta-blockers and ACE inhibitors Doctors are investigating whether blood-pressure medications control hypertension in part by lowering levels of certain inflammatory factors that constrict the blood vessels.

EXERCISE

It should be no surprise that being active is good for you, but the inflammation response may finally explain why. Fat cells are efficient factories for producing key inflammatory elements, and burning calories shrinks those cells. With fewer elements around, inflammation is less likely to flare up or get into the slow burn that contributes to heart disease, hypertension and diabetes.

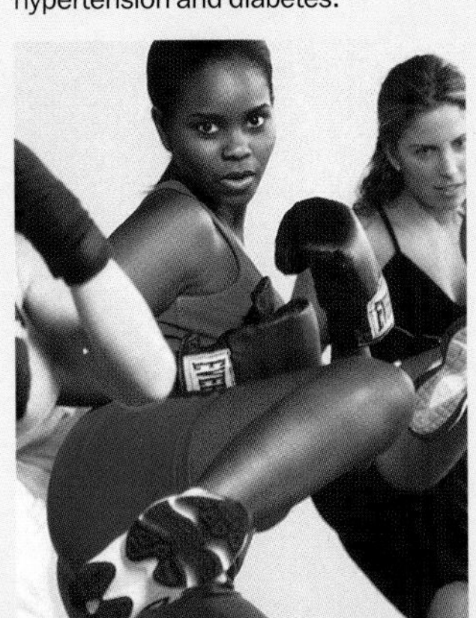

DIET

■ Low fat It's not yet clear which dietary fats fight inflammation best, but it makes sense to avoid the saturated fats in red meat and dairy products and stick with fish and vegetable oils.

■ Fruits and vegetables The richer the color the better, since colorful plants tend to have the most antioxidants—good for mopping up free radicals produced during inflammation.

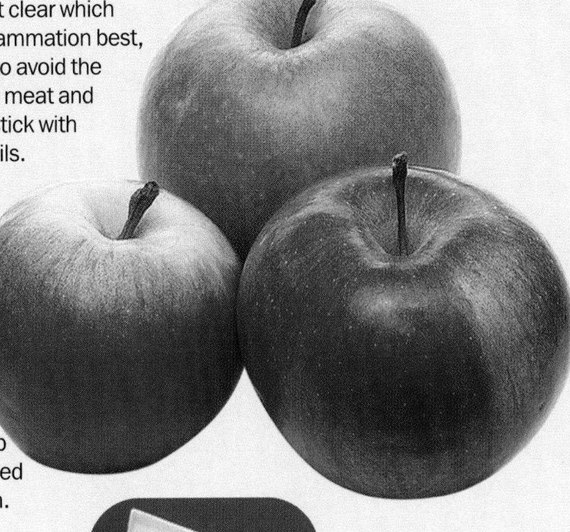

ORAL HYGIENE

■ Floss Keeping your mouth clean by flossing and brushing regularly can reduce the risk of gum disease, a source of chronic inflammation.

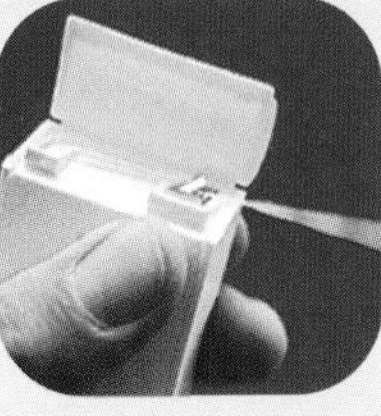

FLOSS: MARCO CAUZ-CORBIS; KICKBOXING: RICK GOMEZ-CORBIS; ASPIRIN: KOOPMAN-CORBIS; APPLES: STEVEN NEEDHAM-ENVISION

Influenza

In 2003 an unexpected strain of the flu stretched resources. But a new nasal vaccine is very promising

Bird-Flu Blues Millions of birds were put to death in Asia as health officials struggled to control a bird-flu outbreak. Early in 2004, federal officials found the flu in U.S. birds

A new nasal flu vaccine, FluMist, was approved by the FDA in the fall of 2003, just in time to help with a

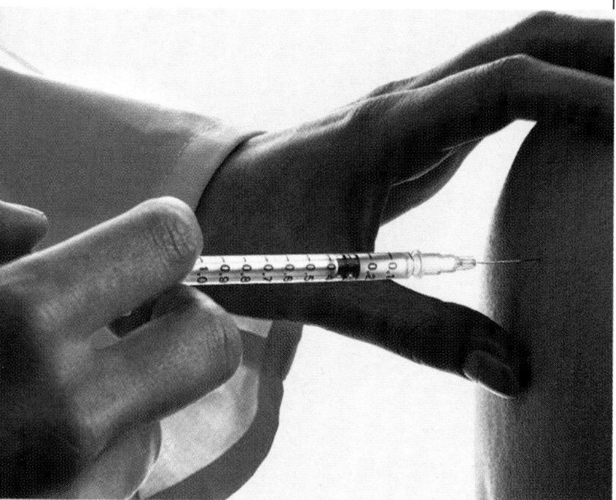
MAURITIUS—PHOTOTAKE

shortage of traditional flu shots prompted by the surprise month-early start of the 2003 flu season and the emergence of a particularly nasty strain of the virus that popped up too late to be included in vaccine preparations. By December, supplies of traditional flu vaccine were gone, CDC officials were referring to flu as "an epidemic," and dozens of children around the country had died from the outbreak.

Yet what really made influenza experts shudder was taking place on the other side of the world. Multiple outbreaks of avian influenza—"bird flu"—in 10 Asian countries resulted in a handful of human deaths, but that may have been only a hint of things to come.

The recent strain of bird flu in Asia has killed thousands of birds (millions more were slaughtered at the order of various governments as a precautionary measure) and seems to have jumped the species barrier, infecting numerous other kinds of animals in zoos and parks. This strain is deadly to humans but doesn't appear to be communicable from one person to another. All cases so far seem to have developed from human contact with animals.

But influenza is a particularly wily bug, constantly transforming itself. And if bird flu does mutate into a form in which human beings can infect one another, that may be the beginning of a crisis for which health experts say we are long over due and not at all prepared—a worldwide flu pandemic. One such outbreak killed at least 20 million people in 1918. Flu watchers estimate that 200,000 Americans would die if a new pandemic were unleashed tomorrow.

Nor is bird flu confined to Asia. In February and March 2004, health officials found the disease among chickens on farms in Texas, Delaware and Maryland, prompting them to order the slaughter of more than half a million birds. Sobered by these close calls, the Federal Government is considering whether to recommend that every American receive a flu shot each year.

In the meantime, the new nasal vaccine has earned some glowing reviews. One study found that FluMist is as safe as a traditional injection of flu vaccine; another found that it may be even more effective, with test subjects who took FluMist showing between 35% and 53% less risk of flu than those who had shots.

COLD—OR FLU?

Flu symptoms
- Fever (can last three days)
- Headache
- General aches, pains
- Fatigue, exhaustion
- Stuffy nose —maybe

Cold symptoms
- No fever
- No headache
- Slight aches, pains
- Slight fatigue
- Stuffy nose—for sure

Resources

NIH WEBSITE:
www.nlm.nih.gov/medlineplus/influenza

ROYALTY FREE—CORBIS

Insurance

Consumer-directed health plans or a health savings account may help you fight soaring insurance costs

Definition These savings accounts allow individuals to sock away money, tax free, to prepare for future medical expenses. The interest on the account also grows tax free

Unhappy about your health insurance (or lack of it)? You're not alone: the Census Bureau reports that more than 43 million Americans have no health coverage. Another report documented that fully half this number are people with jobs—despite the widespread belief that living without insurance is a problem mainly of the poor and

SELF-HELP HEALTH

Consumer-Directed Health Plans

Number of employees enrolled with the nine largest providers, in thousands

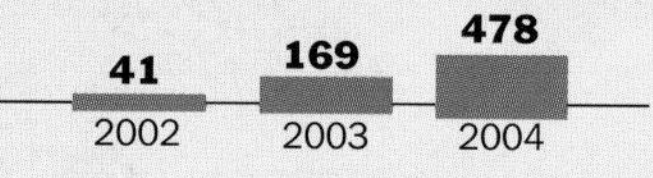

Percentage of large companies offering the plans

21% (2003), 32% (2004)

Facing double-digit increases in health-care costs, more companies are turning to consumer-directed health plans, which transfer control—and much of the responsibility for paying—to workers. In addition to cost sharing with employees, the plans generally feature high deductibles, a strong emphasis on preventive medicine, reimbursement accounts and health savings accounts, which, like IRAs, allow workers to save money tax free.

Sources: National Business Group on Health; Watson Wyatt Worldwide

unemployed. Meanwhile, a team of financial experts testified before Congress in June 2004 that hospitals routinely bill people with no insurance up to four times what they charge patients with coverage.

In a related development, people covered by an HMO no longer have the right to sue in state courts (where jury awards tend to be larger) when the HMO refuses to pay for care that a doctor has recommended. In June 2004, the Supreme Court restricted such litigation to federal court, where awards are severely limited.

As health costs soar and coverage shrinks, businesses and employees are seeking alternatives. Among them are consumer-directed health plans, which transfer control—and most of the payments—to workers. Most such plans feature high deductibles, reimbursement accounts, preventive medicine and health savings accounts, which allow workers to save money tax free to pay future medical bills.

Individual health savings accounts (HSAs) were also authorized by the 2003 Medicare law. Unlike medical savings accounts (MSAs), which are limited to small-business owners and the self-employed, an HSA is open to anyone under 65 covered by a health-insurance policy with an annual deductible of at least $1,000 for singles or $2,000 for families. A family can save up to $5,150 a year, individuals $2,600. Seniors may save an extra $500.

As with a traditional individual retirement account, HSA contributions are tax free and grow tax free. Withdrawals are also tax free, and there are no income limitations. An HSA lets you keep any unused money, accumulating more tax-free savings. The plan's best feature: when you use HSA money, you—and you alone—choose your doctor.

Resources

U.S. TREASURY HSA WEBSITE: *www.treas.gov/offices/public-affairs/hsa/index*

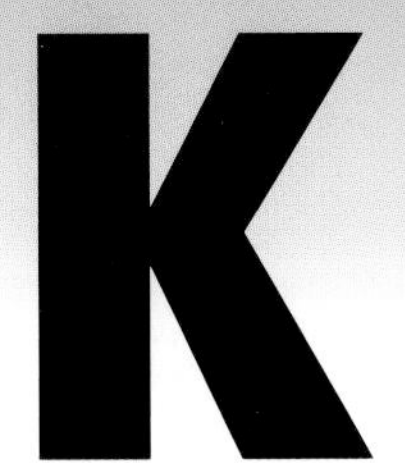

Kidney Disease

High cholesterol counts and long-term use of acetaminophen are seen as potential risk factors for kidney disease, while a new drug offers promise to victims

Blacks at Higher Risk African Americans are five times as likely as whites to suffer from severe kidney disease. One possible reason: blacks receive inferior health care. Another: the fact that two related risk factors—complications from diabetes and from hypertension—are substantially more prevalent among black Americans

Research has identified two new risk factors that can threaten kidney function in the general population: high cholesterol and long-term use of acetaminophen.

One study found that men with elevated levels of LDL ("bad") cholesterol are twice as likely to suffer from kidney malfunction as those with normal readings. A second study suggested that, at least among middle-aged women, 1 in 10 who takes acetaminophen for several years may be at risk for a decline in kidney function of as much as 30%.

Better news: a third team of researchers may have uncovered a way to reduce the health risks associated with kidney failure. Paricalcitol (Zemplar), a drug containing a new formulation of vitamin D, seems to increase long-term survival rates among dialysis patients, compared with test subjects who took calcitriol (Rocaltrol), a more traditional treatment.

Resources

NATIONAL KIDNEY FOUNDATION WEBSITE: *www.kidney.org*

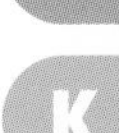
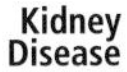

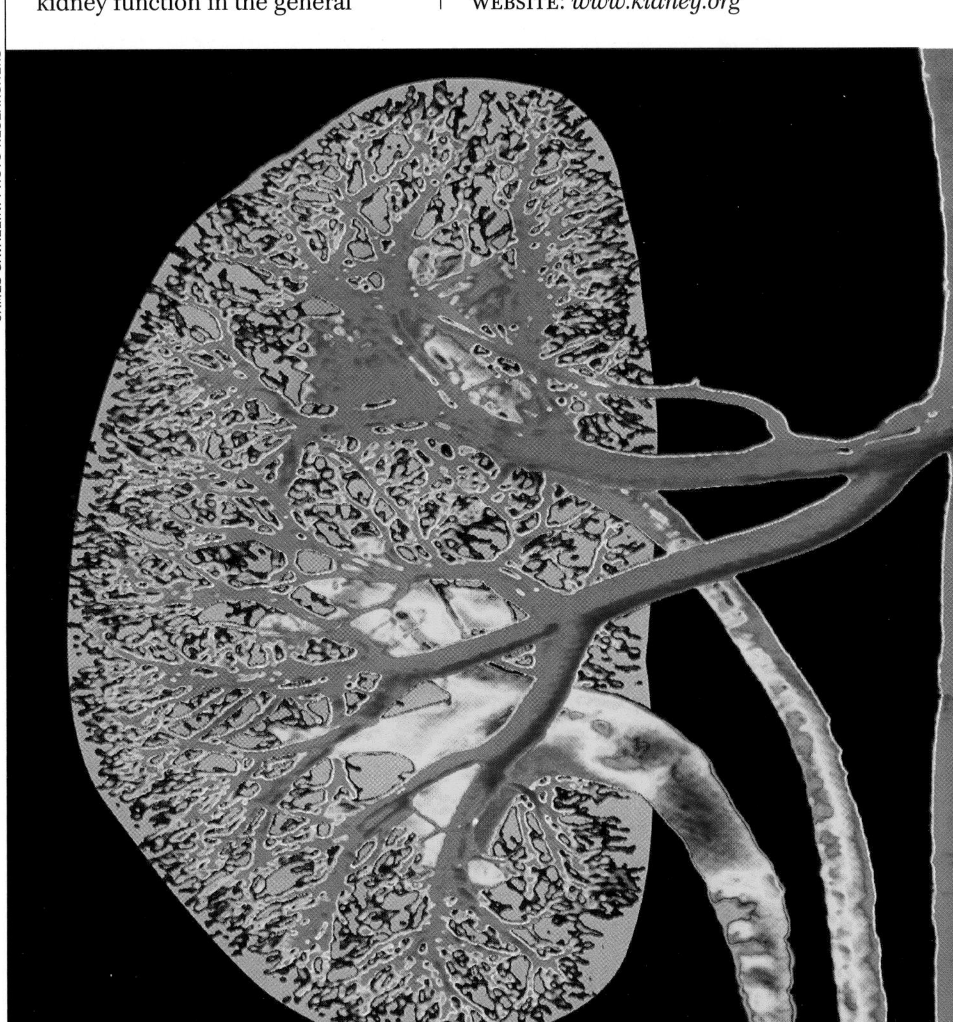
JAMES CAVALLINI-PHOTO RESEARCHERS

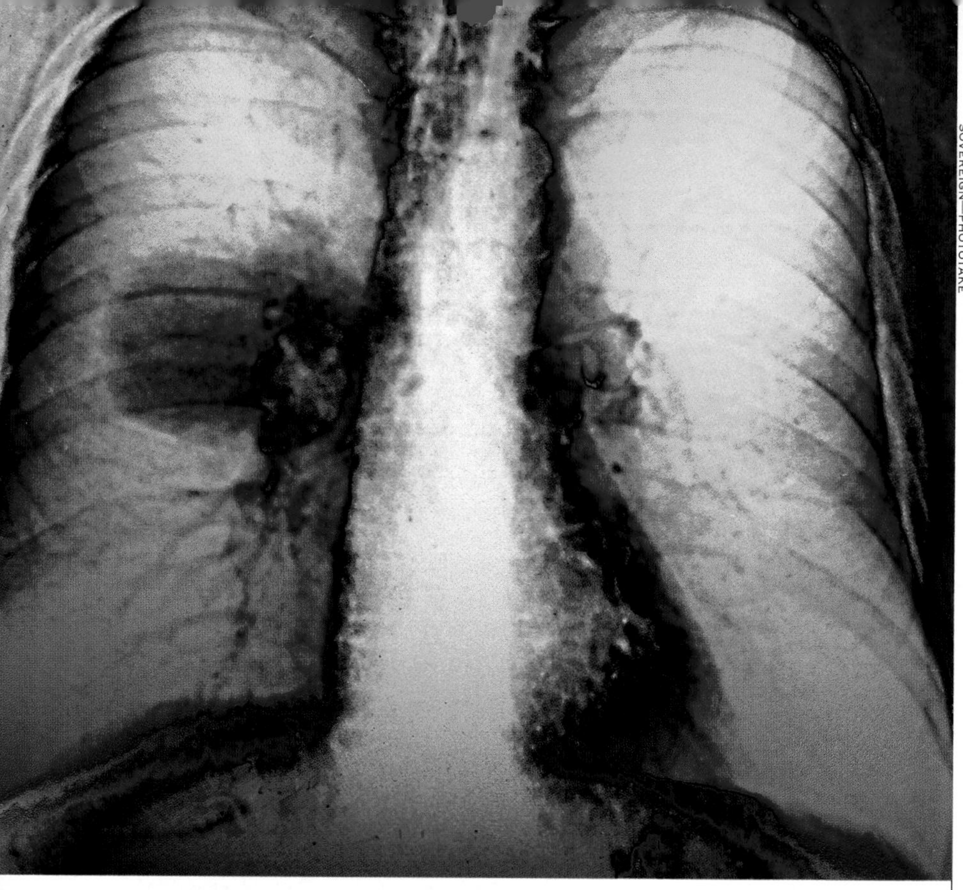

SOVEREIGN—PHOTOTAKE

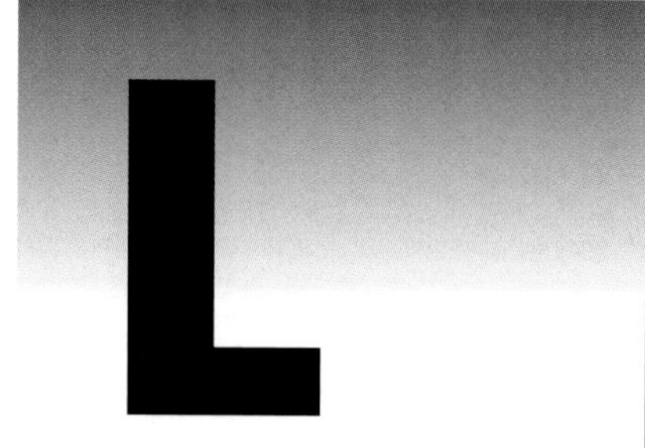

Lung Cancer

New scanning technologies may detect lung cancer earlier, saving many lives, while new drugs may make life easier for its victims

Global Threat Lung cancer remains the single most deadly form of cancer. It claims some 2.7 million lives each year around the world and 150,000 in the U.S.

The battle against lung cancer has proved to be the most frustrating front in the war on cancer. There is no test to screen for this No. 1 killer among all cancers and very little that doctors can do once they have found the disease. But all of this may be changing. A sophisticated new type of CT scan (known as spiral computed tomography) that creates three-dimensional images of the lung is being tested. Some experts believe it may catch lung tumors far earlier than standard X rays. If so, this will be a significant advance, because roughly three-quarters of all lung-cancers currently go undiagnosed until the disease has progressed to a point where it is untreatable.

On the treatment front, clinical trials of a new chemotherapy drug, Alimta, indicated that it may prolong the life expectancy of patients with advanced lung cancer while causing fewer side effects than standard chemo treatments for lung cancer. In July 2004, a panel of experts recommended that Alimta be considered for fast-track approval by the FDA. A final decision may come by 2005.

Two additional studies found that chemotherapy itself is probably more effective for lung-cancer patients than previously believed, raising the possibility that drug treatment after surgery may become as common for lung-cancer patients as it is for breast- and colon-cancer victims.

■ Resources

LUNG CANCER ONLINE:
www.lungcanceronline.org

Lung Diseases

Lung ailments such as emphysema and chronic bronchitis, grouped under the name chronic obstructive pulmonary disease (COPD), are the fourth-largest killer of Americans

Growing pains Chronic obstructive pulmonary disease afflicts some 13 million Americans, causing 120,000 deaths each year. And it's a growing global threat; the number of deaths due to COPD has nearly doubled over the past two decades

The grave threat posed by lung cancer often overshadows chronic obstructive pulmonary disease (COPD), but the "other lung disease" is a major killer. As with lung cancer, the vast majority of COPD cases (around 85%) are caused by smoking. Thus, while COPD isn't curable, it is largely preventable. In COPD, cells lining the lungs swell up, restricting the flow of air. (Living tissues, when exposed for prolonged periods to toxic substances like cigarette smoke, tend to become inflamed and swollen.) The newer treatment options for COPD include lung-volume-reduction surgery, an operation designed to decrease the capacity of the lungs in an attempt to improve their overall efficiency. A major study found in 2003 that this procedure can help some COPD patients breathe more easily and improve their quality of life.

DIVIDE AND CONQUER

Lung-volume-reduction surgery increases the efficiency of the lungs by decreasing their capacity—and it works

■ Resources

THE LUNG ASSOCIATION WEBSITE:
www.lung.ca/diseases

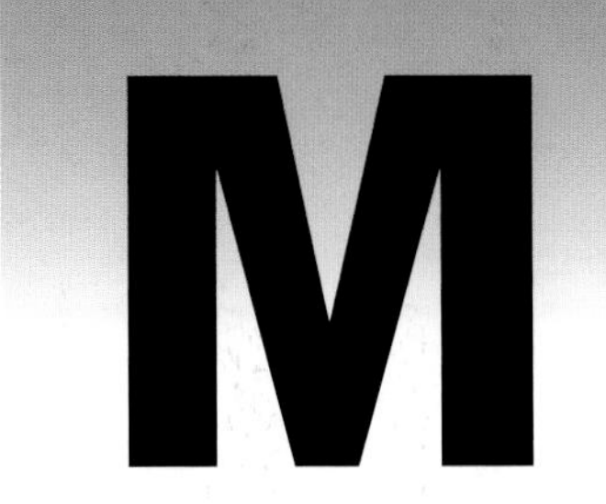

Mad Cow Disease

The disease is caused not by bacteria or viruses but by rogue proteins in the central nervous system called prions. It first turned up in the U.S. at the end of 2003

Silent, Deadly First identified in 1996, the incurable brain-wasting disease has struck more than 150 people, mostly in Europe. But because the disease has an incubation period of 10 to 15 years, scientists don't know how many people are at risk for it

ANDREW HETHERINGTON—PHOTONICA

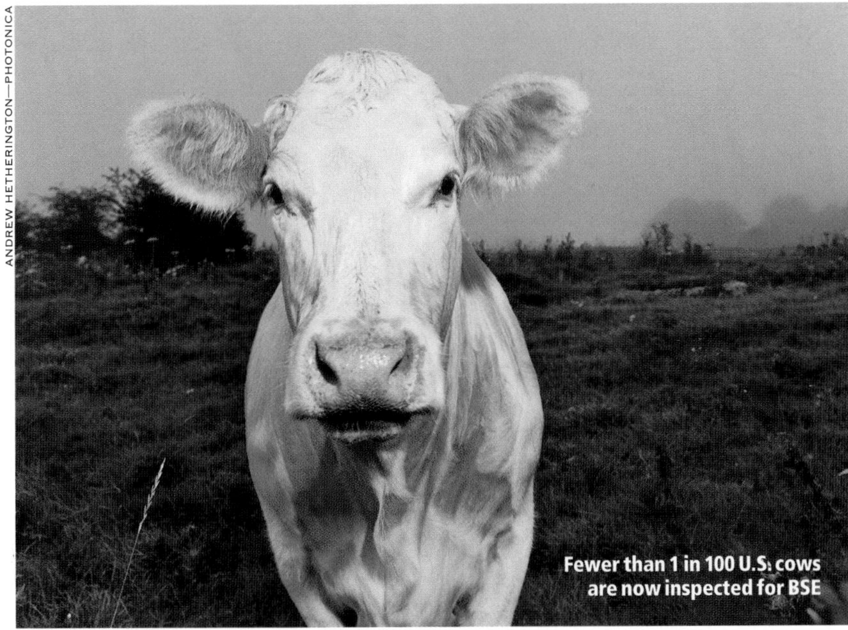

Fewer than 1 in 100 U.S. cows are now inspected for BSE

On June 20, 2004, the first U.S. resident believed to have the human-form variant of Creutzfeldt-Jakob disease (VCJD, also known as mad cow disease) died. Six months earlier, in December 2003, the bovine form of mad cow (bovine spongiform encephalopathy, or BSE) had been found in a slaughtered 6-year-old dairy cow in Washington State. In response, more than 30 countries promptly banned American beef exports, and some of them announced plans to keep the prohibition in place for years, since mad cow disease has a very long incubation period.

The ongoing risks have led to widespread calls for reform in the current procedures for raising, slaughtering and inspecting livestock. Japan now inspects and tests every cow that goes to slaughter, while the European Union checks more than 70% of its herd for mad cow. Both have called upon the U.S. to institute similarly rigorous measures. But government officials argue that testing all 35 million cows slaughtered in the U.S. each year (a number that is more than three times as large as the Japanese and European totals combined) is impractical. As it is, fewer than 1 in 100 U.S. cows is tested. In March 2004, the USDA announced a voluntary program that would temporarily expand screening 10-fold, but critics decried the voluntary approach as both inadequate and ineffective.

In July 2004, a U.S. research team succeeded in manufacturing a synthetic infectious prion, the root cause of the disease, for the first time. This raises the possibility of developing diagnostic tests for mad cow (which can presently be confirmed only by autopsy) and developing a better understanding of why prions, a rogue variant of protein, form in the first place. Until more is known about the disease, more U.S. consumers are buying expensive organic beef, whose feed is certified not to contain any animal by-products.

FROM COW TO TABLE

STEP 1: INFECTION
A cow eats feed contaminated with nervous-system tissue from a diseased cow or sheep. A spontaneous mutation may also create the prions that cause the illness

STEP 2: SPREAD
Prions force proteins to mis-fold throughout the nervous system and bone marrow, eventually ravaging the brain and crippling the afflicted cow

STEP 3: INTO THE FOOD SUPPLY
A "downer" cow is slaughtered for meat. Steaks and chops are presumed to be safe, but careless processing can let bits of nervous-system tissue or marrow get into ground beef

STEP 4: ONTO THE PLATE
Humans eat contaminated tissue. If prions in the meat corrupt human protein molecules, paralysis, dementia and death can follow. The brains of BSE-affected cows have microscopic holes, giving the tissue a spongelike appearance

PROTECTING MEAT

Early in 2004 the USDA announced new safeguards to keep BSE-tainted meat from the dinner table, including:

- **No "downer" cattle—those too sick to walk—will be used for food**
- **High-risk tissues from the heads and spinal columns of cattle 30 months or older won't be allowed in the human food chain**
- **Animals suspected of BSE infection will be held off the market until they test negative**

Resources

FDA WEBSITE: *www.cfsan.fda.gov/~comm/bsefaq*

Malaria

The mosquito-borne disease is one of the world's great killers. New drugs can cure it quickly—if we can get them to those who need them

How To Stop It? The best way to foil this killer is not necessarily through drugs. Low-tech solutions, such as insecticide-laden bed nets, could save millions of lives

Two global epidemics kill millions of people each year, a disproportionately large percentage of them in Africa. But while AIDS garners the lion's share of attention, malaria is doing nearly as much damage. The mosquito-borne illness sickened as many as 300 million people in 2003 and killed almost 3 million, nearly as many as AIDS. Adding to the heartbreak is that most malaria fatalities occur in children under 5. And while sub-Saharan Africa has suffered the brunt of this assault, nations in temperate zones (including the U.S.) are not immune. A malaria outbreak in Florida in the summer of 2003 hospitalized seven people; it was the first extended case of local transmission on U.S. soil in nearly 20 years.

The good news is that malaria can be cured; the bad news is that the resources to provide medicine to those who need it are in many cases not available. Even as malaria parasites have developed resistance to older treatments, several pilot studies conducted in Africa have proved that combination therapy, in which at least one of the medications is derived from a plant called *Artemisia annua*, or sweet wormwood, easily destroys drug-resistant malarial parasites in the bloodstream. Result: more than 90% of malaria patients are cured within three days.

➤**A Suicide Link?** The new treatment may be welcomed by families of U.S. military personnel in Iraq and other regions where malaria is a threat. A rash of suicides among U.S. troops who had been given Lariam, an antimalarial medication that is the Pentagon's standard precaution against the disease, prompted the Defense Department to study a possible link between suicide and Lariam use.

The concerns were not a surprise: earlier reports of psychological disturbances in nonmilitary users of Lariam had led the FDA in 2003 to call on the drug's maker, Roche, to issue a new warning about "certain psychiatric adverse events—anxiety, depression, restlessness or confusion" that the drug may cause.

AN UNWELCOME VISITOR

A 2003 outbreak of malaria in Florida was the first extended case of the disease on U.S. soil in nearly 20 years

■ **Resources**

MALARIA FOUNDATION INTERNATIONAL: *www.malaria.org*

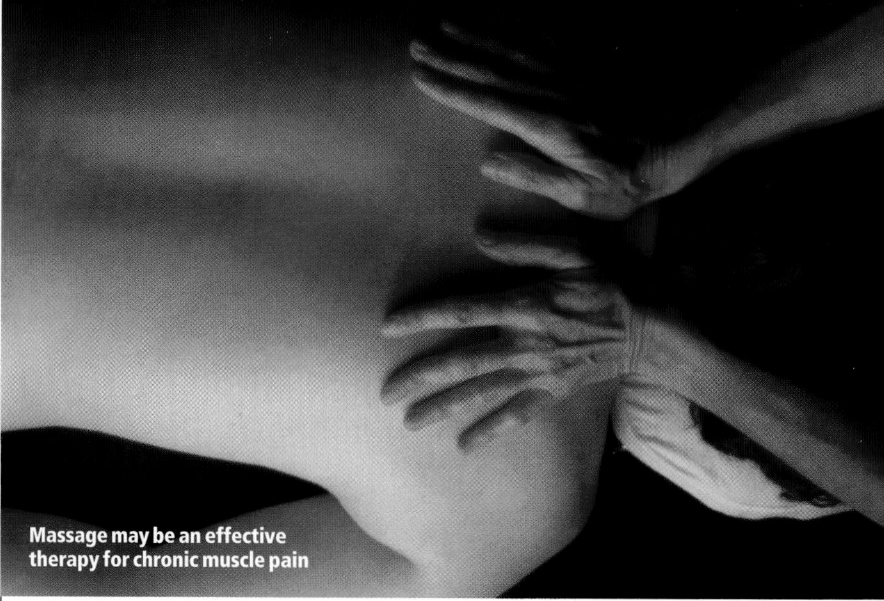
DOUG PLUMMER—PHOTONICA

Massage may be an effective therapy for chronic muscle pain

Massage

No one doubts that massage is a great way to beat stress. Now it seems it may be an effective treatment for chronic muscle pain

Brief Benefits One of the few drawbacks to massage is that its good vibes work best when experienced on a regular basis

Studies have consistently shown that massage can play a useful therapeutic role in a number of situations: treating anxiety and pain in cancer patients; curing sleeplessness in the critically ill; and enhancing relaxation, energy levels and mobility in residents of long-term care facilities.

Now we can add chronic muscle pain to the list of ailments that may benefit from massage. The addition of this ailment is especially good news because such muscle pain is difficult to treat. The new study compared the effectiveness of massage with the value of mental relaxation techniques. The test subjects who were treated with massage showed measurable improvements in overall health as well as in mental energy and muscle pain. The relaxation technique group showed no significant change in these areas.

There are two caveats. The benefits of massage disappeared within three months of the end of massage therapy, which is certainly not surprising. And this study (like many others touting the benefits of massage) was limited in scope. More rigorous verification of the therapeutic benefits of massage awaits further research.

■ **Resources**

AMERICAN MASSAGE THERAPY ASSOCIATION: *www.amtamassage.org*

Memory

A study finds that high blood pressure, or hypertension, is a risk factor for memory loss

Good News and Bad Estrogen therapy may help older women retain their memory. But it may not be worth the risk

Research continues to probe the processes that direct the complex phenomenon of human memory, revealing the factors that influence it. Previous research had shown that test subjects with hypertension scored poorly on memory tests compared with those with normal blood pressure. The new study used brain imaging technology to find that hypertensive patients had less blood flowing to regions of their brains associated with memory while they tried to perform memory-intensive tasks.

A second study showed that postmenopausal women taking estrogen therapy scored significantly better on memory tests than those taking a placebo, suggesting that estrogen therapy may help fend off short-term memory loss. However, because other studies have revealed there are risks of breast cancer and heart disease associated with hormone therapy, most experts recommend avoiding estrogen treatment except for short periods of time to treat the hot flashes of menopause.

■ Resources

NIH WEBSITE: *www.nlm.nih.gov/medlineplus/memory*

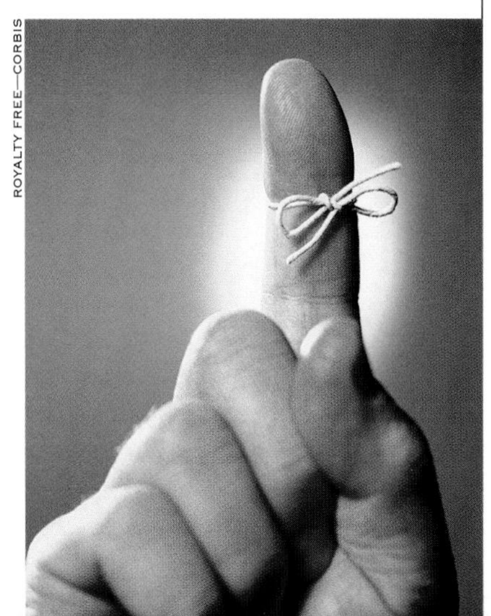

ROYALTY FREE—CORBIS

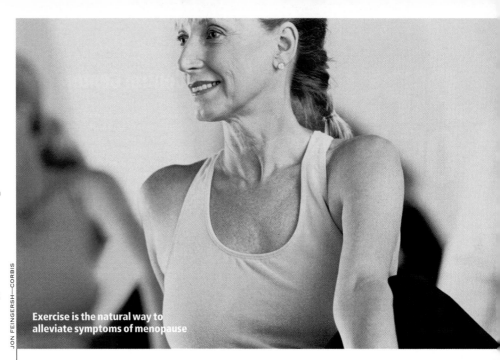

JON FEINGERSH—CORBIS

Exercise is the natural way to alleviate symptoms of menopause

Menopause

You may have heard that women with higher estrogen levels suffer less from hot flashes, and vice versa—but that's an old wives' tale

Turning Down the Heat Tests show that Paxil, a drug used to treat depression, may be an effective aid in helping reduce the number and frequency of hot flashes

Recent research findings have unearthed new treatments to make the symptoms of menopause easier to bear and have put to rest a major myth about this change of life that turns out to be false.

It's no surprise that studies indicate stress can aggravate many symptoms of menopause while exercise can reduce their severity. More specifically, one new study found that a regimen that mixes aerobics, resistance training and stretching can not only help reduce the short-term symptoms of menopause but also diminish its long-term challenges.

Hot flashes, one of the most aggravating side effects of menopause, have long been treated effectively with hormone replacement therapy (HRT). But today's serious doubts about the health risks of HRT have created a demand for alternatives that provide similar relief without the risks. One recent study indicated that the depression drug paroxetine (Paxil) may be effective. Postmenopausal test subjects who were not suffering from depression showed a 63% reduction in hot flashes when taking paroxetine, more than double the reduction observed in a control group.

One common myth about menopause—that women with the highest levels of estrogen suffer less from hot flashes, whereas women with the lowest levels are more prone to them—is falling by the wayside. New research shows that estrogen levels alone don't accurately predict the frequency and severity of flashes, but that race, ethnicity, financial status and lifestyle are better indicators.

The study found that women with low income levels were at greater risk than more affluent women. It also indicated that African-American women are most likely to have hot flashes, while Asians and Hispanics are the least at risk, with white test subjects occupying the center of the spectrum.

■ Resources

NIH WEBSITE: *www.nlm.nih.gov/medlineplus/menopause.*

M

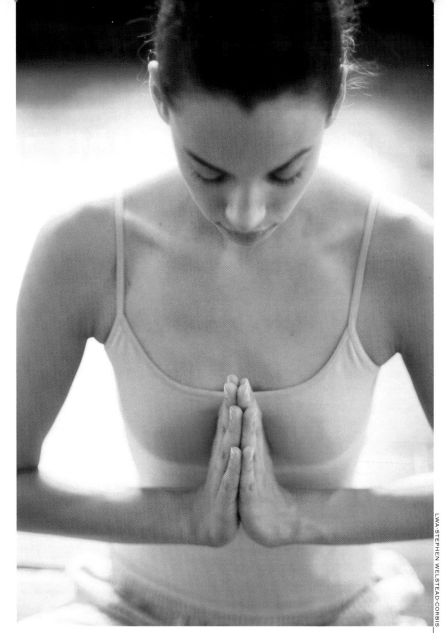

LWA-STEPHEN WELSTEAD-CORBIS

Mind and Body

As studies probe the relationships that link our minds, our social lives and our health, we're learning that the power of positive thinking isn't just good advice—it's good science

Charting Joy Preachers, poets and playwrights have depicted the connections between our mental state and our physical health. Now scientists are studying the physiology of happiness and discovering how our mindsets can affect our bodies

What philosophers and grandmothers have known intuitively for centuries, health-care professionals are now proving with hard science: happiness and health are two sides of the same coin, neither of which can be achieved in significant measure without a generous dose of the other. New research is linking factors like marital status, friendship, personality type, stress level—and even such intangibles as one's ability to forgive—with increased or decreased risk for an astounding variety of ailments, including Alzheimer's, AIDS, heart disease, hypertension, obesity and the common cold.

➤Health and Wealth A study that surveyed 1,500 people repeatedly over a 28-year period found that while healthy people are generally happier than unhealthy ones and married people are happier than unmarrieds, increases in wealth and material goods improve happiness only modestly—and briefly.

Although it's tempting to imagine that the mauve Porsche Boxster with a moonroof you have been dreaming of would actually make you happy, a pair of forces known as hedonic adaptation and social comparison argue otherwise.

Hedonic adaptation is the instinct that drives you to believe that life will be pretty close to ideal and trouble-free once you achieve a certain goal—graduating law school, getting a big promotion at work or marrying the person of your dreams—and it leads to a letdown once the goal is behind you and you realize that your life isn't much different from before.

The good news is that hedonic adaptation also works in reverse: situations that we anticipate as being unbearable—losing a job, getting old or carrying on after the loss of a loved one—turn out be to less awful than imagined once we've made the adjustment.

Social comparison is just what it sounds like: rating yourself against the status and achievement of peers. If Mr. Jones has just installed a swimming pool in the backyard next door, you feel a natural twinge of anxiety about keeping up. But the bottom line seems to be that when you get something new, the thrill quickly wears off, and even if it didn't, there's always someone out there with an even bigger pool than Mr. Jones'.

The answer? Drop out of the status chase—or at least run more slowly—and devote more time to family, friends and home. These lasting pursuits, the study shows, really do pay higher returns in happiness and health.

FEEL IT IN YOUR BONES?

Individuals in happy long-term relationships have higher levels of oxytocin, a hormone with a calming effect

➤Marriage: Risks and Rewards Marriage is the most enduring and complicated of human relationships, so it's not surprising that it can have a favorable impact on one's emotional and physical well-being. But these nuptial benefits are not guaranteed, and they certainly don't come for free.

TWO FOR THE LONG HAUL

Many studies have shown that married people tend to be healthier and live longer than singles

A large body of medical literature shows that married people tend to be healthier and live longer than singles. But newer research adds an important caveat: the quality of the marriage matters. Marital stress, logically enough, is not good for your health.

In one new study, 72 married couples were ranked on a scale of marital stress and tracked for three years. Those with high levels of stress were more likely to have an unhealthy thickening of the walls of the heart's main pumping chamber. The study also found that those in unhappy marriages were able to lower their blood pressure simply by spending less time with their spouses. Other studies have shown that happily married women are likely to have less blockage in their aorta, and that happily married individuals are less likely than the unhappily married to suffer from heart disease.

And that's just the start. People in happy marriages also have less acute and chronic illness; better-functioning immune systems; fewer fatal accidents; less susceptibility to alcohol abuse; and lower rates of depression, schizophrenia and suicide. In stable relationships, studies show, partners help each other's health by encouraging good health habits, such as getting routine mammograms and colonoscopies, while discouraging bad habits like smoking.

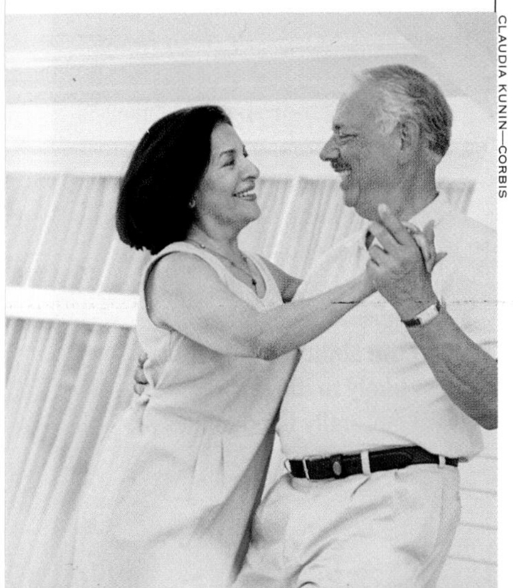

CLAUDIA KUNIN—CORBIS

Someday marital stress may be as important an indicator of health as cholesterol, weight or blood pressure. But like those other health indicators, a marriage needs constant work if you are going to enjoy the benefits.

➤**Unequal Distribution** Although marriage can hold health benefits for both genders, women may reap the larger rewards. A recent study found that episodes of physical and emotional intimacy (such as hugging) not only reduce levels of the stress hormone cortisol in both men and women but also increase levels of a recently discovered hormone, oxytocin, in women. Levels of oxytocin, which has a calming effect, were also found to be higher in both men and women who are involved in happy, long-term relationships.

Separate research showed that women in happy marriages are also significantly less likely to suffer from metabolic syndrome, a group of related symptoms including high blood pressure and high blood triglyceride and sugar levels, which is increasingly recognized as a risk factor for heart disease.

➤**The Benefits of Friendship** A new study finds that heart attack survivors who have at least one close friend with whom they are in regular touch and share personal information are half as likely to have a repeat heart attack as those who lead a more solitary life. The study also suggested that the social loners were more likely to drink heavily and use illegal drugs, both of which are significant risk factors

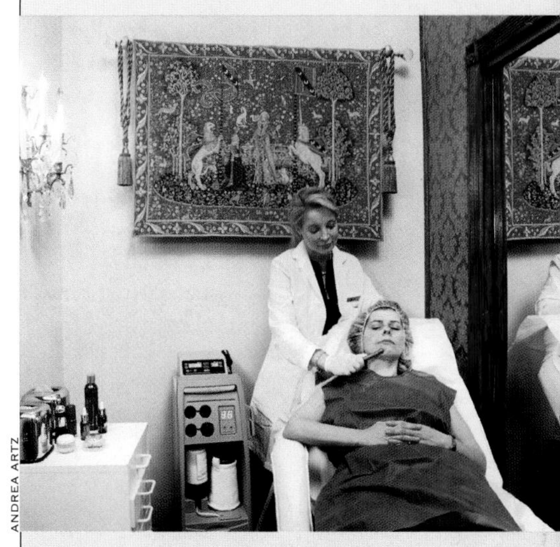

ANDREA ARTZ

Spas Sprout Docs

Medi-spas are day spas that have a doctor on staff, and they're the fastest-growing segment of the spa industry, with estimated annual revenues of $450 million for doctor-run medi-spas and an annual growth rate of 11% to 14%. Although there are some 9,000 spas in the U.S., only about 500 are medical spas, where more complicated and costly procedures can be performed. For plastic surgeons and dermatologists, medi-spas are an opportunity to go retail, with fees determined by the market rather than an insurance company.

Only a doctor can administer such procedures as laser resurfacing to tighten skin, Botox and collagen injections, and write prescriptions for oral hormone-replacement drugs to soften lines and wrinkles. And only a doctor can bill like one. (Prices vary from hundreds of dollars for a Botox injection to more than $1,000 for two laser skin-tightening treatments.)

Despite the potential profits, there is little regulation of medi-spas. Guidelines mandated by the state and protocols for handling people in a medical environment exist, but for the most part professional standards are lacking in the industry. For example, a medi-spa's skin-care products, which generate lots of profit, are not regulated by the FDA.

Some critics warn that if the medi-spa industry doesn't begin to regulate itself, legislators and litigators will take on the job. In the meantime, though, medi-spas are busy catering to—and extracting money from—a youth-obsessed society. ■

medical as it is cultural. Meditation is being recommended by more and more physicians as a way to prevent, slow or at least control stress and the diseases it can lead to, as well as relieve the pain of chronic heart conditions, AIDS, cancer and infertility. It is also being used to restore balance in the face of such psychiatric disturbances as depression, hyperactivity and attention-deficit disorder.

➤Just Say Om The brain, like the body, undergoes subtle changes during deep meditation. In 1967 Dr. Herbert Benson, a professor of medicine at Harvard Medical School, measured the heart rate, blood pressure, skin temperature and rectal temperature of 36 transcendental meditators. He found that when they meditated, they used 17% less oxygen, lowered their heart rates by three beats a minute and increased their theta brain waves—the ones that appear right before sleep—without slipping into the brain-wave pattern of actual sleep.

Studies of the meditating brain became much more sophisticated after brain imaging was developed. At the University of Wisconsin at Madison, Richard Davidson has used brain imaging to show that meditation shifts activity in the prefrontal cortex (the area just behind your forehead) from the right hemisphere to the left. The research suggests that by meditating regularly, the brain is reoriented from a stressful fight-or-flight mode to one of acceptance, increasing contentment. People who have a negative disposition tend to be right-prefrontal oriented; left-prefrontals have more enthusiasms, more interests, relax more and tend to be happier.

More than a decade ago, Dr. Dean Ornish, the low-fat-diet advocate, argued that meditation, along with yoga and dieting, reversed the buildup of plaque in coronary arteries. In April 2003 at a meeting of the American Urological Association, he announced other findings: that meditation may slow the advance of prostate cancer. (It's important to note that those patients were also dieting and doing yoga.)

Jon Kabat-Zinn, who founded the Stress Reduction Clinic at the UMass Medical Center in 1979, has been trying to find a scientific demonstration of the healing power of meditation. He gave a group of newly taught meditators and nonmeditators flu shots and measured the antibody levels in their blood. Researchers also measured their brain activity to see how much the meditators' mental activity shifted from the right brain to the left. Not only did the meditators have more antibodies at both four weeks and eight weeks after the shots, but the people whose mental activity shifted the most had even more antibodies.

The evidence from research into meditation continues to mount. One study, for example, shows that women who meditate and use guided imagery have higher levels of the immune cells known to combat tumors in the breast. This comes after many studies have shown that meditation can significantly reduce high blood pressure. The picture scientists are drawing is taking shape: meditation may be one of the easiest, cheapest ways to make you and your body feel better.

➤Picturing Rejection More news from the mind-body front: the sickening punched-in-the-stomach feeling that comes from painful social snubs and rejection isn't in your imagination, new brain-imaging research finds. In fact, it's

FOUR-STEP PROGRAM

O.K., try this at home, if you want a taste of meditation:

- **Find a quiet place.** Turn out the lights, if you like. The fewer distractions, the easier it will be to concentrate
- **Close your eyes.** The idea is to shut out the outside world so your brain stops processing outside information
- **Pick a word, any word.** Find one that means something to you, whose sound or rhythm is soothing when repeated
- **Say it, again and again.** Try saying the word (or phrase) with every outbreath. The repetitiveness will help you focus

CALMING THE

Wave Change

Even people meditating for the first time will register a decrease in beta waves, a sign that the cortex is not processing information as actively as usual. After their first 20-minute session, patients show a marked decrease in beta-wave activity, shown in bright colors, top.

BEFORE meditation

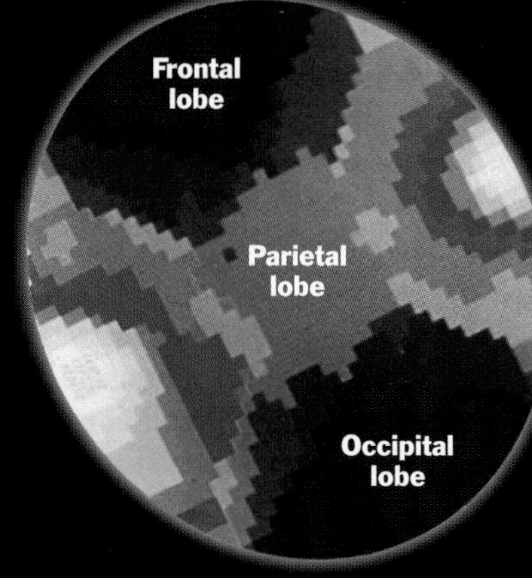

AFTER meditation

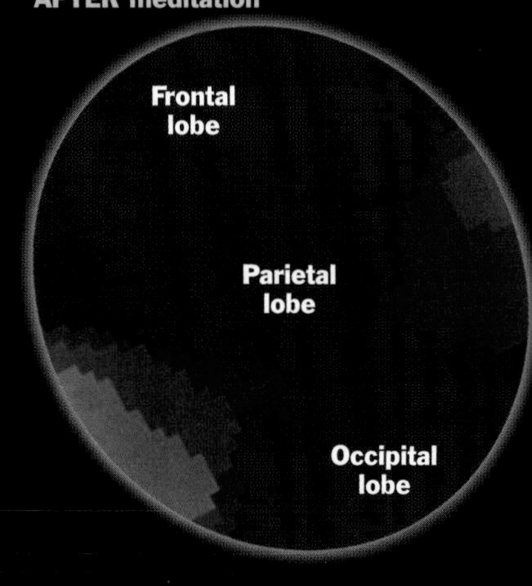

IND Meditation is an ancient discipline, but scientists have only recently developed tools sophisticated enough to see what goes on in your brain when you do it

ide the Meditating Brain

ntal lobe
is the most highly evolved part of brain, responsible for reasoning, nning, emotions and self-conscious reness. During meditation, the tal cortex tends to go offline.

Parietal lobe
This part of the brain processes sensory information about the surrounding world, orienting you in time and space. During meditation, activity in the parietal lobe slows down.

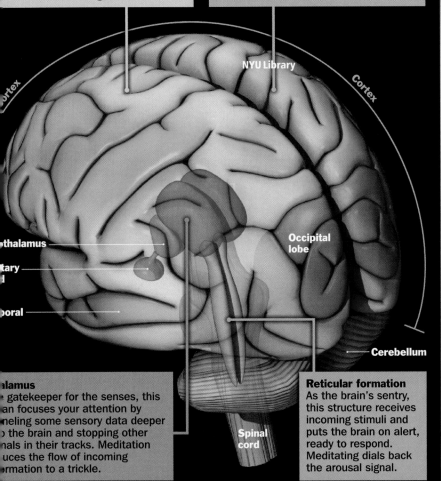

NYU Library

ortex

Cortex

thalamus

tary

oral

Occipital lobe

Cerebellum

Spinal cord

lamus
gatekeeper for the senses, this an focuses your attention by neling some sensory data deeper the brain and stopping other nals in their tracks. Meditation uces the flow of incoming rmation to a trickle.

Reticular formation
As the brain's sentry, this structure receives incoming stimuli and puts the brain on alert, ready to respond. Meditating dials back the arousal signal.

Meditation Training

After training in meditation for eight weeks, subjects show a pronounced change in brain-wave patterns, shifting from the alpha waves of aroused, conscious thought to the theta waves that dominate the brain during periods of deep relaxation

Relaxation increases ...
Power of theta waves as a percentage of total EEG power

26%, 24, 22, 20, 18, 16

Meditation group — Left side of brain; Right side

Control group — Left side; Right side

1 3 5 7 9 11 13 15
Sessions

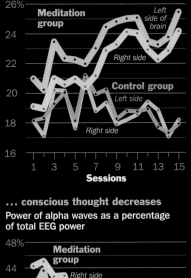

... conscious thought decreases
Power of alpha waves as a percentage of total EEG power

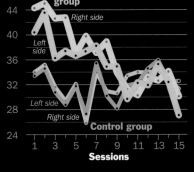

48%, 44, 40, 36, 32, 28, 24

Meditation group — Right side; Left side

Control group — Left side; Right side

1 3 5 7 9 11 13 15
Sessions

r. Gregg Jacobs, Harvard Medical School, author of *The Ancestral Mind.* TIME Graphic by Joe Lertola; text by Alice Park

M

in your anterior cingulate cortex, a region of the brain that manages the emotional response to physical discomfort. Using functional magnetic resonance imaging scans (fMRI), which allow scientists to observe brain activity as it happens, researchers were able to create pictures of test subjects' brains as they experienced painful social rejection—and the images were startlingly similar to the scans of people who were in serious pain.

➤**Stress and Cancer** A new study suggested that two hormones linked to behavioral stress—norepinephrine and epinephrine—can enhance the potential of ovarian cancer cells to become invasive and spread aggressively. The researchers who conducted this study theorize that the same dynamic may be at work in colon and breast cancer, although more research is needed to document this hypothesis.

➤**The Promise** Two conclusions are inescapable from recent research: first, healthy minds, healthy bodies and healthy relationships are one and indivisible. Second, the exploration of the interplay between body and mind may prove to be one of the great moving forces in medicine in the 21st century.

■ **Resources**

TAOIST TAI CHI SOCIETY SITE:
www.taoist.org/english

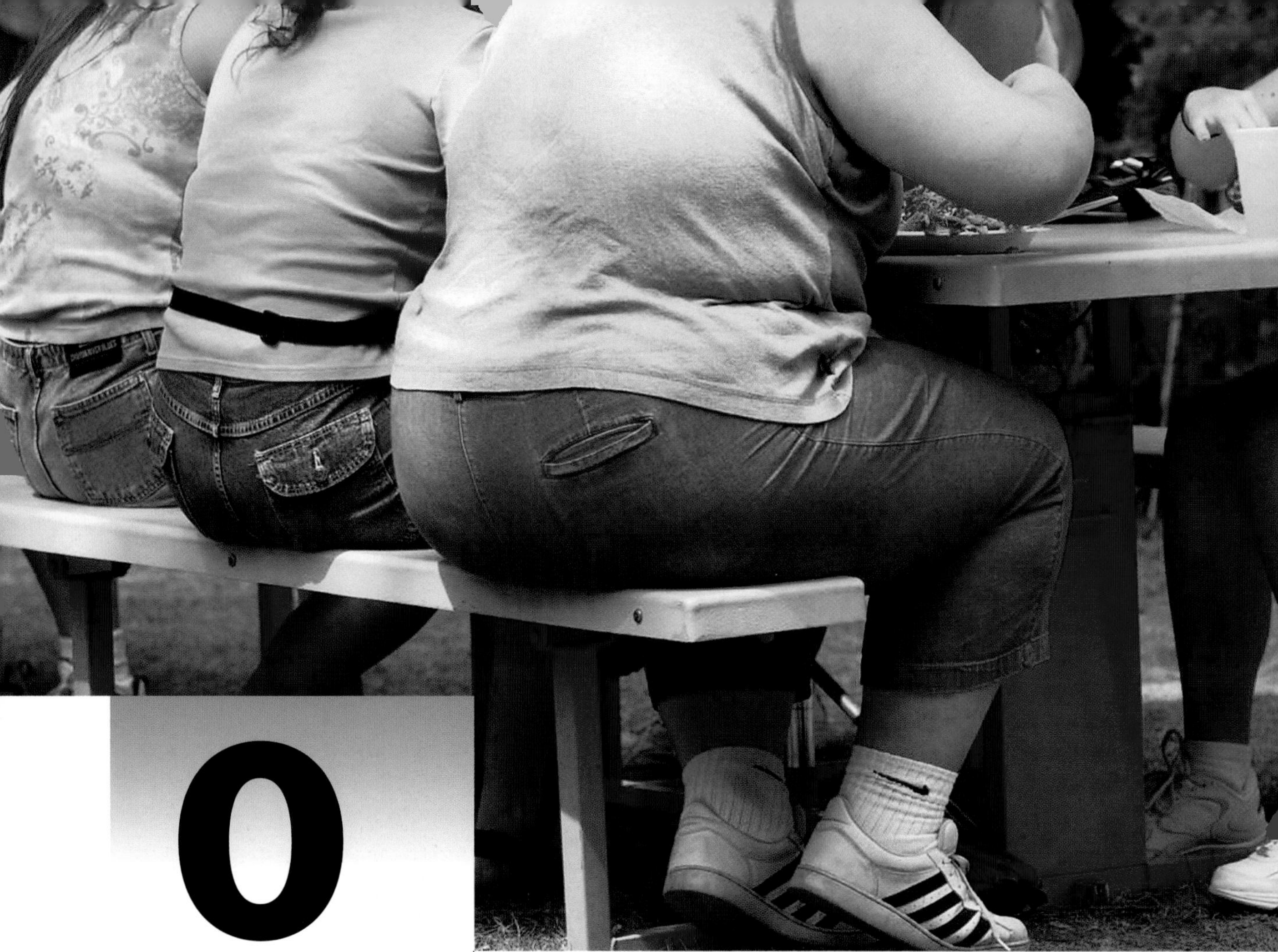

O

Obesity

America's battle with overweight is now at epidemic proportions. There are a number of villains to blame, including ourselves, but the urge to gorge may be a relic of man's past

Diet Coverage This article explores the extent of America's epidemic of obesity and the reasons behind it. The story on Diet covers news of nutrition, while America's current fascination with fast-acting low-carb diets is covered under Carbohydrates

It's hardly news anymore that Americans are just too fat. If the endless parade of articles, TV specials and fad diet books weren't proof enough, a quick look around the mall, the beach or the crowd at any baseball game will leave no room for doubt: our individual weight problems have become a national crisis.

Even so, the actual numbers are shocking. Fully two-thirds of U.S. adults are officially overweight, and about half of those have graduated to full-blown obesity. The rates for African Americans and Latinos are even higher. Among kids between 6 and 19 years old, 15%, or 1 in 6, are overweight.

And things haven't been moving in a promising direction. Just two decades ago, the incidence of overweight in adults was well under 50%, while the rate for kids was only a third what it is today. From 1996 to 2001, 2 million teenagers and young adults joined the ranks of the clinically obese. People are clearly worried. A TIME/ABC News poll released in May 2004 showed that 58% of Americans would like to lose weight, nearly twice the percentage who felt that way in 1951.

GROWING, GROWING ...

Between 1996 and 2001, 2 million U.S. teenagers and young adults joined the ranks of the clinically obese

It wouldn't be such a big deal if the problem were simply aesthetic. But excess poundage takes a terrible toll on the human body, significantly increasing the risk of heart disease, high blood pressure, stroke, diabetes, infertility, gallbladder disease, osteoarthritis and many forms of cancer. The total medical tab for illnesses related to obesity is $117 billion a year—and climbing—according to the Surgeon General, and the *Journal of the American Medical Association* reported in March 2004 that poor diet and physical inactivity could soon overtake tobacco as the leading cause of preventable death in the U.S.

➤**Origins of Obesity** So why is it happening? The obvious answer is that we eat too much high-calorie food and don't burn it off with enough exercise. If only we could change those habits, the problem would go away. But clearly it isn't that easy. Americans pour scores of billions of dollars every year into weight-loss products and health-club memberships and liposuction and gastric-bypass operations—100,000 of the last in 2003 alone. Yet the nation's collective waistline just keeps growing.

SURGICAL SOLUTION?

If you can't beat fat ... Americans underwent 100,000 gastric-bypass operations in 2003

It's natural to try to find villains to blame—fast-food joints or food companies or even ourselves for having too little willpower. But the ultimate reason for obesity may be rooted deep within our genes. Obedient to the inexorable laws of evolution, the human race adapted over millions of years to living in a world of scarcity, where it was wise to eat every calorie-packed and fat-laden thing you could find.

Although our physiology has stayed pretty much the same for the past 50,000 years or so, we humans have utterly transformed our environment. Over the past century especially, technology has almost completely removed physical exercise from the day-to-day lives of most Americans. At the same time, it has filled supermarket shelves with cheap, mass-produced, good-tasting food that is packed with calories. And technology delivers constant, inviting messages that say "Eat this now" to everyone old enough to watch TV.

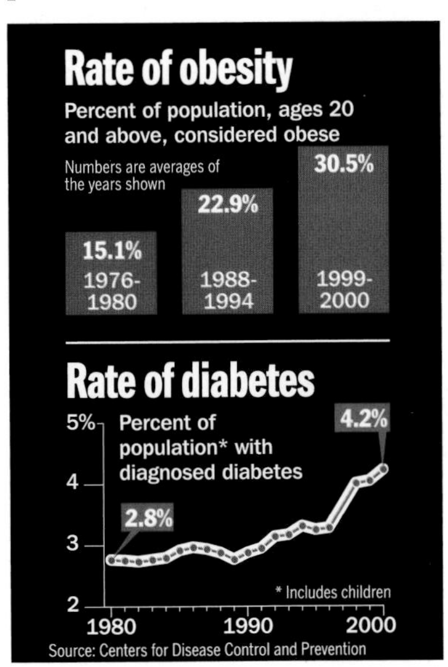

This artificial environment is most pervasive in the U.S. and other industrialized countries, and that's exactly where the fat crisis is most acute. By contrast, among people who still live in conditions most like those of our distant Stone Age ancestors—like the Maku or the Yanomami of Brazil—there is virtually no obesity at all.

That's probably the way it was during 99.9% of human evolution. For most of the 7 million years or so since we parted ways with chimps, life has been harsh—"nasty, brutish and short," in Thomas Hobbes' memorable phrase.

➤Early Diets Our first ancestors probably ate much as their cousins the apes did, foraging for fruits, shoots, nuts, tubers and other vegetation in the forests and savannas of Africa. Because most wild plants are relatively low in calories, it took constant work just to stay alive. Fruits, full of natural sugars like fructose and glucose, were an unusually concentrated source of energy, and the instinct to seek out and consume them evolved in many mammals long before humans ever arose. But humanity's appetite for animal fat and protein is probably more recent.

It was some 2.5 million years ago that our hominid ancestors developed a taste for meat. The fossil record shows that the human brain became markedly bigger and more complex about the same time. Meat provided a concentrated source of protein, vitamins, minerals and fatty acids that helped our human ancestors grow taller.

➤Agriculture The appetite for meat and sweets was essential to human survival, but it didn't lead to obesity for several reasons. The

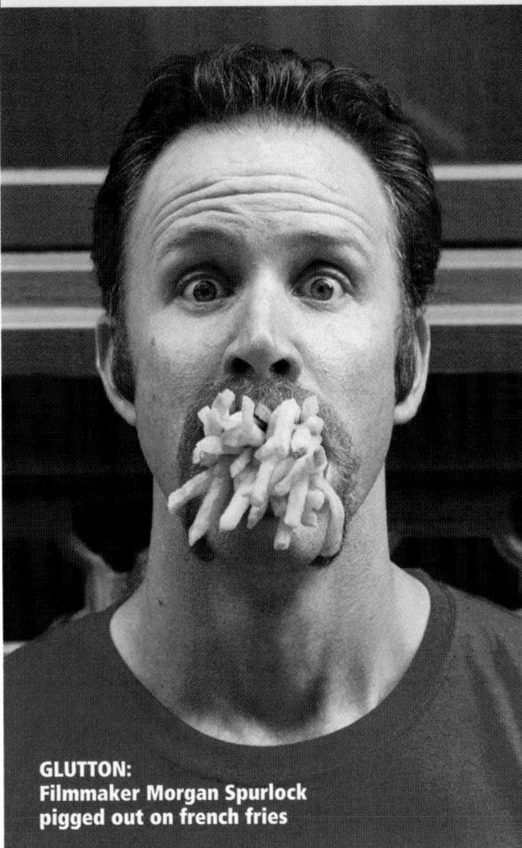

ROADSIDE ATTRACTIONS & SAMUEL

GLUTTON: Filmmaker Morgan Spurlock pigged out on french fries

Fast-Food Frenzy

For 30 days, a trim, fit, politically correct fellow named Morgan Spurlock took all his meals—breakfast, lunch and dinner—at McDonald's while directing film crews who recorded his fast-food feast. Some results of his ordeal, as reported in his documentary *Super Size Me,* are predictable: he gained 24.5 lbs., and his cholesterol count shot up alarmingly. Some are less so: the amount of damage he did to his liver was roughly the same as if he had been on an alcohol binge of a similar duration. There is also evidence that he became something of a fast-food addict, with his sense of well-being increasingly dependent on the rush his fat- and fructose-laden eats provided.

What's best in the film is its depiction of an ugly food chain. A huge American industry seduces the innocent with cheesy toys and free playgrounds. The government ships sloppy-joe makings to grateful school-lunch programs, because it's the cheapest lunch available. School boards sign off on pizza and sodas for lunch, while cutting phys-ed classes. And everyone starts getting fatter younger. ■

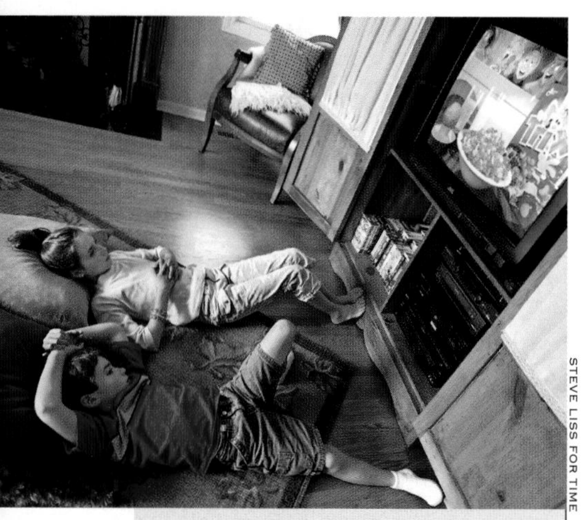
STEVE LISS FOR TIME

Kill the Messenger?

If you can't pry those SpongeBob Cheez-It crackers from your kid's hands, you're not alone. Public-health advocates say food advertising aimed at children has spun out of control—infiltrating schools, sports arenas, the Web and of course TV, by which kids are exposed to 40,000 ads a year, as many as 70% of them for food. Ads for high-fat, high-salt foods have more than doubled since the 1980s, while commercials for fruits and vegetables remain in short supply.

Any attempt to ban junk-food ads from TV is likely to run into resistance from a powerful alliance of food companies, broadcasters and ad agencies, which would brand such a ban as censorship. Norway, Sweden and the province of Quebec, however, have all banned child-targeted TV advertising. For now, the U.S. government's most salient media campaign to reduce childhood obesity is an initiative called Verb, which encourages kids to be more physically active. It does not mention the perils of junk food. ■

wild game our ancestors ate was high in protein but very low in fat—only about 4%, compared with as much as 36% in grain-fed supermarket beef. Beyond that, hunting and gathering took enormous physical work. In essence, early humans ate what amounted to the best of the high-protein Atkins diet and the low-fat Ornish diet and worked out almost nonstop. That was the condition of pretty much the entire human race when anatomically modern humans first arose, between 150,000 and 100,000 years ago, and things stayed that way until what some anthropologists have called humanity's worst mistake: the invention of agriculture.

Nutritionally, the shift away from wild meat, fruits and vegetables to a diet mostly of cultivated grain robbed humans of many of the essential amino acids, vitamins and minerals they had thrived on. Average life span increased, thanks to the greater abundance of food, but average height diminished. Skeletons of the era reveal a jump in calcium deficiency, anemia, bad teeth and bacterial infections.

Most meat that people ate came from domesticated animals, which have more fat than wild game. Livestock also supplied early pastoralists with milk products, which are full of artery-clogging butterfat. But obesity still wasn't a problem, because even with animals to help, physical exertion was built into just about everyone's life.

That remained the case practically up to the present. It's really only in the past 100 years that cars and other machinery have dramatically reduced the need for physical labor. And as exercise has vanished from everyday life, the technology of food production has become much more sophisticated. In the year 1700 Britons consumed about 7.5 lbs. of sugar per capita. Americans now consume more than 150 lbs. of sweetener per capita, nearly 50% of which is high-fructose corn syrup that is increasingly used to replace sugar.

SWEET BUT HARMFUL

High-fructose corn syrup is used to replace healthier ingredients in all kinds of foods, not just your soda pop

Farmers armed with powerful fertilizers and high-tech equipment are raising vast herds of cattle whose meat is laden with the fat that makes it taste so good. They are producing milk, butter and cheese by the tankerload, full of the fat that humans crave.

And thanks to mass production, all that food is relatively cheap. It's also absurdly convenient. In many

The Corn Connection

The U.S. produces so much corn so cheaply that Americans have become quite clever at inventing uses for it, from fuel to power cars and trucks to the polymers in plastics. But most of all, we eat it. And the cattle, hogs, chicken and fish that we eat eat it. In the form of high-fructose corn syrup, it is cheaper than sugar—and, nutritionists say, a primary cause of the obesity epidemic. As much as 57% of the corn we produce becomes inexpensive animal feed that helps keep meat prices down. But it also makes the meat fattier—and consumers fatter—than if the animals were fed grass.

About 5% of our corn is refined to high-fructose corn syrup, which is cheaper, sweeter and easier to transport and mix into foods than sugar. Beverage- and foodmakers use the high-fructose cocktail in place of more nutritious ingredients—not just for sugar—in peanut butter, fruit juices and spaghetti sauce. From 1972 to 2002, the amount of sugar and syrup produced annually per American grew 21%, from 104 lbs. to 126 lbs. In that same time period, the percentage of syrup sweetener in that total grew from less than 1% to nearly 50%.

A battle is looming: nutritionists are calling for warning labels or junk-food taxes, but soft-drink makers and the growers whose corn products are in them will resist any attempt to thwart their sweet deal with thirsty consumers. ■

EISENHUT & MAYER-FOODPIX

United States Of Obesity

Weight is not evenly distributed in the U.S. The highest concentration of obese Americans forms a wide belt across the southern states

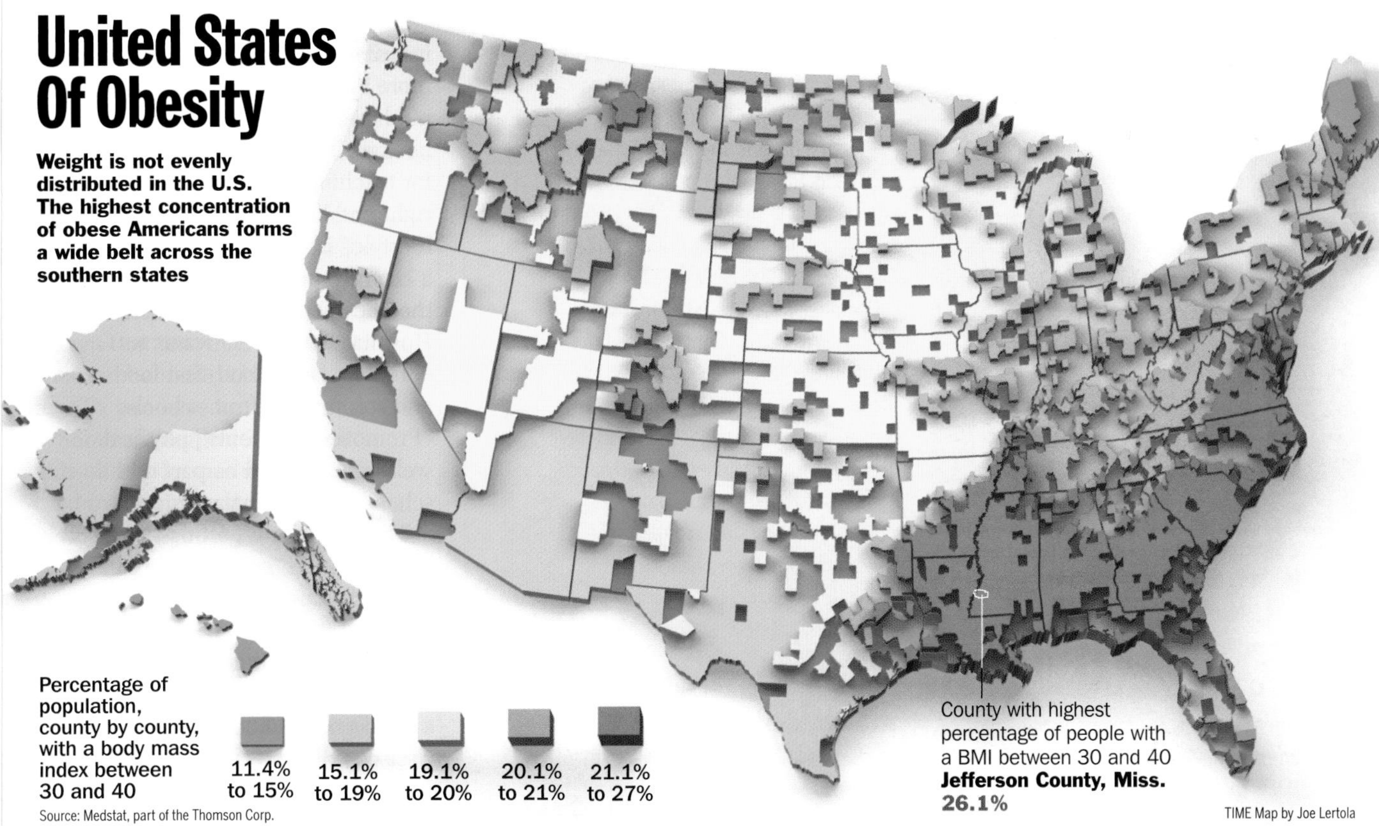

Source: Medstat, part of the Thomson Corp.

TIME Map by Joe Lertola

WHAT IS BMI?

$$\frac{\text{weight in pounds}}{(\text{height in inches})^2} \times 703$$

EXAMPLE:

$$\frac{\text{weight} = 160 \text{ lbs.}}{\text{height}^2 = (69 \text{ in.})^2} \times 703 = 23.6 \text{ BMI}$$

Body mass index is a more accurate measurement than weight because it takes into account that short people tend to weigh less than tall people. It's not perfect, however. The BMI of highly muscular athletes is often in the obese range.

BMI	STATUS
Below 18.5	Underweight
18.5-24.9	Normal
25.0-29.9	Overweight
30.0-39.9	Obese
40 and above	Morbidly obese

O

areas of the U.S., if you had a craving for cookies a century ago, you had to fire up the wood stove and make the dough from scratch. If you wanted a steak, you had to butcher the cow. Now you jump into the car and head for the nearest convenience store.

Evolving during a time of scarcity, humans developed an instinctive desire for basic tastes—sweet, fat, salt—that they could never fully satisfy. As a result, says Rutgers University anthropologist Lionel Tiger, "we don't have a cutoff mechanism for eating. Our bodies tell us, 'Fat is good to eat but hard to get.'" The second half of that equation is no longer true, but the first remains a powerful drive.

➤The Obesity Warriors Despite that truism, some people believe the war on obesity can be won. For a handful of researchers and clinicians, the fight to control obesity has become a crusade to change the way Americans live. The nation's landscape, they argue, is littered with junk food masquerading as health food; candy and candylike cereals featuring kids' favorite cartoon characters and toylike packaging; schools that shamelessly hawk soft drinks and snack foods; and multimillion-dollar advertising campaigns to promote such unwholesome products as beneficial.

HARD-WIRED TO GORGE

"We don't have a cutoff mechanism for eating. Our bodies tell us, 'Fat is good to eat but hard to get'"

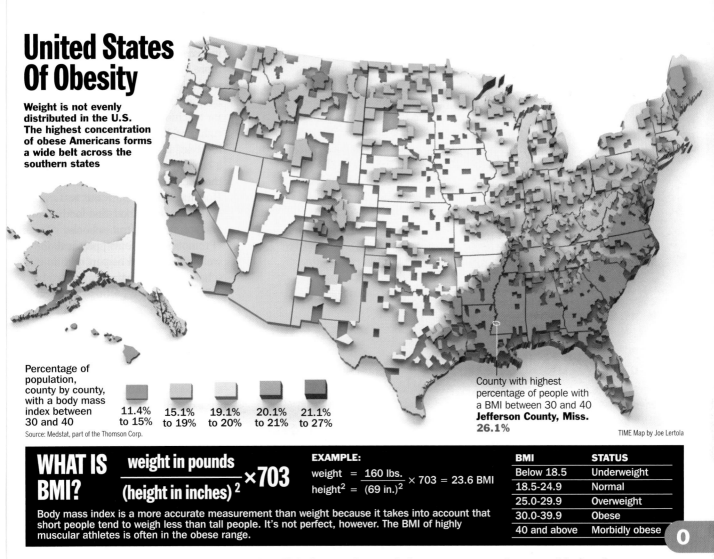

For decades, these scientists say, the country has seen obesity as a personal problem to be solved by each overweight individual waging a lonely war to trim pounds on the diet du jour. While it's true that we are each responsible for what we put in our own mouth, they note that the personal-responsibility approach has been a big, fat flop. In the past 30 years, the percentage of Americans who are overweight has ballooned, from 48% to 65%. The percentage of children who are overweight has tripled, from 5% to 15%, and another 15% are considered borderline.

While biology and personal habits play an undeniable role, there's abundant evidence that environmental factors loom large in the obesity rate. Here are some of the new ideas for cleaning up our fat-friendly society:

➤Start with the Schools Nothing

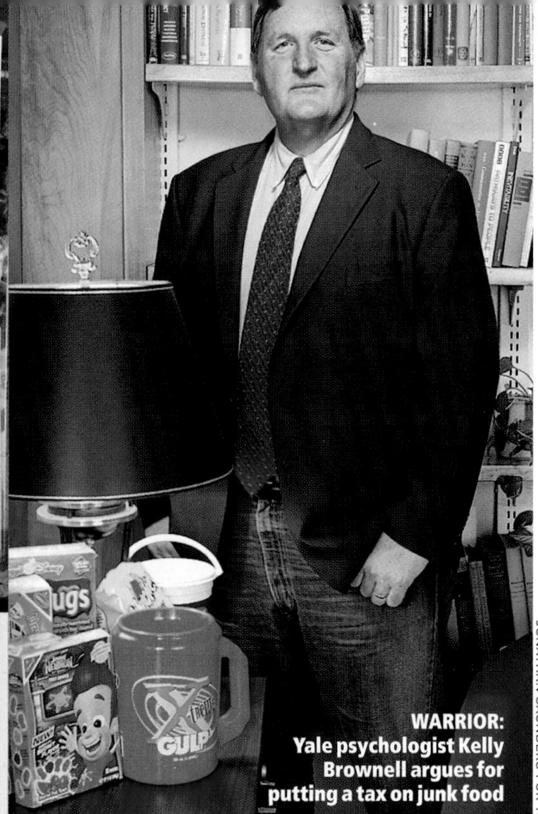
WARRIOR: Yale psychologist Kelly Brownell argues for putting a tax on junk food

JONATHAN SAUNDERS FOR TIME

of one of the few recreational facilities that every community has: schools. "We have many more schools than parks around the country," he says. The challenge is to find funding to keep them open after hours as community centers.

➤A Government Role? The most controversial idea of the nutrition activists calls for a greater role for the Federal Government. Ideally, they are looking for action on the order of the 1964 Surgeon General's report on tobacco, which kicked off a national effort to reduce smoking. Obesity, they point out, is on the verge of supplanting smoking as the nation's No. 1 preventable cause of disease and death. Many of their suggestions for federal intervention come directly from the antismoking playbook.

Idea No. 1 is to ban the broadcasting of junk-food commercials to young children, just as the Federal Government banned cigarette ads from television in 1971. "The average child sees more than 10,000 food commercials a year, and most are for high-calorie foods," says Ludwig.

Although there is popular support for a ban on food ads directed at children—56% of participants in a 2004 TIME/ABC NEWS poll said they favor this—it's difficult to imagine the land of free enterprise following the lead of Norway and Sweden, which have banned advertising aimed at children. The next best thing, says Nestle, would be a federally mandated campaign of public-service ads to promote healthy eating and help balance the effects of junk-food ads.

NO CAPTAIN CRUNCH?

In a 2004 TIME poll, 56% of participants said they favored banning food ads on TV directed at children

Idea No. 2: if you want people to eat less junk food, tax it. Nationally, says Yale psychologist and nutrition advocate Kelly Brownell, "we could raise $1.5 billion from a penny-a-can tax on soft drinks. With $1.5 billion, we could create a 'nutrition Superfund' to clean up the toxic environment. You could get Beyoncé Knowles away from Pepsi and Shaquille O'Neal away from Burger King and have them promote healthy eating instead."

A tax on junk foods? A ban on advertising to tots? A national nutrition campaign advising us all to eat less? Could any of this happen? In the days when the Marlboro Man was riding high on the airwaves, Brownell points out, no one thought you could ban cigarette ads. "I don't know at what point the country will be so desperate," says Nestle, but she thinks that point is coming ever closer. "If you're a family that has kids with Type 2 diabetes, your life is not going to be pretty," she says. "Nobody has a clue how much this overweight business is going to cost us."

➤The Good News Happily, there are glimmers of hope in the war on weight. For the first three quarters of 2003, there was no increase in obesity among adult Americans, according to data from a National Health Interview Survey.

There's no reason to think an anti-obesity campaign uniting the efforts of U.S. schools, communities and federal and local governments can't succeed—as long as everyone involved acknowledges that the problem is real and that solving it will be a long, difficult haul. After all, it's not easy to fight millions of years of evolution.

■ Resources

NIH WEBSITE: *www.nlm.nih.gov/medlineplus/obesity*

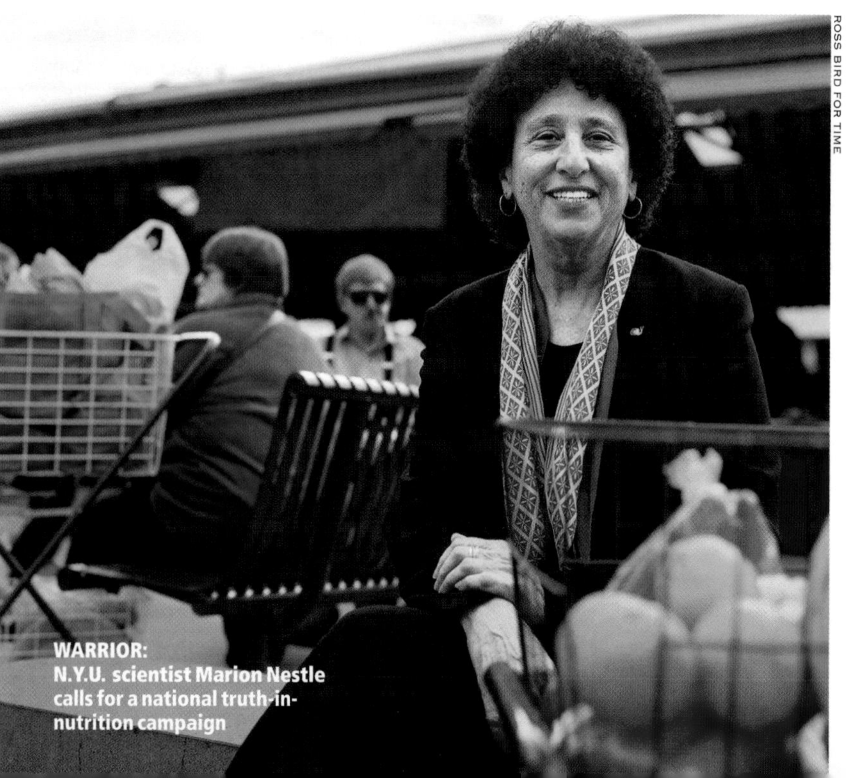
WARRIOR: N.Y.U. scientist Marion Nestle calls for a national truth-in-nutrition campaign

ROSS BIRD FOR TIME

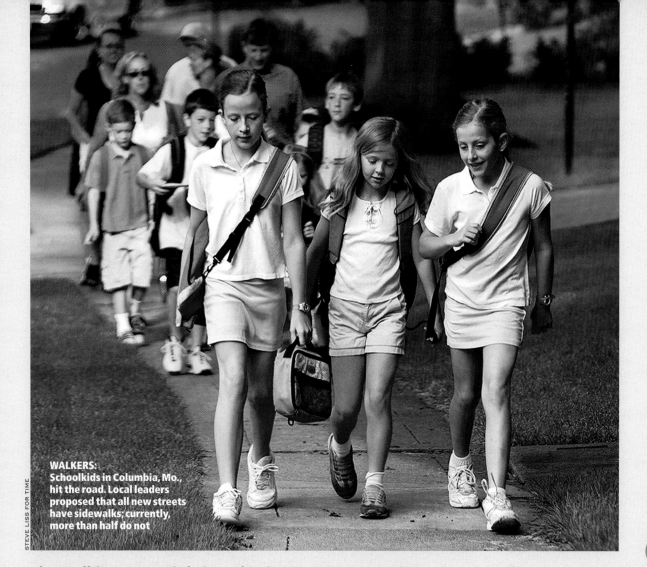

WALKERS: Schoolkids in Columbia, Mo., hit the road. Local leaders proposed that all new streets have sidewalks; currently, more than half do not

STEVE LISS FOR TIME

O

The Walking Cure: Fighting Obesity, One Step at a Time

In Columbia, Mo., a lot of people are trying—really trying—to get their neighbors biking and walking. In case you haven't heard, exercise has many advantages. For anyone trying to keep off weight, the simple activity of putting one foot in front of another is surprisingly useful. So in mid-May 2004, Mayor Darwin Hindman, who at 71 still bikes to work, kicked off Bike, Walk and Wheel Week to coax residents to commute and shop without cars, leading dozens of cyclists on a 4-mile ride. A week later, volunteers were serving breakfast around town for anyone walking, cycling or rolling in a wheelchair.

There's just one problem. If you want to travel by foot or even by bike in Columbia, it's not that easy to get where you need to go. Most of the homes aren't located anywhere near stores. And just walking around the neighborhood can be a challenge, since more than half the streets lack sidewalks. "Everyone is created to walk. But we have designed our streets to create barriers to an obvious, efficient activity," says Mayor Hindman.

Columbia is not alone. Throughout most of the U.S., suburban sprawl has created a nation that has been supersized beyond walking distance. Homes tend to be far removed from shopping; compact, walkable downtowns are rare; traffic is dangerous to pedestrians; and even sidewalks aren't to be taken for granted. Research has found that most Americans will not walk anyplace that's more than a quarter-mile away. In a recent poll, 44% of people questioned said it was difficult to walk to any destination from their home—any destination at all.

In recent years researchers have begun to find a connection between sprawling suburbs and spreading waistlines. Put very simply: people who live in communities where it's hard to get anywhere on foot are heavier than those who live in less car-dependent settings, whether densely settled cities like Boston and Chicago or just pedestrian-friendly towns. While diet remains an important factor in the obesity epidemic, it's becoming increasingly clear that Americans are shaped in part by how America is shaped.

A new study of 11,000 residents of Atlanta conducted by Lawrence Frank, a professor at the University of British Columbia in Vancouver, showed that for every hour people spend in their cars, they are 6% more likely to be obese. For every kilometer—just over a half-mile—they walk in a day, they are 5% less likely to be obese. And if they live in a mixed-use environment (one in which there are shops and services near their homes), they are 7% less likely to be obese—probably because they walk more. Until we change how America is built, it seems, how Americans are built will be a continuing problem. ■

BODY DOUBLE

The Future of Organ Transplants

TIME asked experts in the field to forecast the next advances in organ transplantation. Here's where we are today—and where we may be by the year 2025

HAIR

TODAY: Transplants, hair plugs and scalp grafts

TOMORROW: More permanent approaches, perhaps by stimulating shrunken follicles with growth proteins

EYES

TODAY: Laser surgery or implants to correct near- and farsightedness

TOMORROW: Permanent lens implants to correct vision while leaving the cornea intact

EARS

TODAY: Cochlear implants to replace damaged inner ear

TOMORROW: Implants that can be adjusted to pick up a wider range of frequencies at longer distances

BREAST

TODAY: Breasts are reconstructed with saline sacs or with living tissue, using fat and muscle from the back, buttocks or abdomen

TOMORROW: Breasts may be grown in the lab from a patient's own fat cells and infused back through keyhole slits in the chest

HEART

TODAY: Bypasses, angioplasty and transplants to keep blood flowing to the heart muscle. Doctors are beginning to use gene therapy to grow new blood vessels

TOMORROW: Growing functional patches of heart muscle or coaxing existing heart-muscle cells to repair themselves

ORGANS

TODAY: Small slivers of liver tissue can be grown in the lab from one of the many types of liver cells, but they are not yet ready for transplant

TOMORROW: Heart, liver, kidneys grown from stem cells in vitro and transplanted

TODAY: Grown in the lab from pig cells and synthetic-polymer matrix

TOMORROW: Regenerated from stem or precursor cells in the body

LIMBS

TODAY: Prosthetics wired to peripheral nervous system

TOMORROW: Prosthetics wired directly to motor portions of the brain to improve control and simulate the sensations of touch, pain, etc.

PENIS

TODAY: Penile implants and medication to maintain erection. Surgery to reattach a severed penis; skin grafts to recover urinary, but not sexual, function if penis is not recovered

TOMORROW: Genetically engineered tissue grown in the lab and attached for final growth to form fully functional penis

BONE AND CARTILAGE

TODAY: Injection of bone growth factors into jaw and other fracture areas. Researchers can also grow cartilage in the lab in thin sheets, but it's too weak to be functional in the body

TOMORROW: Coaxing the body to grow bone and cartilage on biodegradable scaffolds infused with a mix of stem cells and growth factors

SKIN

TODAY: Sheets grown in the lab from human and synthetic-polymer matrix

TOMORROW: Grown by the body from stem or precursor cells and growth factors

BLOOD VESSELS

TODAY: Grown in the lab from pig cells and synthetic-polymer matrix

TOMORROW: Grown in the lab from stem or precursor cells to avoid rejection by the immune system

Figure painted by Garrett Garitano

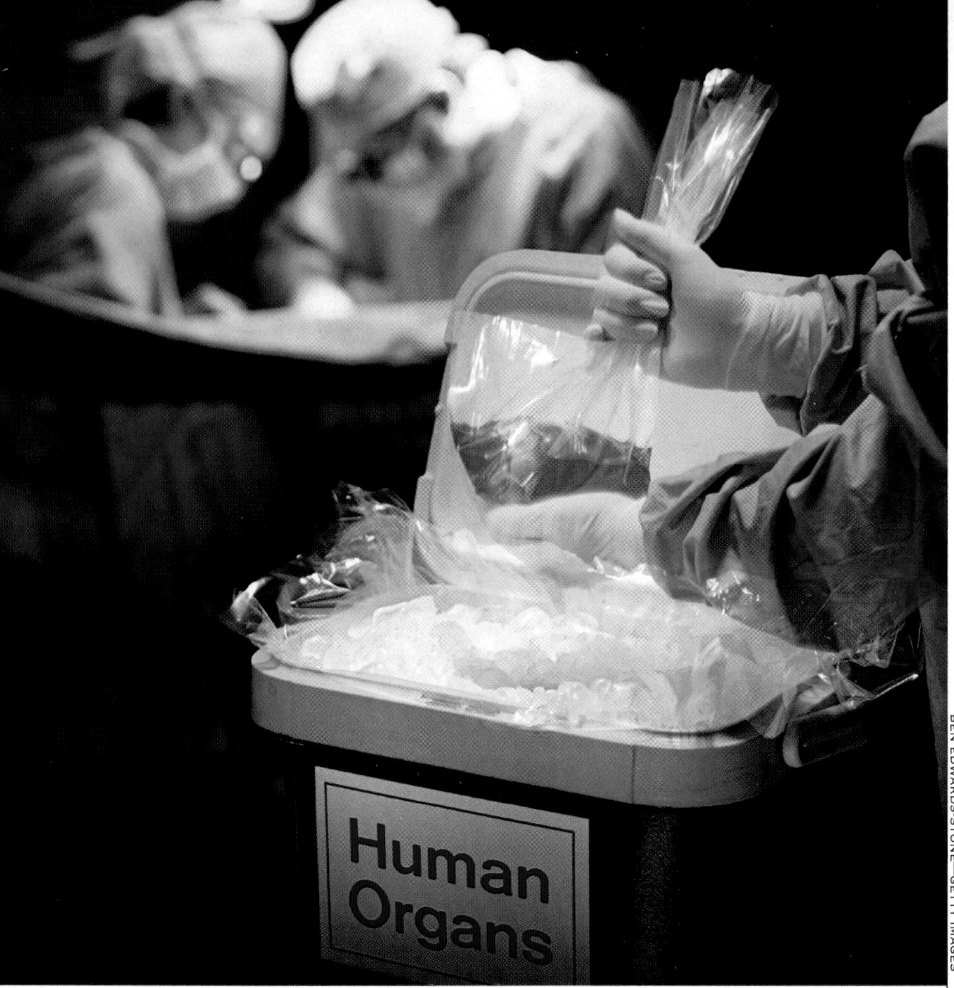

BEN EDWARDS-STONE—GETTY IMAGES

Osteoporosis

One of the great fears of old age is the gradual loss of bone mass we call osteoporosis, which can lead to fractures. And if you think it's only a woman's problem—think again

On the Horizon A natural amino acid that has been implicated in heart disease, homocysteine, is under scrutiny for its possible relationship to osteoporosis. The substance may help us not only diagnose the disease earlier but also treat it in new ways

About 10 million Americans have osteoporosis—a gradual reduction in the density of the bones—and 1.5 million of them will suffer a fracture this year, many of them older folks whose bodies are least able to bounce back from serious injury. That's why doctors were so interested in a pair of new studies on the relationship between osteoporosis and a common amino acid called homocysteine. Not only do the reports suggest an easy way to determine early on which people are most vulnerable to osteoporosis, but they also hint at a totally new way to treat the ailment.

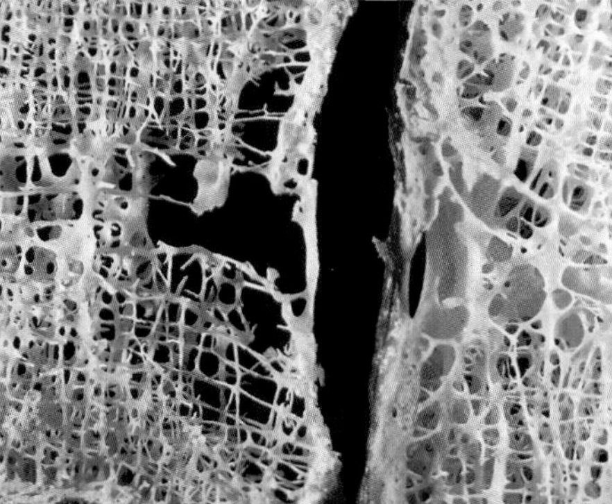
DR. MICHAEL KLEIN—PETER ARNOLD

The normal bone at right is slightly porous, while the osteoporosis-afflicted bone at left is seriously frayed

One study found that men with the highest homocysteine levels were four times as likely to develop hip fractures as men with the lowest levels. The second study found that men and women with the highest levels of homocysteine had twice the risk of suffering a fracture compared with those with the lowest levels.

Organ Replacement

The transplantation of the human lung remains a risky operation, but two experimental approaches promise to help increase the survival rate of lung recipients

Glad Tidings In 2003 the number of people who chose to donate organs after death climbed more than 4%, helping lead to a more than 10% decline in the number of people who died while awaiting organ transplants

In welcome news for lung-transplant recipients, two new approaches to thwarting organ rejection showed great promise in tests. The first involves inhaling a new immunosuppressant drug directly into the lungs (rather than taking the medication in pill form); the second uses standard organ-rejection drugs in far lower doses than were used previously.

SCREENING DONORS

Three people died after receiving rabies-infected organs from a man whose disease was not diagnosed

Transplanted lungs are very susceptible to both rejection and to the infections that often attack a patient taking high doses of drugs that suppress that immune system. As a result, fewer than half of all lung-transplant recipients survive five years, compared with three-quarters of heart, liver and kidney recipients. Both of the new approaches increased survival rates among lung recipients.

A sobering reminder of the need to screen organ donors came in July 2004, when the CDC declared that an Arkansas man who had died of a brain hemorrhage in May had donated his lungs, kidneys and liver—before it was learned he had rabies. The three recipients of his organs all died within weeks.

■ **Resources**

NIH SITE: *www.nlm.nih.gov/medlineplus/organtransplantation*

It turns out that we already know quite a bit about homocysteine. Since an elevated level of the amino acid has been linked to a greater risk of heart disease, many Americans are already getting their homocysteine levels regularly tested. Doctors also know how to treat high homocysteine levels using supplements of folic acid and other B vitamins.

NOT FOR WOMEN ONLY

One in eight men will experience a fracture linked to osteoporosis some time in his life

But don't start popping vitamins just yet. It's still not clear whether homocysteine actually causes bone loss (although there are hints that it may prevent key building blocks of bone from bonding together). So doctors don't know for sure whether lowering your homocysteine level can actually reduce your chances of getting a hip fracture. They also don't yet know how much folic acid and vitamin B are needed to keep bones healthy.

Meanwhile, you have other options for keeping your bones strong. Exercising with weights and making sure you have enough calcium and vitamin D in your diet are good ways to start. Estrogen used to be prescribed to postmenopausal women in part to prevent osteoporosis, but it is no longer recommended because it entails serious risk of breast cancer and other diseases.

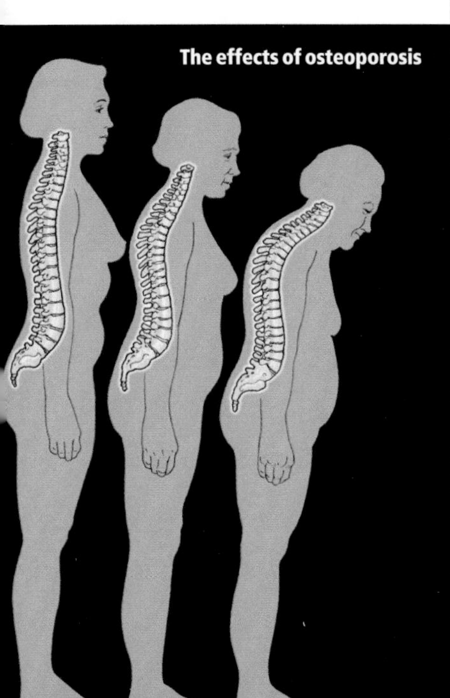

The effects of osteoporosis

DAVID GIFFORD—PHOTO RESEARCHERS

➤A Man's Problem One of the risk groups that is least aware of the dangers of osteoporosis is the half of the population that thinks it is strictly a woman's disease. But what men don't know about osteoporosis definitely can hurt them. This crippling disease is a lot more common in males than they—and their physicians—may realize.

The National Osteoporosis Foundation says 1 in 8 men will experience an osteoporosis-related fracture sometime in their lives. In fact, men older than 50 are at greater risk for such a fracture than they are for prostate cancer.

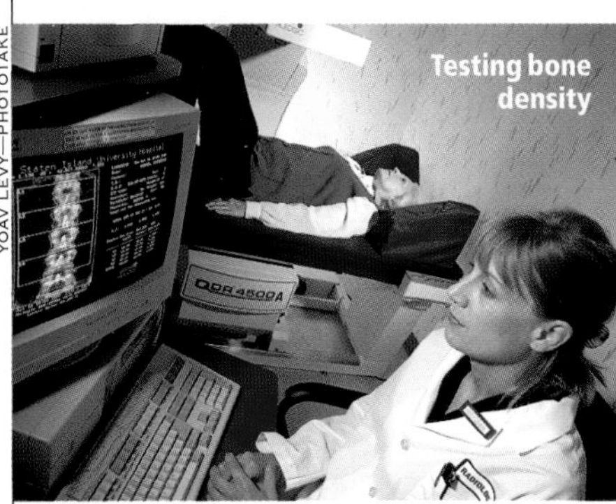

Testing bone density

YOAV LEVY—PHOTOTAKE

➤Testing The most accurate method of diagnosing an osteoporosis problem is with a bone-density test. And while it isn't practical—or even necessary—to screen every man 50 or older, those at highest risk should be tested. Among the signs to watch for: a fracture suffered as an adult, unexplained back pain and the loss of 2 in. or more in height. Also at risk are men with a family history of osteoporosis or a personal history of alcoholism, kidney stones or treatment with cortisone or prednisone for such chronic conditions as asthma and rheumatoid arthritis.

■ Resources

NATIONAL OSTEOPOROSIS FOUNDATION: *www.nof.org; (202) 223-2226*

NIH SITE: *www.osteo.org*

Ovarian Cancer

Cancer of the ovaries takes root stealthily and often isn't detected until it's too far along to treat, but early detection may be on the way

By the Numbers Ovarian cancer strikes more than 26,000 women each year in the U.S., some 16,000 of whom will die

Conventional wisdom holds that ovarian cancer shows no symptoms in its early stages, but that notion is starting to crumble. A new study finds that three symptoms—abdominal swelling, an urgent need to urinate and feelings of bloatedness—occur together in one-half to two-thirds of all women who have ovarian tumors but in fewer than 1 woman in 10 who is free of the disease.

When such symptoms arise, especially if they are severe and frequent, women should get tested for ovarian cancer. And don't assume the worst: tests show that these symptoms are associated with benign tumors about as often as they indicate malignancies. The cancer is almost always curable when caught early, but in two of three cases it goes undiagnosed until it has reached an advanced stage that defies treatment.

■ Resources

NIH ALTERNATIVE MEDICINE WEBSITE: *www.nccam.nih.gov*

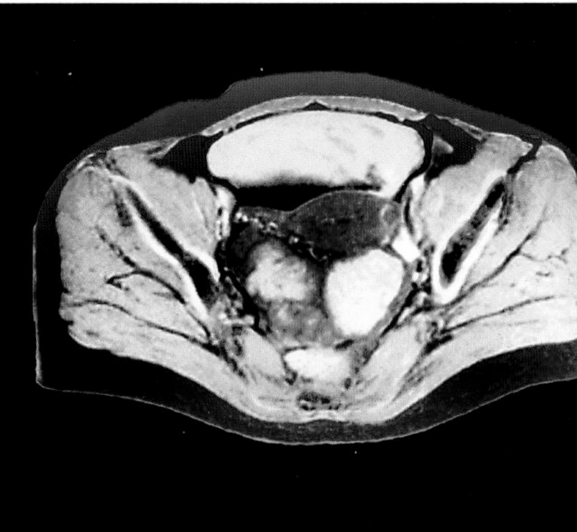

ZEPHYR—PHOTO RESEARCHERS

Ovaries infected by cancer are indicated in blue

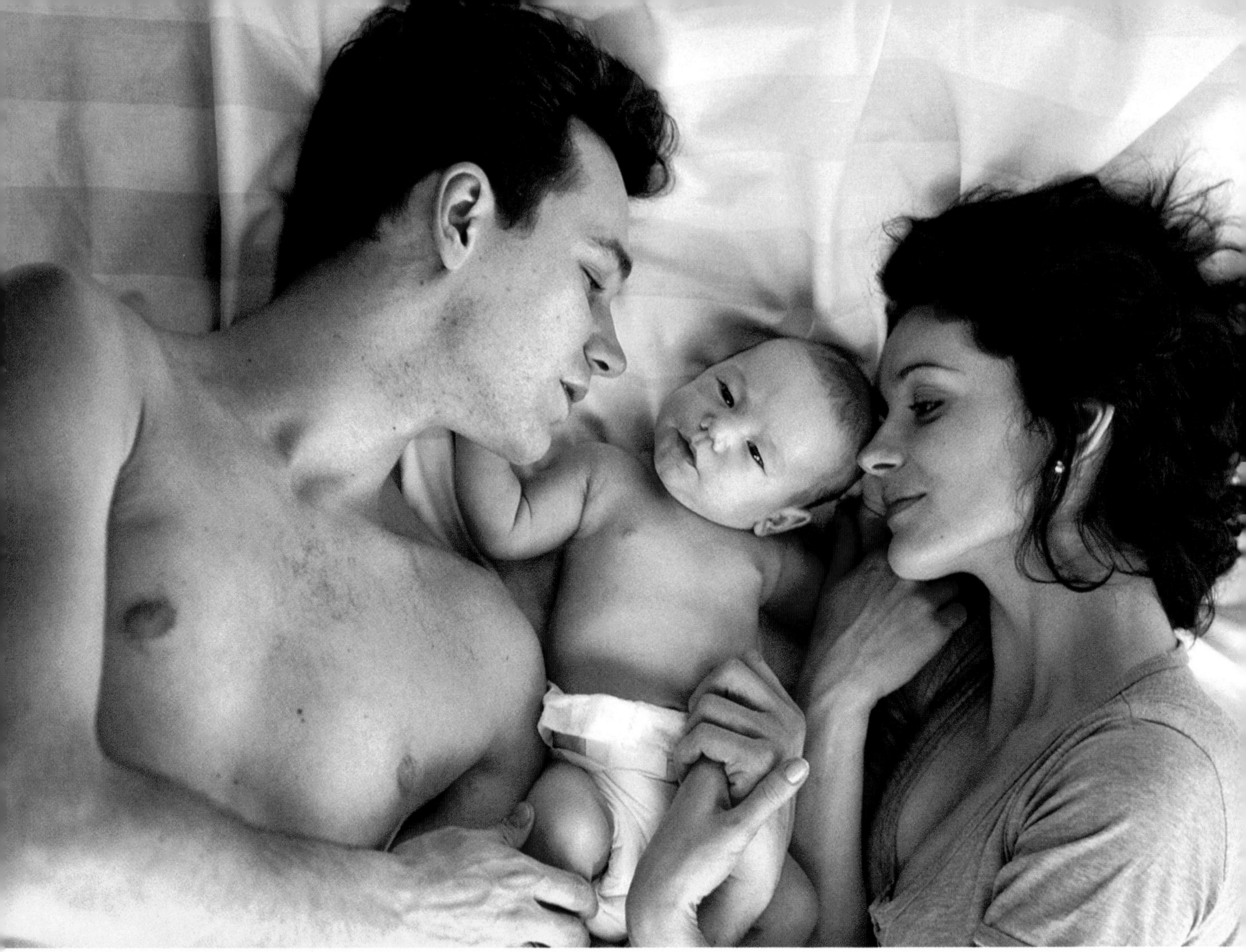

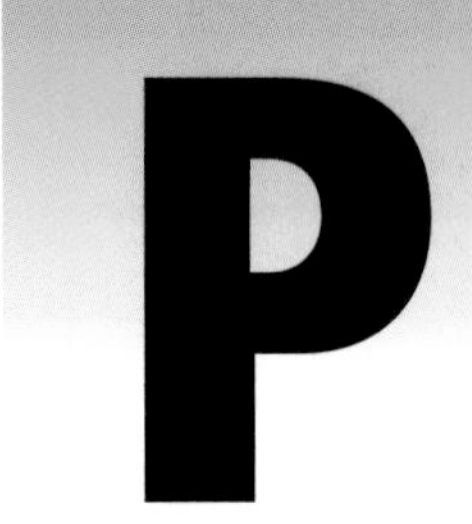

Parenting

Sorry, Mom, you can't have it all. Why more women are dropping out of the workplace to stay at home

By the Numbers Some 72% of mothers with children under 18 are in the work force, compared with 45% who were working in 1975. But the numbers aren't rising

It's 6:35 in the morning, and Cheryl Nevins, 34, dressed for work in a silky black maternity blouse and skirt, is busily tending to Ryan, 2½, and Brendan, 11 months, at their home in the leafy Edgebrook neighborhood of Chicago. Both boys are sobbing because Reilly, the beefy family dog, knocked Ryan over. In a blur of calm, purposeful activity, Nevins, who is eight months pregnant, shoves the dog out into the backyard, changes Ryan's diaper on the family-room rug, heats farina in the microwave and feeds Brendan cereal and sliced bananas while crooning *Open, Shut Them* to encourage the baby to chew.

Cheryl's husband Joe, 35, who is normally out the door by 5:30 a.m. for his job as a finance manager for Kraft Foods, makes a rare appearance in the morning muddle. "I do want to go outside with you," he tells Ryan, who is clinging to his leg, "but Daddy has to work every day except Saturdays and Sundays. That stinks."

At 7:40, Vera Orozco, the nanny, arrives to begin her 10½-hour shift at the Nevinses'. Cheryl, a labor lawyer for the Chicago board of education, hands over the baby and checks her e-mail from the kitchen table. "I almost feel apprehensive if I leave for work without logging on," she confesses. In between messages, she helps Ryan pull blue Play-Doh from a container, then briefs Orozco on the morning's events: "They woke up early. Ryan had his poop this morning; this guy has not." Throughout the day, Orozco will note every meal and activity on a tattered legal pad on the kitchen counter so Nevins can stay up to speed.

MORE WORKING MOMS

Women with kids under 18 now make up 72% of the work force, up from 47% of moms with kids in 1975

Suddenly it's 8:07, and the calm mom shifts from cruise control into hyperdrive. She must be out the door by 8:10 to make the 8:19 train. Once on the platform, she punches numbers into her cell phone, checks her voice mail and then leaves a message for a co-worker. On the train, she makes more calls and proofreads documents. "Right now, work is crazy," says Nevins, who has been responsible for negotiating and administering seven agreements between the board and labor unions.

Nevins is "truly passionate" about her job, but after seven years, she's about to leave it. When the baby arrives, she will take off at least a year, maybe two, maybe five. "It's hard. I'm giving up a great job that pays well, and I have a lot of respect and authority," the attorney says. The decision to stay home was a tough one, but most of her working-mom friends have made the same choice. She concludes, "I know it's the right thing."

"I'M AT THE OFFICE"

Dual-career couples with kids under 18 now spend a combined 91 hours a week at work, up from 81 in 1977

➤**Juggling—and Struggling** Ten or 15 years ago, playing the double role of Mom and career woman all seemed so doable. Bring home the bacon, fry it up in a pan, split the second shift with some sensitive New Age man. Yet slowly the snappy, upbeat work-life rhythm has changed for women in high-powered jobs. E-mail, pagers and cell phones promised to allow execs to work from home. Who knew that would mean that home was no longer a sanctuary? Today BlackBerrys sprout on the sidelines of Little League games. Cell phones vibrate at the school play. And it's back to the e-mail after *Goodnight Moon.* "We are now the workaholism capital of the world, surpassing the Japanese," laments sociologist Arlie Hochschild, author of *The Time Bind: When Work Becomes Home and Home Becomes Work.*

The U.S. workweek still averages around 34 hours, thanks in part to a sluggish manufacturing sector. But for those in financial services, it's 55 hours; for top executives in big corporations, it's 60 to 70. For dual-career couples with kids under 18, the combined work hours have grown from 81 a week in 1977 to 91 in 2002.

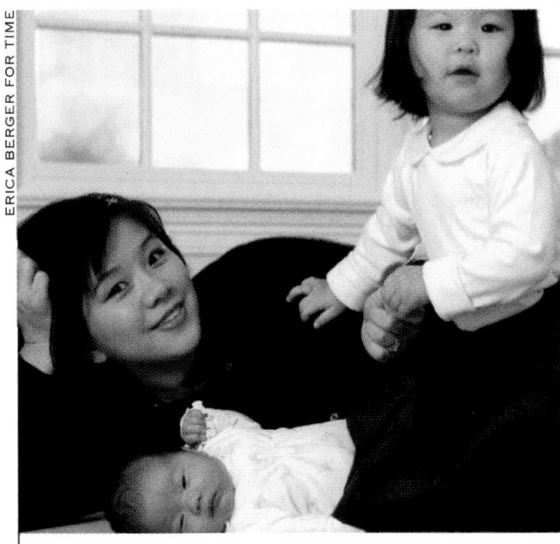

ERICA BERGER FOR TIME

Dropping Out: Jisoo Im

Five months pregnant, exhausted from 12-hour workdays and worried that the stress would affect her first baby, Im, 34, quit her job as an advertising vice president. Her husband Yongin's income as a corporate lawyer allows her to stay at home in Chappaqua, N.Y. with Ines, 18 months, and Isabel, 5 weeks (as of March 2004). Im told TIME that she misses working but not the stress at work. She may start her own business when she feels like returning to work, in order to create a job that will offer her maximum flexibility. ■

Meanwhile, the pace has quickened on the home front, where a parent's job has expanded to include managing a packed schedule of child-enhancement activities. Yet for most mothers—and fathers, for that matter—there is little choice except to persevere on both fronts to pay the bills. Indeed, 72% of mothers with children under 18 are in the work force—a figure that is up sharply from 47% in 1975 but has held steady since 1997. And thanks in part to a dodgy economy, there's growth in another category: working women whose husbands are unemployed, which has risen to 6.4% of all married couples.

But in the professional and

Dropping Out: Cheryl Nevins

Although she continued working as a lawyer for the Chicago board of education when her sons Ryan, 2½, and Brendan, 11 months, were born, Nevins, 34 (who was eight months pregnant in the picture at right, taken in March 2004) and her husband Joe decided that she would leave work and be a fulltime mom when their third child arrived. Nevins told TIME "I have a great job that pays well." But she also is eager to be home with her children. "I have such limited time with my kids now," she says. ■

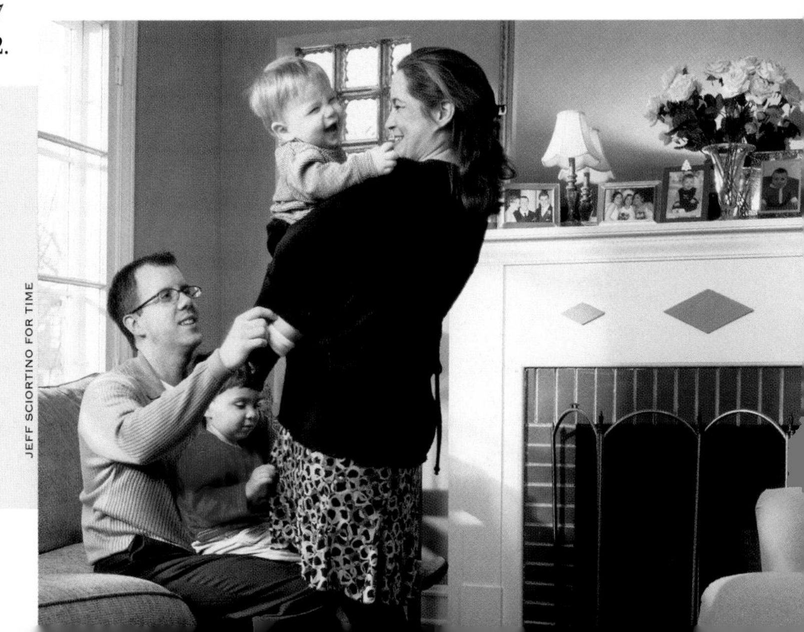

JEFF SCIORTINO FOR TIME

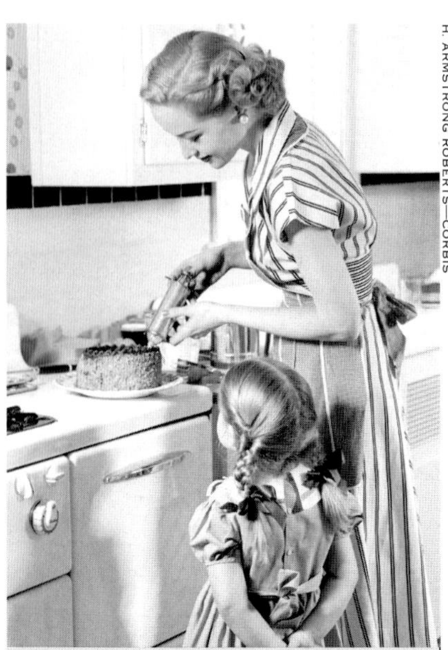

H. ARMSTRONG ROBERTS—CORBIS

Follow the Money

Why are today's mothers working so hard, putting in long hours at home and at the office? For the money. Oh, sure, those ladies who took their grandmother's advice and married a doctor, a lawyer or an Enron executive may show up for work to "fulfill themselves." But for most women who came of age in the '90s, it comes down to dollars and cents, and the calculation is brutal.

Anyone who hasn't been hiding under a rock in Montana knows that it costs more to purchase a house than it used to. Since the mid-'70s, the amount of the average family budget earmarked for the mortgage has increased a whopping 69% (adjusted for inflation). At the same time, the average father's income increased less than 1%. How to make up the difference? With Mom's paycheck, of course.

Then there is preschool. No longer an optional enterprise, preschool is widely viewed as a prerequisite for elementary school. A full-time preschool program can cost more than $5,000 a year. Add the cost of health insurance (for those lucky enough to have it) and the eventual price of sending a kid to college, and most middle-class moms find they have no choice but to get a job if they want to make ends meet. ■

—By Amelia Warren Tyagi, co-author of *The Two-Income Trap: Why Middle-Class Mothers & Fathers are Going Broke*

managerial classes, where higher incomes permit more choices, a reluctant revolt is under way. Today's women execs are less willing to play the juggling game, especially in its current high-speed mode, and are more willing to sacrifice paychecks and prestige for more time with their family.

MORTGAGES AND MOM

Since the mid-1970s, the amount of family income earmarked for the mortgage has increased 69%

➤Stopping Out or Dropping Out?

Like Cheryl Nevins, most of these women are choosing not so much to drop out as to stop out, often with every intention of returning. Their mantra: You can have it all, just not all at the same time. Their behavior, contrary to some popular reports, is not a June Cleaver–ish embrace of old-fashioned motherhood but a new, nonlinear approach to building a career and an insistence on restoring sanity to their lives.

"What this group is staying home from is the 80-hour-a-week job," says Hochschild. "They watched their mothers and fathers be ground up by very long hours, and they would like to give their own children more than they got. They want a work-family balance."

Because these women represent a small and privileged sector, the dimensions of the exodus are hard to measure. What some experts are zeroing in on is the first-ever drop-off in workplace participation by married mothers with a child less than 1 year old. That figure fell from 59% in 1997 to 53% in 2000. Significantly, the drop was mostly among women who were white, over 30 and well educated.

Census data reveal an uptick in stay-at-home moms who hold graduate or professional degrees—the very women who seemed destined to blast through the glass ceiling. Now 22% of them are home with their kids. A study by research firm Catalyst found that 1 in 3 women with an M.B.A. was not working full-time (it's 1 in 20 for their male peers). Economist and author Sylvia Ann Hewlett, who teaches at Columbia University, says she sees a brain drain throughout the top 10% of the female labor force (those earning more than $55,000). "What we have discovered in looking at this group over the past five years," she says, "is that many women who have any kind of choice are opting out." Other experts say the drop-out rate isn't climbing but is merely more visible now that so many women are in high positions. In 1971 just 9% of medical degrees,

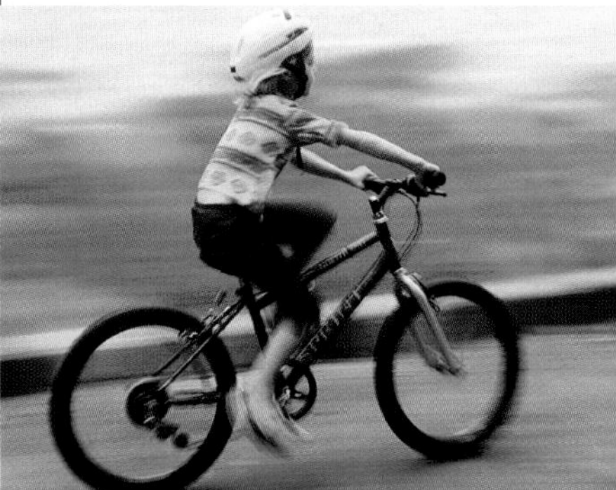

LWA—JDC—CORBIS

Parents, Use Your Heads

The protective helmet for mobile sports may the most cost-effective safety device ever made, and yet only 41% of kids ages 5 to 14 wear one while riding on bikes, scooters or skates, according to a study by the National Safe Kids Campaign. And even among those kids who don the headgear, 35% wear it improperly—a tragic lapse, considering that head injuries account for 80% of bike-related fatalities.

Why the concern? In 2001, according to the Safe Kids website, 134 children ages 14 and under died in bicycle-related crashes. In 2002, nearly 288,900 children were treated in hospital emergency rooms for bicycle-related injuries.

Meanwhile, a 2004 study reported that wrist fractures among kids and teens have risen dramatically during the past three decades. The highest fracture rates—a 60% jump from 1974—were found in girls ages 8 to 11 and boys ages 11 to 14. ■

7% of law degrees and 4% of M.B.A.s were awarded to women; 30 years later, the respective figures were 43%, 47% and 41%.

Generation Gap? For an older group of female professionals who came of age listening to Helen Reddy roar, the exodus of younger women can seem disturbingly regressive. Fay Clayton, 58, a partner in a small Chicago law firm, watched in dismay as her 15-person firm lost three younger women who left after having kids, though one has since returned part time. "I fear there is a generational split and possibly a step backward for younger women," she says.

Others take a more optimistic view. "Younger women have greater expectations about the work-life balance," says Joanne Brundage, 51, founder and executive director of Mothers & More, a mothers' support organization with 7,500 members and 180 chapters in the U.S. While boomer moms have been reluctant to talk about their children at work for fear that "people won't think you're a professional," she observes, younger women "feel more entitled to ask for changes and advocate for themselves." That sense of confidence is reflected in the evolution of her organization's name. When she founded it in Elmhurst, Ill., 17 years ago, Brundage called it FEMALE, for Formerly Employed Mothers at Loose Ends.

FLEEING THE FAST LANE

"We are talking about how to create off-ramps and on-ramps, slow lanes and acceleration ramps"

Maternal Desire Despite misgivings, most women who step out of their careers find expected delights on the home front, not to mention the enormous relief of no longer worrying about shortchanging their kids. Psychologist Daphne de Marneffe speaks to these private joys in her book, *Maternal Desire* (Little Brown). De Marneffe argues that feminists and American society at large have ignored the basic urge felt by most mothers to spend meaningful time with their children. She decries the rushed fragments of quality time doled out by working moms trying to do it all. She writes, "Anyone who has tried to 'fit everything in' can attest to how excruciating the five-minute wait at the supermarket checkout line becomes, let alone a child's slow-motion attempt to tie her own shoes when you're running late getting her to school." The book, which puts an idyllic gloss on staying home, could launch a thousand resignations. De Marneffe largely omits, however, the sense of pride and meaning that women often gain from their work.

Building On-Ramps Hunter College sociologist Pamela Stone has spent the past few years interviewing 50 stay-at-home mothers in seven U.S. cities for a book on professional women who have dropped out. "Many of the women I talked to have tried to work part time or put forth job-sharing plans, and they're shot down," she says. "Despite all the family-friendly rhetoric, the workplace for professionals is extremely inflexible."

In April 2004, Columbia's Hewlett convened a task force of leaders from 14 companies and four law firms to discuss what she calls the hidden brain drain of women and minority professionals. "We are talking about how to create off-ramps and on-ramps, slow lanes and acceleration ramps" so that workers can more easily leave, slow down or re-enter the work force, she explains. One reason businesses are getting serious about the brain drain is demographics. With boomers nearing retirement, a shortfall of perhaps 10 million workers appears likely by 2010.

Will these programs work? Will part-time jobs really be part time, as opposed to full-time jobs paid on a partial basis? Will serious professionals who shift into a slow lane be able to pick up velocity when their kids are grown? More important, will corporate culture evolve to a point where employees feel genuinely encouraged to use these options? Anyone who remembers all the talk about flextime in the 1980s will be tempted to dismiss the latest ideas for making the workplace family-friendly. This time, perhaps, the numbers may be on the side of working moms—along with many working dads who are looking for options as well.

Spanking: Just Say No

A 2000 survey found that 61% of parents of young children condoned spanking as a regular form of punishment for young children, and 37% thought spanking was O.K. for children under 2 years of age. Yet parents who spank their under-2 kids can expect them to get into trouble at school, a 2004 study in the medical journal *Pediatrics* concluded. Compared with kids who were never hit, white non-Hispanic toddlers who were spanked five times a week were four times as likely to have behavioral problems later. No significant link was found between spanking and later misbehavior in black and Hispanic children. ■

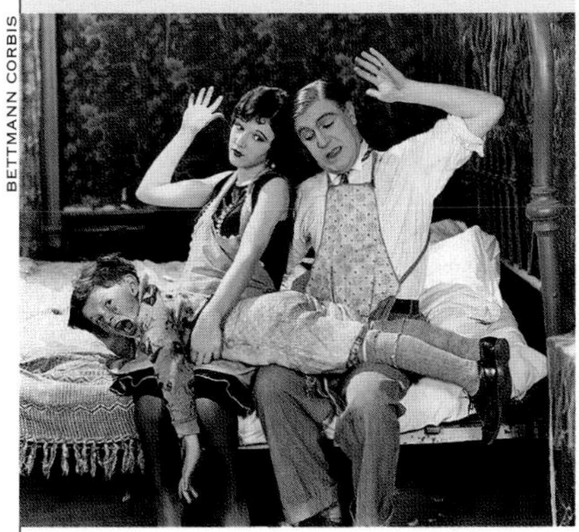

BETTMANN CORBIS

■ **Resources**

NATIONAL SAFE KIDS CAMPAIGN SITE: *www.safekids.org*

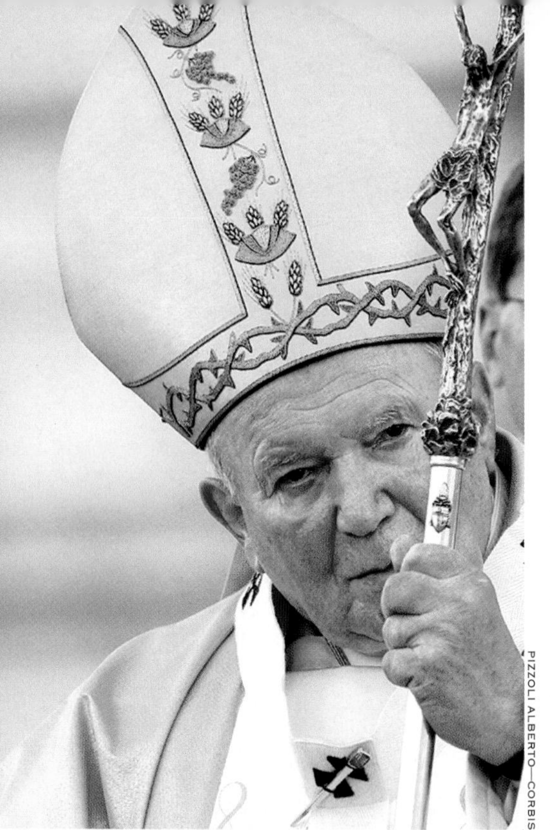

PIZZOLI ALBERTO—CORBIS

Parkinson's Disease

There is no cure for this neurological ailment that often afflicts the elderly, but new strategies are helping us understand its causes

Special Delivery Scientists applied genetic engineering to make new viruses that may be able to place therapeutic genes into the brains of Parkinson's patients

As the once famously robust Pope John Paul II wages a gallant struggle against Parkinson's disease, the world is reminded of how debilitating this ailment can be. Once acquired, the disease can be slowed but not cured, which makes preventing it the most promising approach to treatment. Currently, some 1.5 million Americans suffer from its quaking, shaking symptoms.

One new study suggested that nonsteroidal anti-inflammatory drugs (NSAIDS), such as ibuprofen, do offer some protection against Parkinson's disease when used regularly. The study found that the risk of developing Parkinson's was 45% lower among men and women who regularly used NSAIDs than among nonusers.

PREVENTION AID?

A study found that a regular regimen of a drug like ibuprofen may help reduce one's risk for Parkinson's

Two separate studies also suggest the possibility of fine-tuning the use of levodopa, the standard drug treatment for the symptoms of Parkinson's. Levodopa, however, can also cause dyskinesia (involuntary and uncontrollable jerking movements in the limbs and face) in people who take it. One two-year study found that ropinirole (Requip) may be a beneficial alternative to levodopa: patients who took it experienced one-third slower loss of nerve function than those on levodopa, and reported a better than 90% reduction in jerking movements. But these benefits may come at a price: the research also showed that patients taking levodopa had better overall movement ability than the group using ropinirole.

A second study found that the schizophrenia drug clozapine (Clozaril) taken in combination with levodopa may significantly reduce the duration and intensity of dyskinesia episodes. Several of the test subjects, however, had to stop taking clozapine when they developed a dangerous rise in their white blood cell counts.

Meanwhile, a separate team of researchers announced in June 2004 that they had genetically engineered three new viruses that may be able to deliver therapeutic genes into the brains of Parkinson's patients. Eventually, the doctors hope to be able to switch the genes on and off at appropriate times, allowing them to regulate precisely the production of brain chemicals that control the nerve functions related to Parkinson's.

Resources

PARKINSON'S DISEASE FOUNDATION SITE: *www.pdf.org*

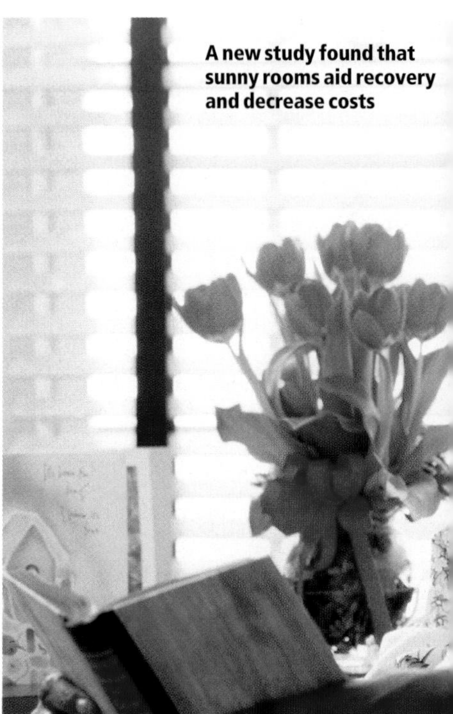

A new study found that sunny rooms aid recovery and decrease costs

Patient Care

Who said a hospital stay had to resemble a prison stay? (Well, aside from the cook). Professionals are taking a new look at how our surroundings influence our recovery

On the Sunny Side Even simple matters, like ensuring your room is sunny, can make a big difference in your recovery process

New attention is being paid to the unglamorous, nuts-and-bolts basics of how health professionals care for patients. Doctors and nurses are learning to admit mistakes, and patients are learning to inquire about down-to-earth subjects like hand washing. The common goal: improved patient care and more effective treatment of illnesses.

➤Owning Up Health professionals are only human, and in the interest of preventing errors, the private nonprofit organization U.S. Pharmacopeia has begun issuing annual reports on hospital medication errors. Contributions are voluntary and anonymous. The idea is catching on: the 2004 report catalogs 192,000 admissions of error at more than 500 hospitals, whereas

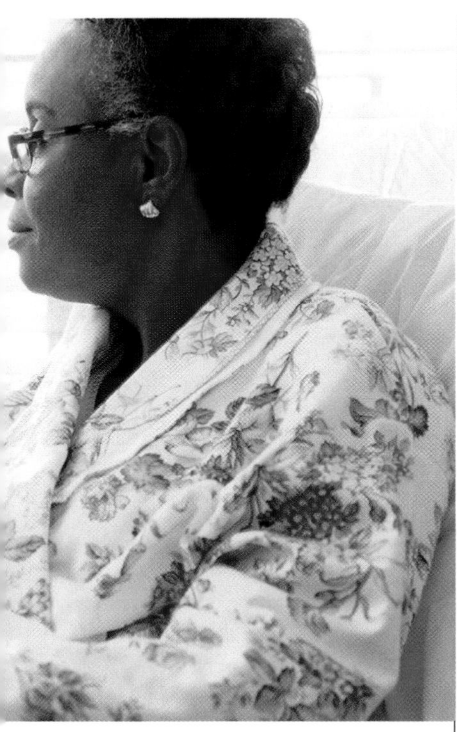

JOHN HENLEY—CORBIS

in the first report, in 1999, professionals from only 56 hospitals participated, admitting to some 40,000 mistakes.

USP's database tries to identify patterns of errors in hopes of preventing future mistakes. Common examples include administering the wrong drug—or administering the right drug the wrong way (say, by an intravenous tube instead of a feeding tube).

➤Scrubbing Up Nearly 10% of Americans who are admitted to a hospital pick up an infection while they are there, most of them transmitted by doctors, nurses and other health-care workers. In fact, hospital infections contribute to the deaths of nearly 90,000 patients in the U.S. each year. Yet the solution can be as simple as a bar of medicated soap. Sadly, study after study has shown that hospital staff generally follow hand washing guidelines less than 40% of the time—and sometimes less than that.

In January 2004, researchers at the Mayo Clinic recommended that health-care workers carry alcohol hand rubs in their pockets to make disinfecting easier. Some experts suggest that patients quiz doctors and nurses to see if they've washed their hands before an examination begins—smile when you ask!

➤Lightening Up Prescription: keep on the sunny side. Sunlight may play a key role in easing surgical pain and saving millions of dollars in hospital pharmacy costs, according to a 2004 study. It found that surgery patients in rooms with lots of natural light took less pain medication, and their drug costs ran 21% less than those of equally ill patients assigned to darker rooms.

LIFETIME LEARNING

Some 10 percent of all Americans who visit hospitals pick up an infection, often from doctors and nurses

■ Resources

U.S. AGENCY FOR HEALTHCARE RESEARCH AND QUALITY: *www.ahcpr.gov*

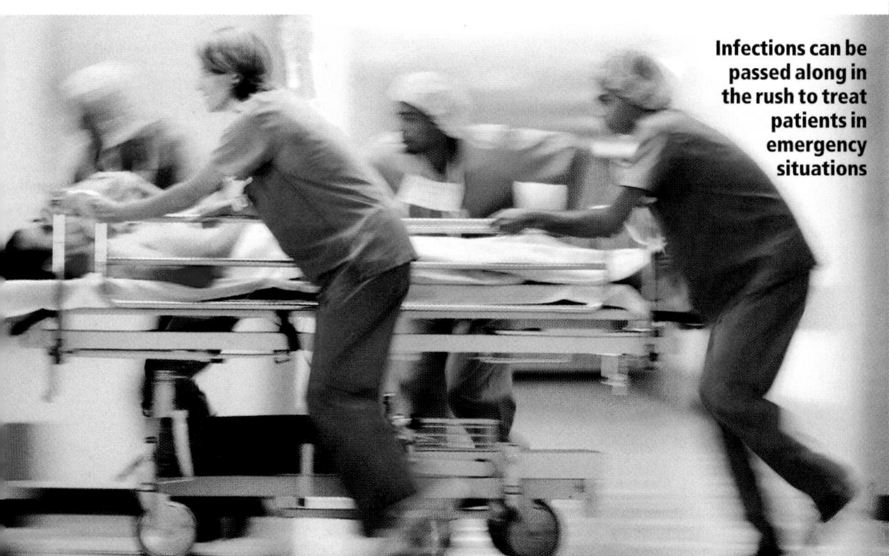

Infections can be passed along in the rush to treat patients in emergency situations

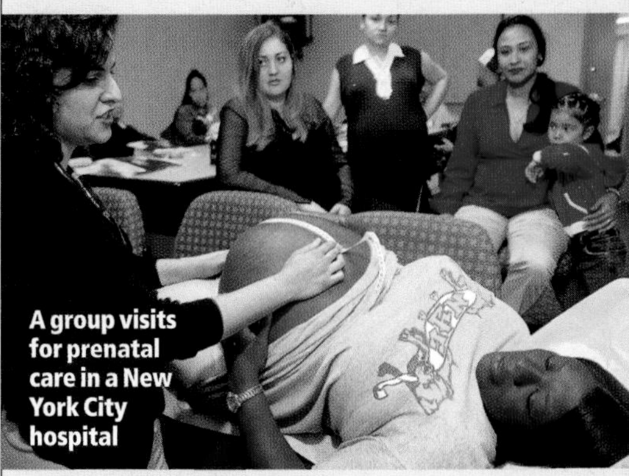

MARK PETERSON—REDUX

A group visits for prenatal care in a New York City hospital

Safety in Numbers

Patients tired of waiting forever to see the doctor are now making appointments en masse. For people accustomed to thinking of a doctor's visit as a private, one-on-one affair, the idea of a roomful of strangers discussing something as intimate as the progress of one's pregnancy may seem strange. Yet look at it this way: Would you rather wait an hour or two to see your doctor for 10 minutes—or meet at a prearranged time and see the doctor, along with up to 25 other patients, for two hours?

More and more doctors and patients are opting for the latter course. It works particularly well in cases where the doctor is providing basic health information, such as prenatal care for mothers-to-be, health tips for the elderly, or immunization schedules for young patients. Patients enjoy the support of people who are in the same boat; doctors savor the efficiency of providing better care to many more patients than they could see one at a time.

The idea is catching on. The VA Medical Center in Bay Pines, Fla., began making group appointments in 2002 to combat a backlog of 17,000 patients waiting to be inducted into its primary-care system. Today that waiting list hovers at about 100, and the group model is being extended to VA centers around the country.

Proponents argue that the group approach also provides superior care. One study randomly allocated elderly patients to group or individual care and found that, after two years, those who attended the groups regularly had 18% fewer emergency-room visits and a 12% decrease in hospital admissions; were more likely to get flu and pneumonia shots; and cost health insurers about $50 less per patient each month. ■

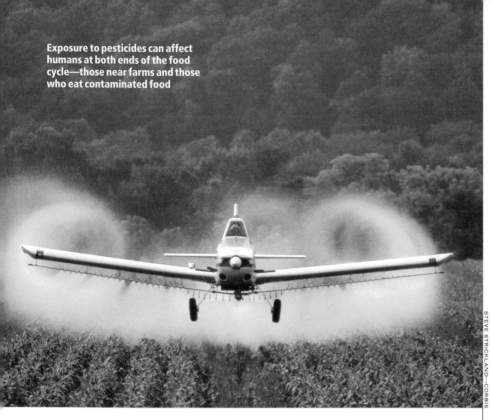
Exposure to pesticides can affect humans at both ends of the food cycle—those near farms and those who eat contaminated food

STEVE STRICKLAND—CORBIS

Pesticides

Four decades after Rachel Carson's *Silent Spring* first warned of the danger of pesticides, we're still learning about their harmful effects

Good News Controlling pesticides that have proved harmful to humans can begin to show positive effects within a few years

Although government scientists and medical researchers have been investigating the health effects of pesticides for decades, new information continues to document the prevalence and impact of the chemicals used to keep harmful insects away from plants and people.

A 2003 study conducted in Missouri found that men who lived in communities where the agricultural pesticides diazinon and atrazine were widely used (and whose urine showed traces of these chemicals) were up to 16 times more likely than a control group to suffer from low sperm counts and poor sperm quality, both of which can contribute to male infertility. In an especially sobering finding, only two of the men whose urine samples indicated the presence of these pesticides were farmers, leading researchers to theorize that the others were exposed through drinking water that had been contaminated through farm runoff.

On the consuming side of the pesticide chain, in July 2004 a team of British researchers reported that pesticide residues in fresh fruit can expose children to amounts of agricultural chemicals that exceed recommended maximum levels.

SORRY SIDE-EFFECT

A study found that men living in areas where pesticides were widely used suffered from low sperm counts

The good news: scientists are also finding that decisive action to control pesticide contamination can have a positive impact on health almost immediately. In March 2004—four years after the EPA banned the pesticides chlorpyrifos and diazinon from household products—researchers announced that the rate of low-birth weight babies, a key predictor of later health problems, had dropped dramatically in communities where these products had been used widely. Before the ban, roughly one baby in three in urban communities where these pesticides were frequently used tested positive for exposure; after the ban, fewer than one in seventy tested positive. Researchers estimated that exposure to the pesticides reduced the birth weight of babies within the test group by an average of six ounces.

■ Resources

EPA WEBSITE: *www.epa.gov/pesticides/health/index.htm*

Pets

Studies continue to document the positive power of pets, which offer health benefits to young and old

Moods and Mutts Interacting with pets can increase the levels of brain chemicals that affect our sense of well-being

Three cheers for Fido! Researchers are now quantifying what animal lovers have long believed: pets offer health benefits to humans of all ages. Studying children, doctors have discovered that proximity to family pets exposes infants to the microbes that make their home in

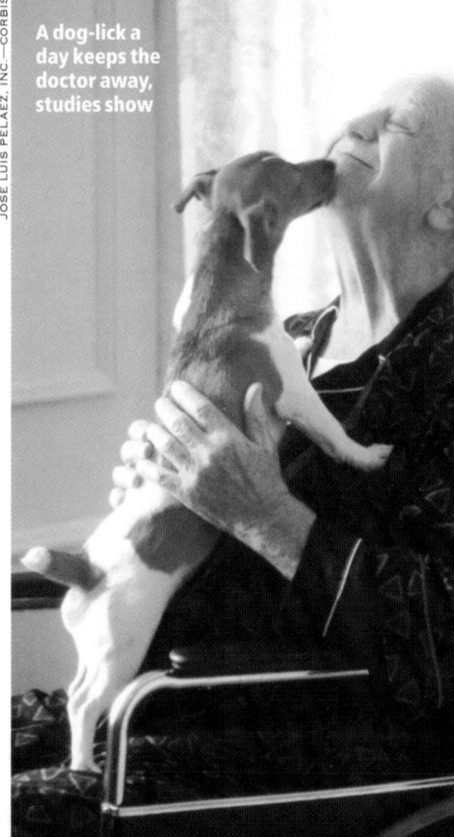
A dog-lick a day keeps the doctor away, studies show

JOSE LUIS PELAEZ, INC.—CORBIS

animal fur; the experience helps prime infants' immune system to recognize common allergens as harmless, short-circuiting later allergy attacks (*see* Allergies).

Scientists are also finding that owning and caring for a pet may improve the quality and duration of an older person's life. In one simple study of pet owners who were 65 and older, researchers found they visited the doctor 16 percent less frequently than seniors without pets in their homes.

In 2003 a separate team of researchers presented findings suggesting that interaction with pets may minimize or even reverse some of the damaging cell changes that occur naturally with aging. According to this study, levels of endorphins, serotonin and prolactin—substances that can enhance feelings of well-being—increased in study participants during interaction, while cortisol levels (stress hormones) decreased. Separate research, also published in 2003, suggested that in addition to these other upsides, older pet owners are considerably less likely to be confined to bed.

The power of pets comes with a pricetag, however. Of the 1,400 or so recognized human pathogens, 61 percent are naturally communicable between animals and people. Experts advise that a few precautions can reduce the risk. First, acquire your animal friends from reliable sources and adhere to a regular schedule of veterinary visits and vaccinations. Second, wash your hands after handling pets (particularly reptiles) and get immediate treatment for any parasites that show up. Third, don't let your pet scavenge, hunt or eat raw meat. And finally, avoid contact with your pet's feces, urine and other body fluids—and clean up your kitty's litter boxes daily.

Resources

CDC PET WEBSITE:
www.cdc.gov/healthypets

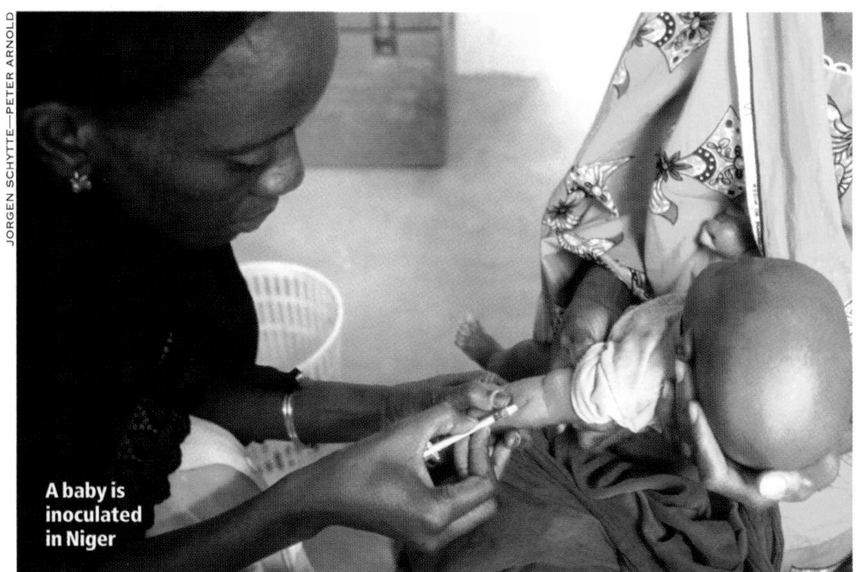

JORGEN SCHYTTE—PETER ARNOLD

A baby is inoculated in Niger

Polio

In the spring of 2004, even as world health officials were poised to announce the global eradication of polio, fresh outbreaks of the disease spread misery in nine African nations

Definition Polio is a highly contagious virus-borne infection that attacks the nervous system and spinal cord. It can result in muscle weakness or paralysis

The year 2004 marked a milestone in the fight against polio, the crippling disease that once affected more than 50,000 Americans and untold millions of others around the world each year. It has now been exactly half a century since the first effective vaccine against the disease, developed by Jonas Salk, was successfully tested. In those five decades, the disease has been wiped out in the U.S. (where the last case of infection was reported in 1979) and has been almost completely eradicated around the world.

The goal of stamping out polio (which would make it only the second disease, after smallpox, to be made extinct by human hands), is so close that U.S. and world health officials announced in late 2003 that it would be accomplished sometime in the following 24 months. But they spoke too soon: an outbreak in Western Africa hit Nigeria and Sudan's war-ravaged Darfur region in the spring of 2004. Relief workers moved quickly to put out both fires, but to little avail. In Nigeria, a culture clash led to the mistaken belief among the nation's Muslims that polio shots were part of a Western plot to cause infertility and spread HIV and AIDS, while in Sudan the chaos of civil war hampered efforts to vaccinate at-risk refugees. By June 2004 polio had re-emerged in nine African countries and the worldwide tally of cases for the year was double 2003's mid-year total—all before polio's "high season" began in September.

A SAD MILESTONE

Fifty years after the first effective polio vaccine was launched, a fresh outbreak of the disease hit Africa

The news sent chills down the spines of health officials in developed nations, where polio has not been seen for decades, because many of them no longer bother to immunize children against the disease. Sadly, doctors working to put polio in the history books may have miles to go before they sleep.

Resources

POLIO ERADICATION INITIATIVE SITE:
www.polioeradication.org

P

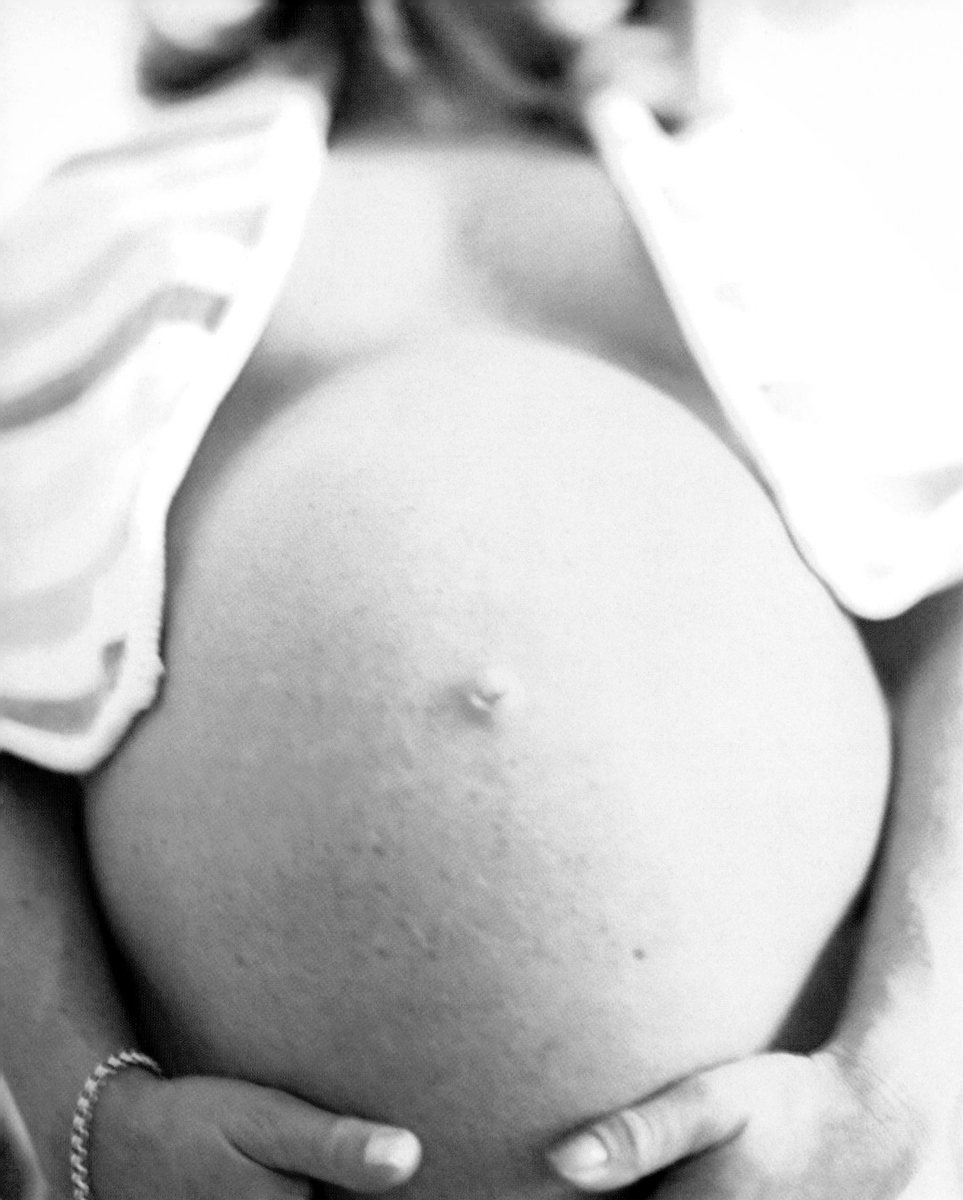

ERIK RANK—PHOTONICA

Pregnancy and Birth

The news for expectant moms is good: dangers like sudden infant death syndrome are receding, and new therapies are helping mothers-to-be cope with problems ranging from nausea to premature birth

Surge in C-Sections

A major increase in the number of women choosing voluntary C-sections has some doctors concerned

Does the C in C-section stand for convenience? More and more women today are voluntarily choosing nonvaginal birth. These are not the emergency caesareans that have been performed for hundreds of years to rescue babies from women in medical crisis, but an increasingly popular modern variation: planned, scheduled operations for all sorts of less-than-critical reasons. In the U.S., according to the CDC, at least 1 in 4 babies is now born by C-section—the highest rate since the government began keeping track—up from 10.4% in 1975. And more than 20% of these are purely by patient choice, a 20% increase since 1999.

All of which puts the obstetrics community in an uneasy ethical position. Although C-sections are safer than ever—thanks to improvements in anesthetics, antibiotics and operating techniques over the past few decades—they still carry real risks. In 1% to 2% of cases, C-sections lead to infection, damage to other organs during surgery or severe bleeding in the mother. They can also endanger the baby if the infant's gestational age has been miscalculated and the child is removed from the womb too soon. Risks to the mother increase with each C-section, and the procedure isn't recommended for women who plan to have more than two children.

So the question for doctors is this: Should women be allowed to have C-sections just because they can? Many doctors believe that a woman should have the right to choose for herself how she wants to have her child, as long as she is fully informed of the risks and benefits. Officially, the American College of Obstetricians and Gynecologists (ACOG) agrees. In November 2003, an ACOG ethics committee issued its opinion on the debate, finding it ethical for doctors to perform elective C-sections so long as the procedure doesn't imperil the health of the mother or child. But the committee fell short of offering guidelines, citing lack of evidence.

One common belief about such deliveries—that once you've given birth by caesarean, it becomes risky to deliver subsequent babies vaginally—may be falling by the wayside. A large-scale four-year study concluded that the risk of complications in so-called VBAC cases (vaginal birth after a C-section) is actually quite small.

IT'S ALL IN THE WRIST

Wrist bands designed to help quell motion sickness are turning out to help pregnant women handle nausea

➤Coping with Nausea

A new study shows that a battery-powered wrist band originally developed to help with motion sickness (by stimulating a particular nerve in the lower arm) may be able to help fight nausea associated with pregnancy. Researchers found that pregnant women who wore the

Clearing the Air

Pregnant women who suffer from allergies have long been wary of taking antihistamines, for fear of endangering the health of the unborn child. But two recent studies failed to find any link between this group of drugs (and in particular the widely used antihistamine Claritin) and birth defects. In the first, more than 1,400 mothers were divided into three test groups: those who had taken Claritin, those who had taken other antihistamines and those who had used no antihistamines.

The study found a virtually identical rate of birth defects (around 3%) across each of these populations, suggesting that Claritin does not measurably increase the risk of birth defects. The study's authors cautioned however, that more research is needed before definitively ruling out such a link.

A second study looked at the possible relationship between Claritin use and a common genital birth defect in boys. Previous research (published in 2002) had suggested that Claritin use during pregnancy might increase the risk of hypospadias (a deformity in which the urethra opening is along the shaft of the penis, instead of at the tip), which occurs in approximately 4 out of every 1,000 boys and requires surgery to correct. The newer study, which was sponsored by the CDC, found no link between Claritin (which is used by approximately 3% of American women of child-bearing age) and the occurrence of hypospadias.

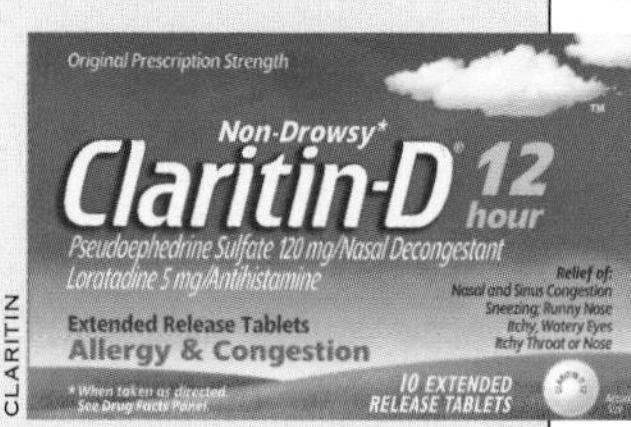

CLARITIN

In a related development, a new study has shown that pregnant women who suffer from asthma may be able to breathe a little bit easier. Research that looked at more than 2,200 pregnant women (one-third of whom showed symptoms of asthma or took asthma medications) found that neither a diagnosis of asthma nor treatment with bronchodilator medications such as epinephrine increased the risk of preterm delivery. The study did find, however, that women who took oral steroids were at increased risk of delivering their babies early—usually by a week or two. ■

watch-size ReliefBand experienced fewer and less intense bouts of nausea and vomiting than test subjects who wore a placebo device. Women who wore the ReliefBand also measured less dehydration than those who didn't.

JUST-IN-TIME DELIVERY

Hormone injections may help reduce the chance of premature delivery by as much as one-third, a study said

➤How to Prevent Preemies Taking weekly doses of the naturally occurring hormone progesterone may reduce by as much as one-third the chance that a woman at high risk for preterm delivery will give birth early, a new study found. This is significant because as many as 12% of all U.S. births are now premature (meaning they occur before 37 weeks of gestation), and progesterone therapy is the first clearly effective means of preventing the problem. Researchers deemed the progesterone injections so effective, in fact, that the study was ended early, because it would have been considered unethical to continue giving some of the test subjects a placebo.

➤How Not to Prevent Preemies Expectant mothers deemed to be at risk of preterm delivery are sometimes advised by their doctors to undergo cerclage—a procedure in which the cervix is stitched closed—during the last weeks before delivery, as a way of preventing premature birth and miscarriage. Although the procedure is commonly used (doctors perform it in up to 2% of all pregnancies), previous research has offered conflicting evidence on its effectiveness. But a new study, involving more than 2,100 women who were at risk for premature delivery, found that cerclage has no measurable effect on when a baby is born. A second study examined more than 47,000 pregnant women in several countries and yielded similar results.

While the first study found no link between the cerclage procedure and serious complications for the mother or child, it did suggest that mothers who undergo cerclage are more likely to develop infections and need drugs to prevent contractions.

■ Resources

NIH WEBSITE: *www.nlm.nih.gov/medlineplus/childbirth.html*

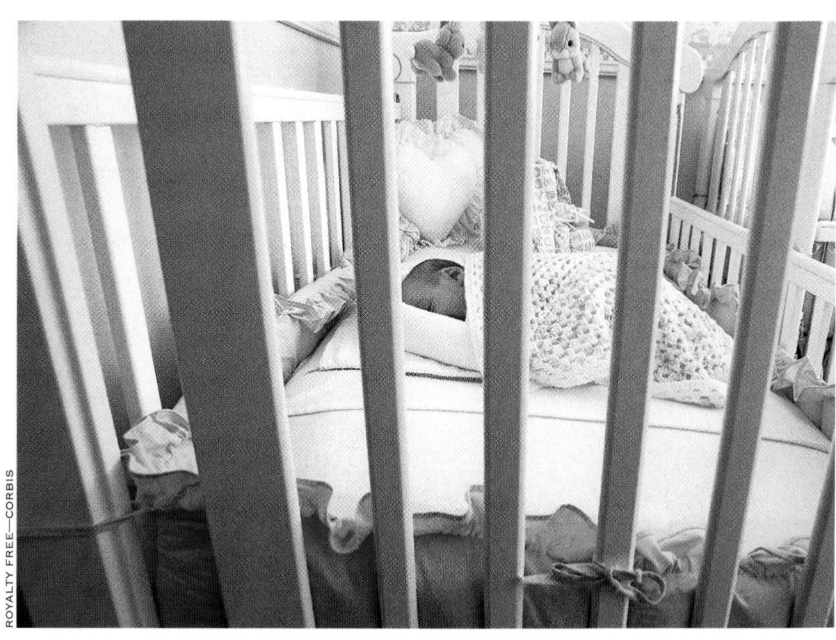
ROYALTY FREE—CORBIS

P

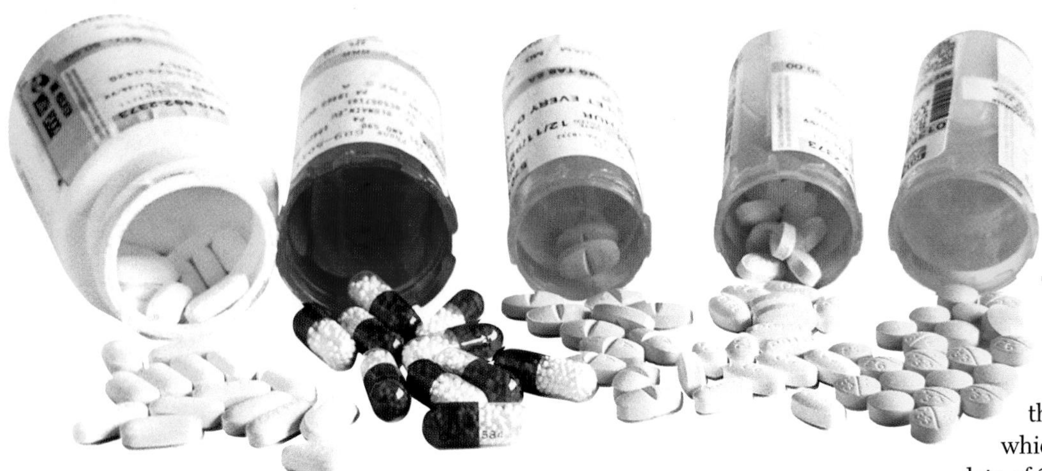

MICHAEL P. GADOMSKI—PHOTO RESEARCHERS

Prescription Drugs

The high price of today's powerful new drugs is driving everyone who needs them—especially older Americans on fixed incomes—to seek lower costs any way they can

Remedy—or Not? Under a 2003 law passed by the Bush Administration, the U.S. Medicare program is now offering a new discount card intended to help enrollees cut the high cost of drugs. But many seniors call the program confusing and ineffective

In December 2003 the Bush Administration and Congress succeeding in passing a long-sought bill to provide a prescription drug benefit for American seniors on Medicare. But the first stage of the overhaul, a discount card that became available in June 2004, got off to a slow, troubled start. (The second stage—insurance coverage for prescription drugs—is not scheduled to begin until 2006.)

Although more than 3 million people were enrolled in the new program by the time the discount cards became effective, most of them were signed up automatically through their health-care providers, such as state welfare organizations. Fewer than half a million people who were not enrolled automatically took the trouble to sign up—far short of estimates that more than 1 million users would enroll on their own. The shortfall was due in part to confusion among some low-income seniors that other benefits (like food stamps) would be reduced if they applied for the card, as well as the mistaken belief that assets like insurance or personal heirlooms (such as wedding rings) would have to be sold in order to qualify for the benefit.

Medicare officials took steps to remedy these misperceptions, with the result that several hundred thousand more seniors began to enroll in the program. By August, however, a report indicated that 47% of Medicare recipients had retained a negative view of the program, while only 26% regarded it as beneficial.

Although most Medicare beneficiaries surveyed believed that the program would help some people on Medicare, fewer than one-third believed it would benefit them personally. More than half felt that the discount cards were not worth the trouble it would take to enroll in the program, because of a perception that the discounts were modest and the program confusing. More than 80% of those surveyed called for two changes in the law: permission to buy lower-cost drugs from Canada and removal of the law's ban on the Federal Government's negotiating with drug companies to pay lower prices.

BORDERS AND ORDERS

In one survey, more than 80% of Medicare recipients called for the right to buy their drugs from Canada

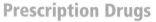

➤Medicare's Future The prognosis for Medicare took a turn for the worse in March 2004, when the program's trustees revised their predictions about when the health-care system would exhaust its funds. The new estimate, 2019, is much sooner than the 2003 official estimate of 2026 (and earlier too than the 2002 estimate, which called for a doomsday date of 2030). The trustees also reported that Medicare will have to begin draining its trust fund to meet expenses no later than 2013—three years sooner than envisioned in the 2003 report.

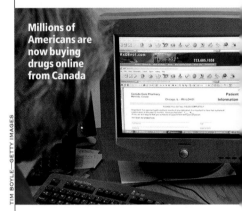

Millions of Americans are now buying drugs online from Canada

TIM BOYLE—GETTY IMAGES

Experts cited three reasons for the new estimate. First, an ever larger number of baby boomers will be reaching retirement. Second, the new prescription drug benefit will vastly increase the program's costs. Finally, payments to private insurers will grow, for they will play an increasingly important role in Medicare under the 2003 reorganization of the plan.

➤Price Tags In June 2004, the AARP (formerly the American Association of Retired Persons) published a study showing that prices for drugs used most often by elderly Americans rose dramatically in the months after the Bush Administration enacted the new law, climbing 3.4% in the first three months of the year—about three times the rate of inflation. This followed a previous AARP report showing that drug prices for the elderly had risen 6.9% in 2003.

Among the drugs most widely used by seniors, Plavix (an anti-blood-clotting drug) showed one of the most dramatic price surges, jumping 7.9%, while Pravachol (a cholesterol-fighting medicine) rose 7%. At a single company, Pfizer, prices for a range of eight medicines often used by elderly Americans, including Lipitor and Celebrex, rose between 2.9% and 6.4%.

UNLIMITED CEILING?

Over the first three months of 2004, prices for prescription drugs rose at three times the rate of inflation

A separate study published by a consumer advocacy group, Families USA, noted that the gap between the general rate of inflation and the faster rate at which drug prices are rising is especially harmful to older Americans, whose Social Security benefits are indexed to the Consumer Price Index, a broad-based measure of inflation. As a result, increases in Social Security payments are not keeping pace with the steeper rate at which drug prices are climbing.

➤Hidden Costs Higher drug prices can lead to serious medical consequences. For example, many Americans are now skimping on (or skipping entirely) medications for which they have a serious medical need. A study published in May 2004 showed that when insurance companies raised co-payments on eight types of prescription medicines (for conditions ranging from asthma to depression to allergies), patients sharply reduced their use of these drugs. The study found that patients were most likely to cut back on prescription drugs that could be replaced by over-the-counter medications that treat the symptoms of a disorder rather than the underlying disease.

These data are sobering enough, but analysts point out that when patients cut back on prescription drugs for chronic conditions like asthma and diabetes, it often leads to more costly medical problems and more expensive forms of treatment (like an increased number of emergency room visits), further taxing an already overburdened health-care system.

■ Resources

MEDICARE PRESCRIPTION DRUG BENEFIT HOTLINE: *800-633-4227*

FDA WEBSITE ON ONLINE BUYING: *www.fda.gov/oc/buyonline*

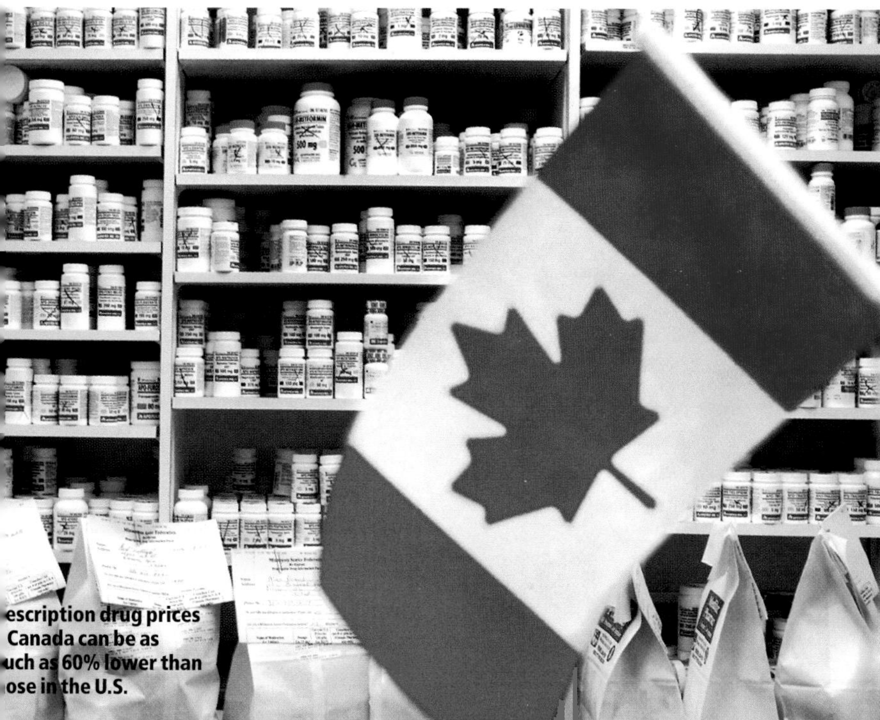

escription drug prices Canada can be as uch as 60% lower than ose in the U.S.

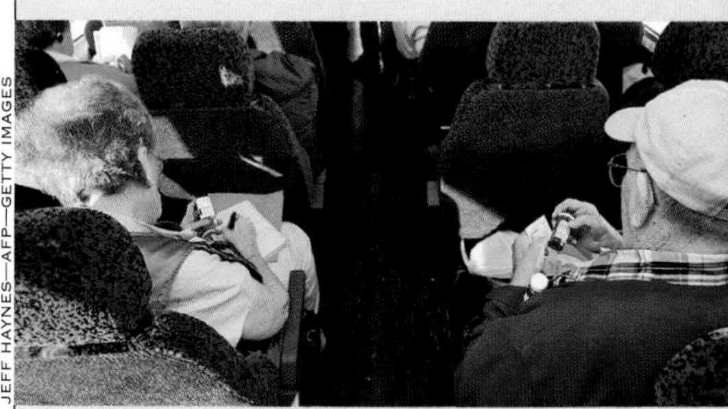

JEFF HAYNES—AFP—GETTY IMAGES

Canadian Connection

It is technically illegal by federal law for Americans to bring prescription drugs meant for sale in other countries into the U.S. But the FDA has long looked the other way as individual U.S. citizens have carried across the border (or had delivered by mail) small quantities of drugs that a doctor has prescribed for them.

Now an increasing number of Americans are trying to save money by purchasing medicine from foreign countries (mainly Canada) where price controls keep drugs costs down. Why defy Uncle Sam? Because drug prices inside the U.S. are often double what the same medicines fetch in Canada. A three-month supply of the blood thinner Plavix costs around $400 in Detroit yet would be little more than half that in Toronto. As border-crossing buyers are being urged on by dozens of local and state U.S. governments, however, the feds are taking a harder line.

In August 2004, Illinois Governor Rod Blagojevich gave up on getting a federal O.K. for residents of his state to buy cheaper drugs from abroad. He declared that in September, state health officials would begin helping Illinois residents purchase such drugs, whether the FDA liked it or not.

The Bush Administration has sided with the U.S. pharmaceutical industry in resisting imported drugs. But Illinois is just one of six states now encouraging foreign drug purchases. Factor in the many individuals and Web-based businesses that are doing the same, and you realize that even the Federal Government has a finite number of fingers with which to plug holes in this dike. In May 2004, Health and Human Services Secretary Tommy Thompson described the eventual passage of legislation permitting prescription drug imports as "inevitable." The White House quickly dialed back that statement. If drug prices remain high, however, a showdown is sure to come. ■

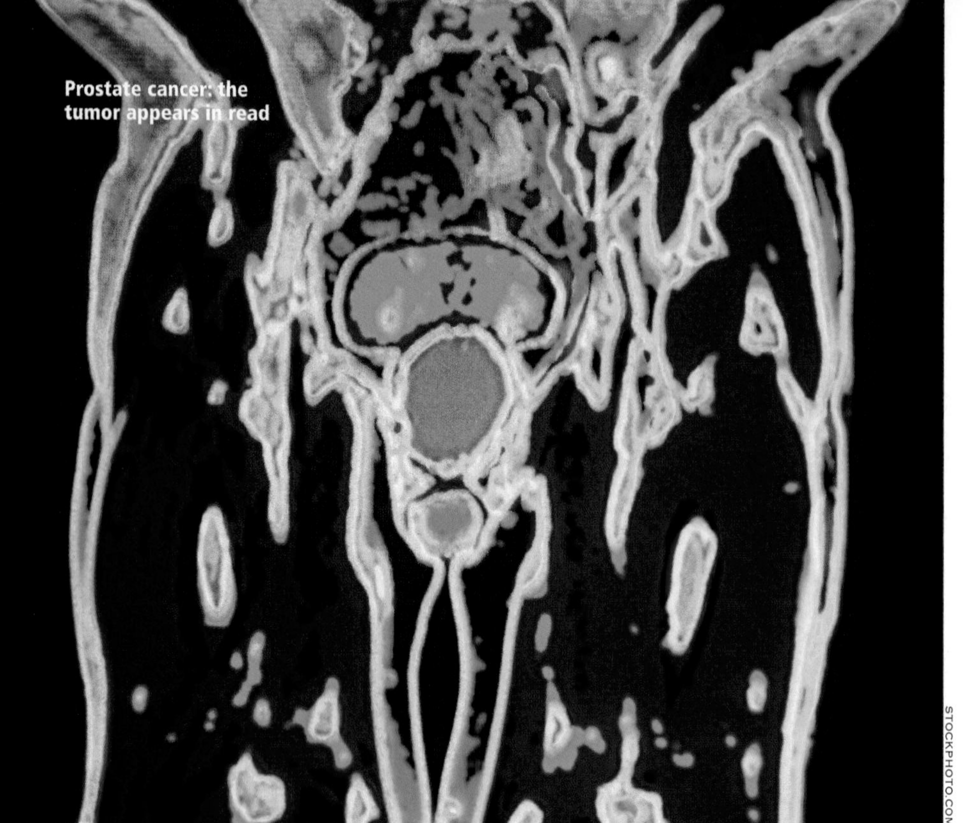
Prostate cancer: the tumor appears in read

STOCKPHOTO.COM

Prostate Cancer

Over the past 10 years, the PSA test has helped lower the number of deaths from prostate cancer. But it needs to be made more precise

By the Numbers The PSA test misses 82% of cancers in the prostate gland of men under 60, according to one study

Slow but steady progress is being made against prostate cancer, a disease that afflicts 221,000 American men each year and takes the lives of more than 29,000, making it the second leading cause of cancer deaths in men. Deaths from prostate cancer have fallen dramatically (about 20% among white men and 16% among blacks) since testing for prostate-specific antigen (PSA) became common in the mid-1990s. Most of the good news in recent years has come in the form of new insight into how to interpret exams that screen for prostate cancer—and the prospect of making those tests more precise in years to come.

➤A Test Under Fire The PSA blood test measures levels of a protein released by the prostate. It is increasingly coming under question because the early detection it offers has not necessarily translated into saved lives. A study published in the summer of 2003 reported that the test, which recommends biopsies for men with PSA blood levels of more than 4 nanograms per milliliter, misses 82% of cancers in men under 60. Lowering the threshold for biopsy to 2.6, the study's authors suggested, would double the cancer-detection rate. Critics, however, cautioned that lowering the biopsy threshold could result in over-diagnosis and needless anxiety.

In a study that raised more questions than it answered, researchers reported in May 2004 that they had discovered another major problem in the PSA test. For years doctors had assumed that a reading lower than 4 ng/mL of blood meant the patient was cancer free. But a study of 2,950 men published in the *New England Journal of Medicine* found that 15% of those with PSA levels less than 4 actually did have the cancer, and almost 15% of these men had "high grade" tumors, which can become aggressive. Doctors fear that the news will trigger a flood of requests for unnecessary biopsies.

Although more biopsies will lead to more early diagnoses, most prostate cancers grow so slowly that it's hard to say whether early detection is worth it. The study's authors recommend that men also consider their age, ethnicity and family history of disease before opting for a biopsy—or for treatment.

➤Too Many False Positives Doctors have long been challenged by the fact that the PSA test yields a high return of false positive tests. Three-quarters of the more than 1 million men who have prostate biopsies each year (after a PSA test

A Paradoxical Drug

Imagine there was a drug that could significantly lower your risk of prostate cancer. Say it could also increase your chance of growing particularly aggressive tumors—those most likely to spread and kill—if you do get cancer. Should you take it?

That's the question doctors and patients have been wrestling with since the results of a National Cancer Institute–sponsored trial were published in the summer of 2003. Compared with a placebo, Merck's finasteride—a drug currently marketed to treat baldness and benign prostate enlargement—apparently reduced one's risk of getting prostate cancer by 25%.

However, in the seven-year study, involving more than 9,000 men age 55 and older, the finasteride group also had a slightly higher rate of aggressive, "high grade" tumors, which are harder to treat. Finasteride also caused loss of libido and impotence. It's not clear that this is a drug that should be taken to prevent prostate cancer. ■

ROYALTY FREE—CORBIS

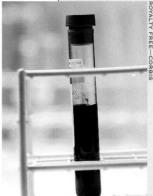

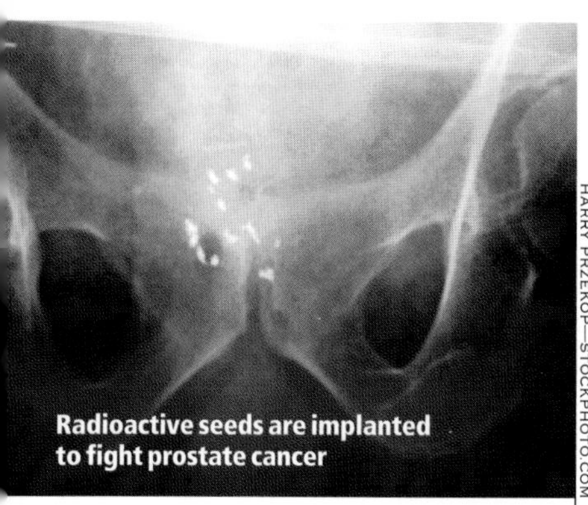
Radioactive seeds are implanted to fight prostate cancer

HARRY PRZEKOP—STOCKPHOTO.COM

indicates the possible presence of cancer) turn out not to have the disease. But a new study suggests that interpreting PSA results in combination with four other risk factors may help physicians refine this approach and cut the number of unnecessary biopsies dramatically. The other indications that doctors need to consider, the study suggested, are a rectal exam in which a doctor probes with a finger to feel for the presence of a tumor; a rectal ultrasound, to spot tumors visually; PSA density (the relationship between the size of a patient's prostate gland and his PSA level); and age, since the vast majority of prostate cancer cases are found in men age 65 or older.

ROOM TO IMPROVE

The PSA test saves lives, but it can fail to detect cancer, even while reporting false positives too often

➤Better Tests Ahead? Why does the PSA test yield so many false positives, even while giving a clean bill of health to a significant number of men who actually have prostate cancer? In the summer of 2003, a team of researchers helped illuminate this problem when they found three variations in part of the gene that controls prostate-specific-antigen levels. Together, these variations can contribute to an increase of as much as 30% in PSA levels. It was long assumed that the level of PSA in a man's bloodstream was a direct indicator of the presence of cancer, but it is now known that these genetic variations—single nucleotide polymorphisms—can boost PSA levels even in cases when cancer is not present.

➤A Superior Gauge Some new research suggests that the level of PSA itself is far less important than the rate at which it increases. A study published in July 2004 suggested that the rate at which PSA levels climb can predict the presence of deadly tumors nearly 10 times more accurately than PSA levels alone. The research, which followed more than 1,000 prostate cancer patients, found that more than 1 in 4 whose PSA levels rose more than two points in 12 months before diagnosis died of prostate cancer within seven years, despite aggressive surgery to remove their tumors.

HORMONE THREAT

Men age 50 or older who have high levels of testosterone face an elevated risk of prostate cancer

➤Reviewing Radiation A study published in January 2004 raises questions about the effectiveness of low-dose radiation therapy for men with prostate cancer. The study examined four treatment strategies: low-dose radiation, high-dose radiation, surgery to remove the prostate and the implantation of radioactive "seeds" within the prostate. It found that in more than 2,900 men with early-stage prostate cancer, the last three therapies led to five-year survival rates (without relapses) of around 80%, while low-dose radiation yielded a relapse-free survival rate of only 51% over the same period of time.

➤A Testosterone Link Men age 50 or older who have high levels of testosterone face an elevated risk of prostate cancer, according to research published in May 2004. The news raises questions about testosterone-replacement therapy, a new kind of treatment currently being tested in older men who suffer from symptoms of andropause (the male equivalent of menopause), which include decreased energy, depression, muscle loss and diminished physical performance.

■ Resources

PROSTATE CANCER RESEARCH INSTITUTE: *www.prostate-cancer.org*

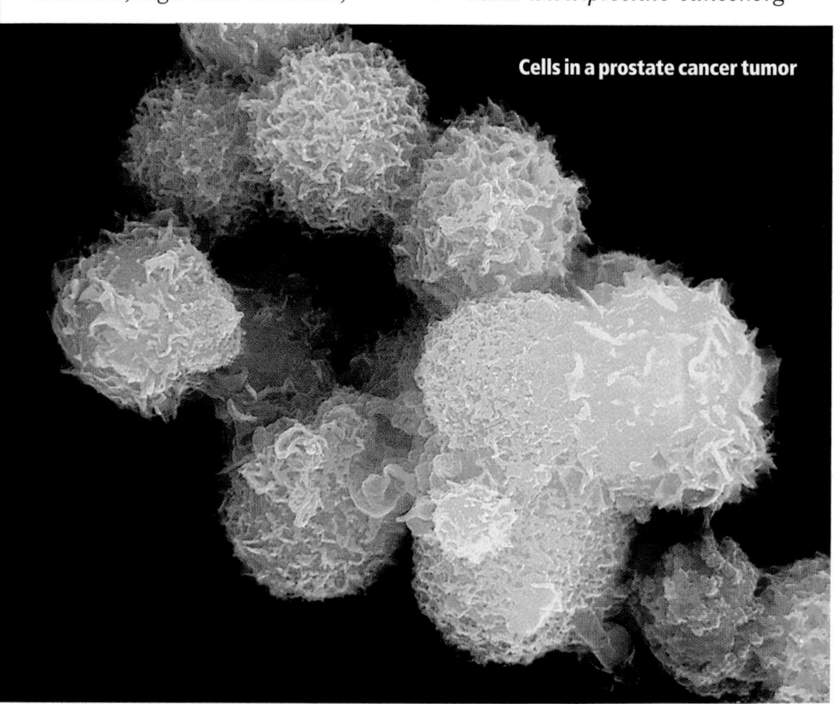
Cells in a prostate cancer tumor

MICROWORKS—PHOTOTAKE

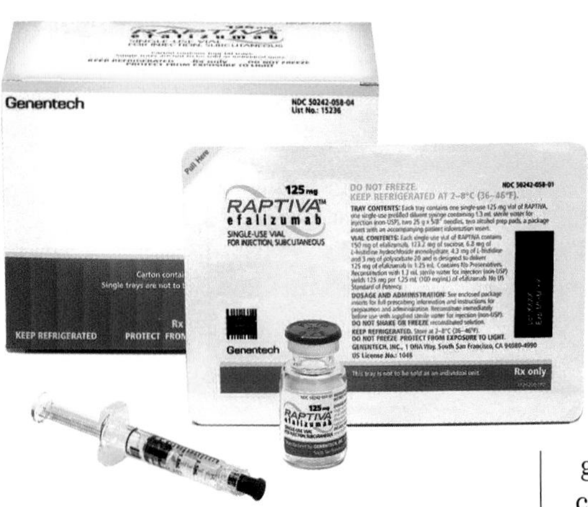

RAPTIVA

Psoriasis

New drugs offer better treatment for this condition that turns the skin scaly, while molecular research may finally help put an end to it

A Cancer Link? Research has connected psoriasis to lymphoma, but the tie may be the result of treatments used in the past

New drugs are offering relief to the more than 4 million Americans who suffer from psoriasis. In October 2003, the FDA approved Raptiva (whose generic name is efalizumab) as an effective new treatment for the irritating, unsightly ailment, which is characterized by scaly patches of inflamed skin. The bad news: a year's worth of the weekly injections costs more than $14,000.

Coming on the heels of the FDA's January 2003 approval of another drug, Amevive, the decision ushered in a new era in psoriasis treatment. Both medicines work by interfering with immune-system cells that grow out of control in psoriasis patients and migrate to the skin's surface, where they trigger abnormal growth and create the disease's hallmark lesions. And more therapies are on the way: Enbrel, Remicade and Humira—drugs already approved to treat other conditions—are being studied as psoriasis therapies.

On a different front, a German research team announced in August 2004 that they had discovered molecular switches, metalloproteinase inhibitors, that may be able to block the out-of-control cell growth that causes the major symptoms of the disease.

The arrival of these drugs is good news in more ways than one. Researchers announced in November 2003 that they had discovered a troubling link between psoriasis and lymphoma: psoriasis patients are three times as likely as the general population to develop cancer of the immune system. The scientists theorized that the increased risk is not due to psoriasis itself but to the previous generation of drugs used to treat it, which worked by suppressing the patient's immune system—a strategy recognized as a risk factor for lymphoma.

■ **Resources**

NATIONAL PSORIASIS FOUNDATION: *www.psoriasis.org/home*

Psychotherapy

Cognitive therapy continues to prove its effectiveness; now it appears to be helpful in relieving post-traumatic stress disorder

Alzheimer's Warning Family members who act as caregivers for Alzheimer's patients are at high risk for depression

Cognitive therapy, a treatment technique used by some psychologists that aims to help patients reframe their view of the world so that setbacks and losses are put in less catastrophic perspective, may be more effective than previously thought in treating chronic post-traumatic stress disorder (PTSD). A study published in November 2003 involving survivors of traumatic auto accidents suggested that cognitive therapy may be nearly 90% effective in relieving the symptoms of PTSD, while alternative strategies were effective in little more than 50% of the cases studied.

BEARING THE BURDEN

If you're helping take care of a relative with Alzheimer's disease, don't forget to look after your own health

A second study found that people who provide care for a family member suffering from Alzheimer's disease are themselves especially vulnerable to depression, but it also said that counseling can make a significant difference in maintaining a steady mood. The study looked at more than 400 caregivers and found that rates of depression fell by as much as one-fourth among those who received family counseling or attended support group meetings with other caregivers, whereas the incidence of depression among those who received no treatment remained largely the same.

■ **Resources**

AMERICAN INSTITUTE FOR COGNITIVE THERAPY: *www.cognitivetherapynyc.com*

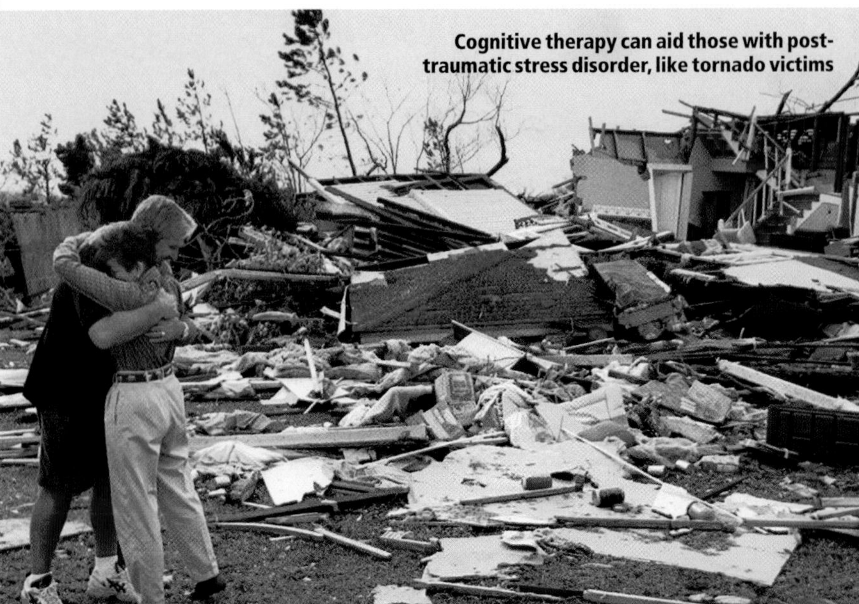

ALBANY HERALD—CORBIS SYGMA

Cognitive therapy can aid those with post-traumatic stress disorder, like tornado victims

R

Race and Health Care

The gap is shrinking, but black Americans remain more at risk than whites of suffering from diabetes or cancer or even dying in infancy

The Culprit? A new study blames higher rates of smoking among blacks for their heightened risk of dying from cancer

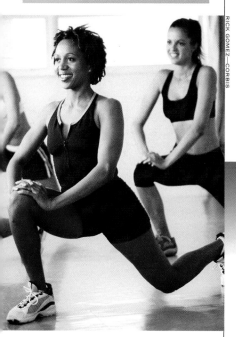

RICK GOMEZ—CORBIS

The relationship between race and health remains troubling: recent research has confirmed that black Americans are still twice as likely to die from diabetes as whites and one-third more likely to die of cancer, while infant mortality among African Americans is more than double the rate among whites. (A genetic predisposition is largely responsible for the high rate of diabetes in blacks.)

Some progress is being made. The introduction in 2000 of a new vaccine, Prevnar, which fights *Streptococcus pneumoniae* bacteria (a cause of pneumonia, ear infections and meningitis), has narrowed the racial gap among young victims of these diseases. Before Prevnar became available, the incidence of invasive pneumococcal infections was 3.3 times as high in black children under age 2 as it was in whites. By 2002, that figure had thinned to 1.6.

Another new study found statistical evidence for why cancer deaths are so much higher among black men than white men: smoking. The research team determined that nearly all the disparity between white and black cancer rates can be attributed to higher tobacco use among blacks.

■ Resources

NATIONAL CANCER INSTITUTE SITE: *crchd.nci.nih.gov/chd/racial_ethnic_disparities*

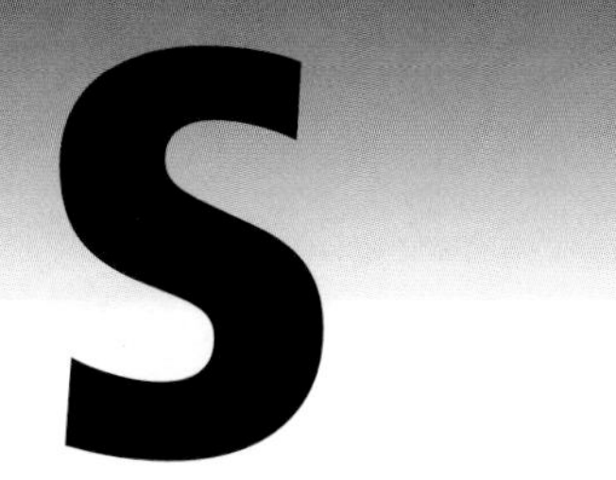

SARS

Epidemiologists braced for a storm when the first SARS victims of 2004 were reported in China, but the cases seem to have been confined

Danger: Deadly The highly contagious disease killed nearly 10 percent of those it infected when it first broke out in 2003

In April 2004, Beijing's Ministry of Health reported the first death of the year from severe acute respiratory syndrome (SARS) and announced four other confirmed cases (plus four additional possible cases) of the disease. SARS infected

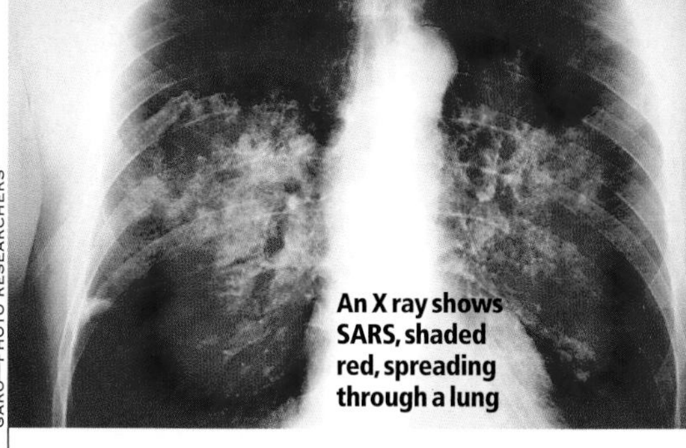

GARO—PHOTO RESEARCHERS

An X ray shows SARS, shaded red, spreading through a lung

more than 8,000 people around the world between November 2002 and July 2003, killing nearly 10 percent of its victims. This time around, the disease was safely contained—for now.

SARS SCORECARD

Chinese health officials fumbled the SARS outbreak in 2003 but seem to have confined the few cases of 2004

Also in April, China began human trials on a vaccine designed to fight SARS. By August, 36 healthy human volunteers had been injected with the vaccine, which contained the genetic sequence for a protein belonging to the SARS virus; none of the volunteers had shown signs of adverse effects to the innoculation. Meanwhile, two more experimental vaccines developed by American and European scientists showed promising results in animal tests, raising the hope that new immunization agents could be tested on humans as early as 2005.

Researchers at the Mayo Clinic announced in August 2004 that they had constructed a three-dimensional computer model of the enzyme that allows the SARS virus to replicate itself, raising the possibility of using genetic engineering to develop new drug treatments for the contagious killer.

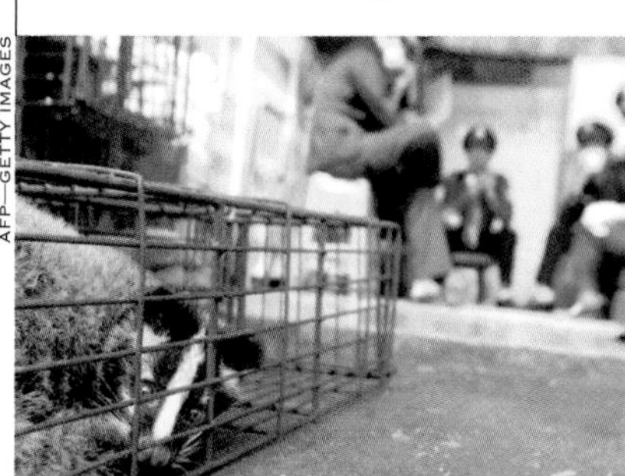

AFP—GETTY IMAGES

Chinese officials round up civet cats, eaten as a delicacy in Asia, because the small mammals can spread SARS

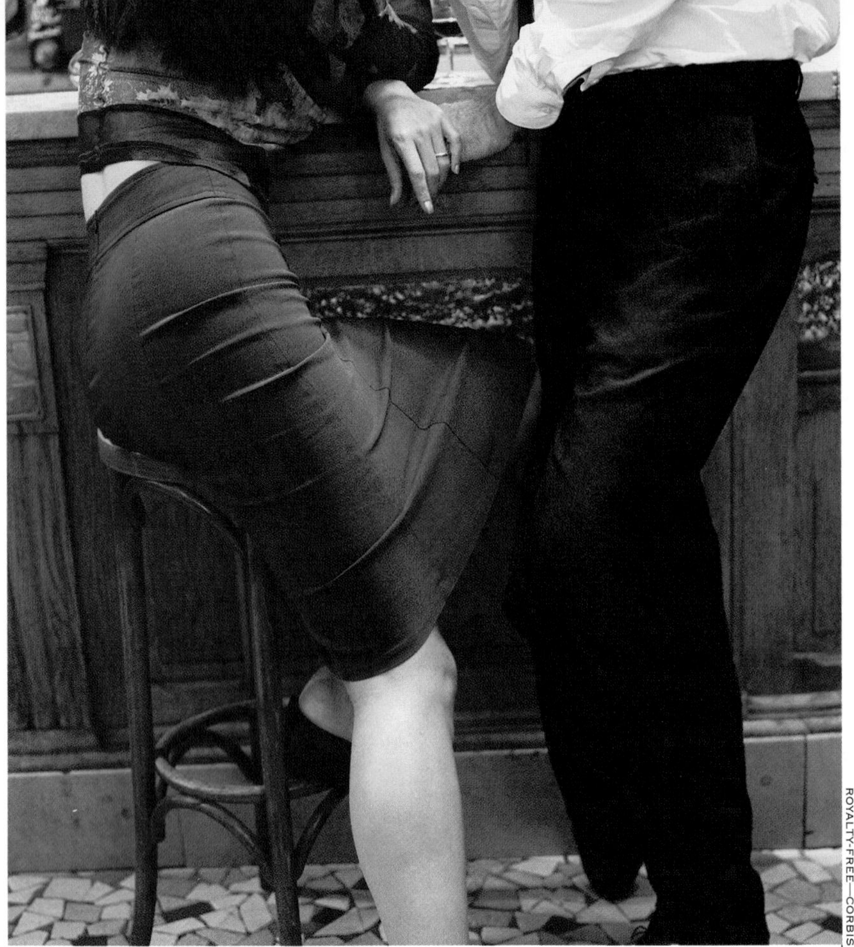

ROYALTY-FREE—CORBIS

Sexuality

The good news: an active sex life can lead to a longer life, healthier heart and improved ability to ward off pain. The bad news? ... Hey, we're still absorbing the good news!

Workout During orgasm, heart rate and blood pressure double. Intercourse burns about 200 calories, the equivalent of running vigorously for 30 minutes

The "sex glow." Carrie Bradshaw and her *Sex and the City* sidekicks may be the champions of detecting it, getting it and keeping it, but you don't need a closetful of Prada to appreciate the rosy radiance that follows a pleasant sexual encounter. The fact is, sex leaves its mark, not just on the mind but on the body as well. Researchers have begun to explore its effects on almost every part of the body, from the brain to the heart to the immune system. Studies are showing that arousal and an active sex life may lead to a longer life, better heart health, an improved ability to ward off pain, a more robust immune system and even protection against certain cancers, not to mention lower rates of depression.

But finding mechanisms for these benefits and proving cause and effect are no easy matter. "The associations are out there, so there has to be an explanation for it," says Dr. Ronald Glaser, director of the Institute of Behavioral Medicine Research at Ohio State University. In this article, we'll trace those associations, first discussing the biology of desire, then exploring how an active sex life benefits the body.

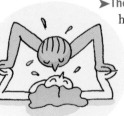

A HORNY HORMONE?

Oxytocin, a hormone released in the brain, may turn out to play a key role in the biology of sexual arousal

➤The Chemistry of Desire In human sexuality, mind, body and experience are endlessly intermingled. People find themselves turned on in obvious situations—slow-dancing together, seeing someone with a sexy body, finding a member of the opposite or same gender to be excitingly sharp-witted or funny. Yet no matter how lust is triggered, sex, like eating or sleeping, is ultimately biochemical, governed by hormones, neurotransmitters and other substances that interact in complicated ways to create the familiar sensations of desire, arousal, orgasm.

In the past decade or two, scientists have identified many of the pieces of this complex puzzle. It clearly involves testosterone, along with other hormones, including estrogen and oxytocin, and brain chemicals such as dopamine, serotonin and norepinephrine.

Scientists have also learned that the old notion that 90% of sex is in the mind is literally true: the parts of the brain involved in sexual response include, at the very least, the sensory vagus nerves, the midbrain reticular formation, the basal ganglia, the anterior insula cortex, the amygdala, the cerebellum and the hypothalamus (*see chart,* p. 129).

Desire is complex. Arousal, by contrast, is pretty straightforward: fill the penile arteries with blood or divert blood to the vagina and clitoris, and you're there. In men, a chemical that facilitates the blood flow is vasoactive intestinal polypeptide, a hormone that also directs the expansion and contraction of smooth muscles in the gastrointestinal tract.

But the primary chemical in charge of that function is nitric oxide. It's a vascular traffic cop, activating the muscles that control the blood vessels. If the mind is in the mood, or if a nitric-oxide-boosting drug such as Viagra or Levitra is in your body—you will respond.

Yet if there's one substance that

ultimately makes it possible to get turned on in the first place, testosterone is probably it. "When testosterone is gone," says Dr. Jennifer Berman, a urologist and director of the Female Sexual Medicine Center at UCLA, "for whatever reason—aging, medication—men experience erection and libido problems." Restore the testosterone and you usually fix those problems.

Women too seem to have problems getting interested in sex when their testosterone levels are too low, which is why Procter & Gamble is experimenting with testosterone patches. But estrogen may also be crucial to female desire, especially when used in tandem with testosterone.

Both testosterone and estrogen trigger desire by stimulating the release of neurotransmitters in the brain. These chemical are ultimately responsible for our moods, emotions and attitudes. And the most important of these for the feeling we call desire seems to be dopamine, which is at least responsible in part for making external stimuli arousing.

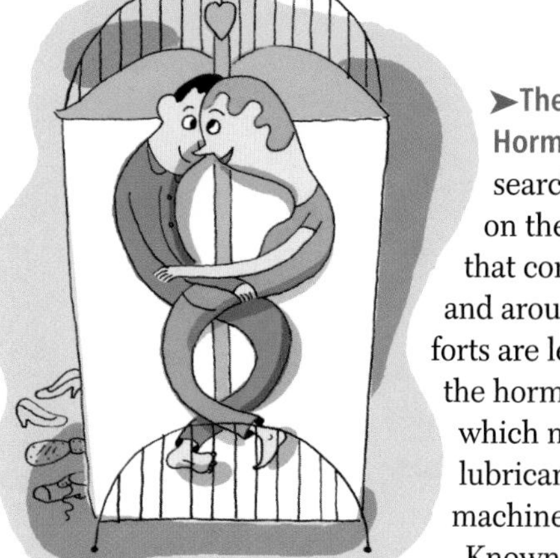

Another neurotransmitter almost certainly involved in the biochemistry of desire is serotonin, which, like dopamine, plays a role in feelings of satisfaction. Antidepressants like Prozac, which enhance mood by keeping serotonin in circulation longer than usual, can paradoxically depress the ability to achieve orgasm.

➤The Cuddle Hormone As researchers close in on the chemicals that control desire and arousal, their efforts are leading them to the hormone oxytocin, which may be the key lubricant for the machinery of sex.

Known for controlling the muscles of the uterus during childbirth, oxytocin surges up to five times as high as its normal blood level during orgasm. Studies in animals have also revealed oxytocin's softer side. It is responsible for helping individuals forge strong emotional bonds, earning its moniker as the cuddle hormone.

Released in the brain, oxytocin works in the blood, where it travels

LOVE POTIONS

Sex may be a natural act, but for the millions who suffer from sexual dysfunction, it can be vexingly unattainable. Below, a guide to some of the medical treatments available for what ails our libidos

OPTIONS	MEN	WOMEN
PRESCRIPTION THERAPIES JEAN PAUL CHASSENET—PHOTO RESEARCHERS	■ **Viagra, Levitra and Cialis** All these drugs work the same way, by relaxing smooth-muscle cells and widening blood vessels, primarily in the penis. Cialis stands out as more long-acting—up to 36 hours, compared with four or five hours for the others ■ **Testosterone** For men who don't produce enough, patches (Androderm, Testoderm) and gels (Androgel) deliver extra hormone through the skin ■ **Alprostadil** This vasodilating drug can be self-administered as an injection (Caverject) in the penis or inserted into the urethra as a suppository (MUSE)	■ **Testosterone** Doctors prescribe the hormone in lower doses than typically used for men, though it is not approved for this use by the FDA. Women can also take under-the-tongue drops specially formulated by pharmacies or use patches and gels ■ **Estrogen** Tablets (Vagifem), creams (Estrace, Premarin) and a silicone ring (FemRing) inserted into the vagina release estrogen to alleviate such symptoms of menopause as vaginal dryness ■ **Viagra and Levitra** Initial trials are not promising, but the drugs appear to work for some women
NONPRESCRIPTION THERAPIES	■ **Ginkgo Biloba** Better known as a memory enhancer, this herb is believed by some to improve blood flow to the body, including the penis. Conclusive scientific proof is lacking ■ **Ginseng** In the lab, ginseng has been shown to release nitric oxide, but there's no evidence to suggest that it improves erectile function ■ **L-Arginine** This naturally occurring amino acid is a precursor to nitric oxide and is believed to improve the flow of blood to the genitals	■ **Avlimil** The pill contains various plant leaves and roots and is touted as the female Viagra, but experts question its effectiveness ■ **Zestra** A botanical-oil lotion applied to the genitals can create a tingling sensation and enhance orgasm (breath mints or a few drops of Binaca on your partner's tongue during oral sex do the same) ■ **Xzite** A daily capsule, manufactured in Marina Del Rey, Calif., containing Chinese plant bark, flowers and roots; doctors at UCLA's Female Sexual Medicine Center say it works for many of their patients
DEVICES	■ **Penile Prostheses** These surgically implanted devices are still used by men who, for medical or physical reasons, don't respond to drugs	■ **Slightest Touch** UCLA doctors express high hopes for this device, which uses a set of electrodes to stimulate nerve pathways

S

to tissues as distant as the uterus, as well as along nerve fibers, where it regulates body temperature, blood pressure, wound healing and even relief from pain.

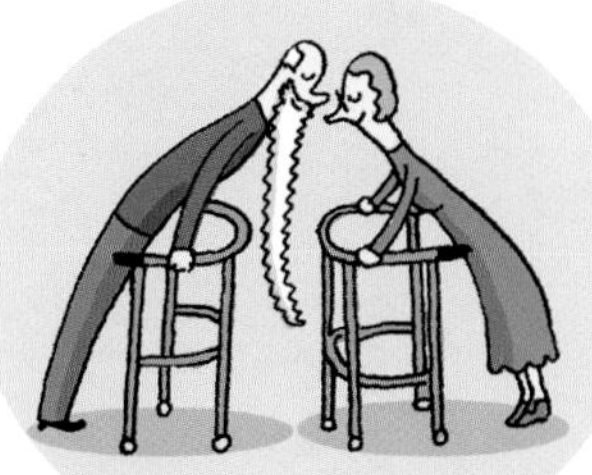

Although it is unlikely that oxytocin alone is responsible for sex's wide-ranging effects on the body, researchers hope that by tracking the hormone they can expose the network of body systems affected by sexual activity and clarify the connection between sex and good health. Here's what they have learned so far.

➤Sex and Fitness The single strongest case that can be made for the benefits of sex come from studies of aerobic fitness. The act of intercourse burns about 200 calories, the equivalent of running vigorously for 30 minutes. During orgasm, both heart rate and blood pressure typically double, all under the influence of oxytocin. It would be logical to conclude that sex, like other aerobic workouts, can protect against heart disease, but studies in support of this link have yet to be done. "Can we make the claim that having sex is equal to walking a mile or bicycling? We don't know," says Robert Friar, a biologist at Michigan's Ferris State University. "The data don't really exist."

At least not yet. A study conducted in Wales in the 1980s showed that men who had sex twice a week or more often experienced half as many heart attacks after 10 years as men who had intercourse less than once a month. The trial, however, did not include a parallel group of randomly chosen control subjects, the scientific gold standard. So it's unclear whether frequent intercourse was responsible for the lower rate of heart attacks or whether, for example, the men who were sexually active were healthier or less prone to heart disease to begin with.

Recent research has focused on the hormones dehydroepiandosterone and testosterone, both important for libido. They have been linked to reducing the risk of heart disease as well as protecting the heart muscle after an attack. That may explain why doctors maintain that sex after a heart attack is relatively safe.

➤Pain Control In the 1970s Dr. Beverly Whipple of Rutgers University identified the female G spot, the vaginal on-switch for female arousal, and stumbled upon one of oxytocin's more potent effects: its ability to dull pain.

Whipple showed that gentle pressure on the G spot raised pain thresholds 40% and that during orgasm women could tolerate up to 110% more pain. But she could not explain the link until the advent of

HOW YOUR BODY BENEFITS FROM SEX

Sexual activity affects you from head to toe. Here's what doctors have learned about its positive effects on health:

Heart Disease Lovemaking is good aerobic exercise that improves the circulation and works the heart. Sexually active people tend to have fewer heart attacks, possibly owing to their better fitness

Weight Intercourse can burn around 200 calories, not bad for a few minutes' work and far more entertaining than a 15-minute churn on a treadmill at the gym

Pain Endorphins released during orgasm can dull the chronic pain of backaches and arthritis as well as migraines

Depression Sexually active people appear to be less vulnerable to depression and suicide, perhaps because they are more comfortable with their sexuality

Anxiety Hormones released during arousal can calm anxiety, ease fear and break down inhibitions

Immunity Frequent intercourse may boost levels of key immune cells that help fight off colds and other infections

Cancer Early studies hint that oxytocin and the hormone DHEA, both released during orgasm, may prevent breast-cancer cells from developing into tumors

Longevity Frequent orgasm has been linked to longer life; this finding may have something to do with sex's beneficial effects on the heart and immune system

WHERE OUR SEX DRIVE COMES FROM

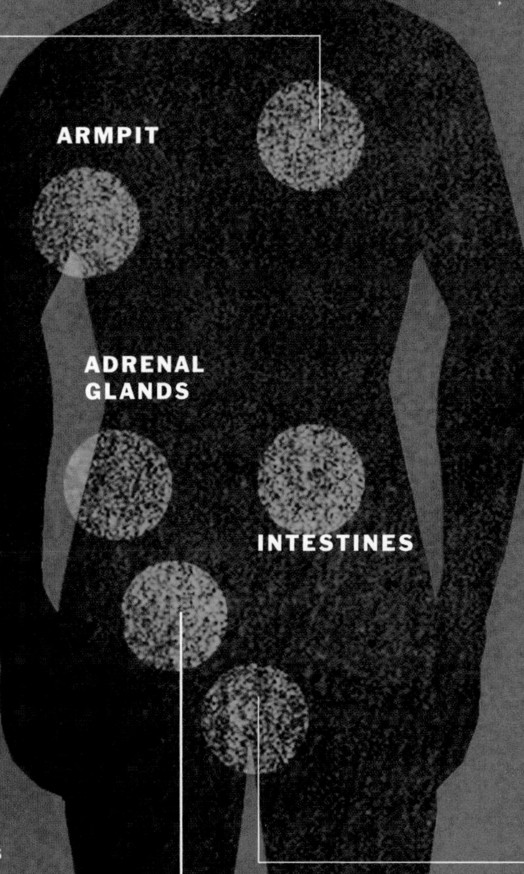

HEART AND BLOOD

Nitric Oxide

When you're turned on, cells in the genital area release this chemical, which causes blood vessels to dilate, increasing the flow of blood. Drugs like Viagra artificially stimulate nitric oxide release

Vasoactive Intestinal Polypeptide

Found in a man's intestines and brain, this protein works much like nitric oxide: it opens blood vessels to enhance erection and stimulate libido

Pheromones

Scientists believe these chemicals, produced in glands in the armpits, carry sexually stimulating signals that can be picked up—but only unconsciously—by others. Pheromones have been found in animals but have not yet been isolated in humans

Epinephrine/Norepinephrine

Found in the adrenal glands above the kidneys, in the nerves of the spinal cord and in the brain, these neurotransmitters play an important role in facilitating arousal and orgasm. They excite the body by giving it a shot of natural adrenaline, causing the heart to beat faster and blood pressure to rise

OVARIES

Estrogen

A hormone produced in the ovaries and the brain, estrogen regulates ovulation. It is also involved with making women, and maybe even men, feel desire, possibly by stimulating the release of the neurotransmitter dopamine

CENTRAL/MIDBRAIN

Dopamine

This is probably the most important neurotransmitter involved in desire. Dopamine-producing neurons in the central part of the brain color one's perception of the outside world, creating what is experienced as a sexy mood. Dopamine levels are highly correlated with desire

Serotonin

This neurotransmitter is produced in the midbrain and brain stem and helps one experience satisfaction, including the kind people feel after an orgasm. Serotonin can increase desire—most likely by working in concert with dopamine—but, paradoxically, serotonin-boosting drugs like Prozac can also make orgasm harder to achieve

Alpha Melanocyte Polypeptide

Produced in the pituitary gland, this hormone also acts as a neurotransmitter. Injecting one version of the chemical into male test subjects triggers erections

Oxytocin

Another hormone released by the pituitary gland, oxytocin helps activate milk production, uterine contractions during childbirth and pelvic shudders in orgasms. It also contributes to the feelings that bond parents to their children

TESTES

Testosterone

Small quantities of this hormone are made in the brain, but most of it is produced in the testes and ovaries; in women it is quickly converted into estrogen. For men, it's the key hormone of desire, creating feelings of positive energy and well-being. When it's depleted, both men and women experience low libido

Porn by the Numbers

Pornography was once furtively glimpsed at dimly lighted newsstands or seedy adult theaters. Today it is easily available, and while that has helped fostered a less repressive view of sexuality and put the spark back in many marriages, a growing number of psychologists and sociologists are concerned that porn's pervasiveness is transforming sexuality and relationships for the worse. Experts say men who frequently view porn may develop false expectations of women's appearance and behavior and have difficulty forming and sustaining relationships and feeling sexually satisfied. Meanwhile, porn exposes youngsters to false ideas about sexuality at a formative age. Some measures of our demand for porn:

■ Porn amounts to some 7% of the 3.3. billion Web pages indexed by Google

■ Americans rent upwards of 800 million pornographic videos and DVDs a year. Nearly 1 in every 5 rentals is a porn flick

■ Hollywood produces 400 feature films a year; the porn industry churns out 11,000

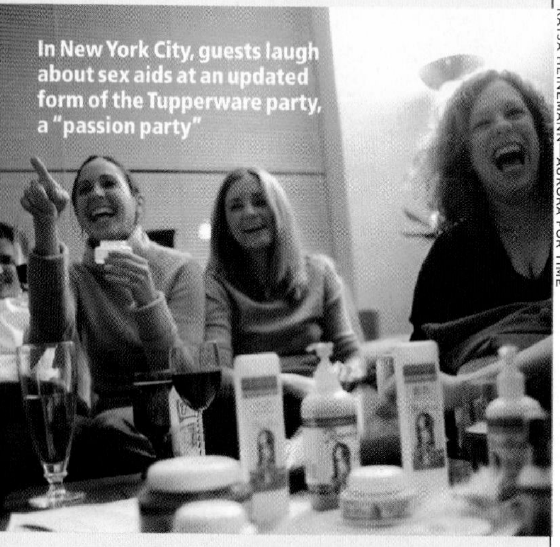

In New York City, guests laugh about sex aids at an updated form of the Tupperware party, a "passion party"

KATJA HEINEMANN—AURORA FOR TIME

■ In a 2001 poll by the Kaiser Family Foundation, 70% of 15-to-17-year-olds said they had accidentally found porn online

■ In the same poll, 59% of 15-to-24-year-olds said they believe seeing porn on the Internet encourages young people to have sex before they are ready; 49% said it promotes bad attitudes toward women and encourages viewers to think unprotected sex is O.K.

functional magnetic resonance imaging (fMRI). Using fMRI to view the brains of easily orgasmic women as they climaxed, either with visual stimuli or by self-stimulation, Whipple found that the body's pain-killing center in the midbrain is activated during peak arousal. Signals from this part of the brain instruct the body to release endorphins and corticosteroids, which can temporarily numb the raw nerve endings responsible for everything from menstrual cramps to arthritis and migraine for several minutes. Activating this region also reduces anxiety and has a calming effect.

LONGER LIFE VIA SEX?

A study of 3,500 Scottish men found a link between frequent intercourse and greater longevity

➤**Healing Power** A trial involving more than 100 college students in 1999 found that levels of immunoglobulin, a microbe-fighting antibody, in students who engaged in intercourse once or twice a week were 30% higher than in those who were abstinent. Curiously, those who had sex more than twice a week had the same levels as those who were celibate. Could there be an optimal rate of sexual frequency for keeping the body's defenses strong?

Researchers in Sweden are meanwhile exploring how sex affects another immunological function: the healing of wounds. Here again, oxytocin may lead the way. Using injections of oxytocin as a surrogate for arousal, Swedish investigators have found that sores on the backs of lab rats heal twice as fast under the influence of the hormone as without it.

To find out whether oxytocin has the same healing effect in people, Ohio State's Glaser and his wife Janice Kiecolt-Glaser, a psychologist at the same institution, are enrolling married couples in an unorthodox study in which each spouse's arm is blistered and then covered with a serum-collecting device. Over a 24-hour observation period, the couples discuss positive aspects of their marriage and mates as well as points of contention, such as finances and in-laws. The Glasers will analyze how levels of oxytocin change during these discussions, along with rates of healing.

➤**A Long, Happy Life** It's well known that married folk tend to live longer and suffer less depression than singles do. But is this because of more frequent sex, simple companionship or some benign aspect of personality that lends itself to marriage?

Teasing apart such matters is difficult, but sex itself appears to be a factor. A study of 3,500 Scottish men, for example, found a link between frequent intercourse and greater longevity. A much smaller study of elderly men found that those who masturbated appeared to experience less depression than those who did not.

In addition, frequent sexual activity has been tied to lower risk of breast cancer in women and prostate cancer in men. This relationship is still not fully understood but may involve some interaction between oxytocin and the sex hormones estrogen and testosterone and their roles in cell signaling and cell division. "Scientifically, it's an exciting time that will lead to a lot of rethinking and reconceptualizing of human sexuality," says Dr. John Bancroft, director of the Kinsey Institute. As the answers to the questions surrounding the biology of desire and the benefits of sex come in, we may begin to appreciate that the "sex glow" stays with us a lot longer than we realized.

■ **Resources**

NIH WEBSITE: *www.nlm.nih.gov/medlineplus/sexualhealthissues*

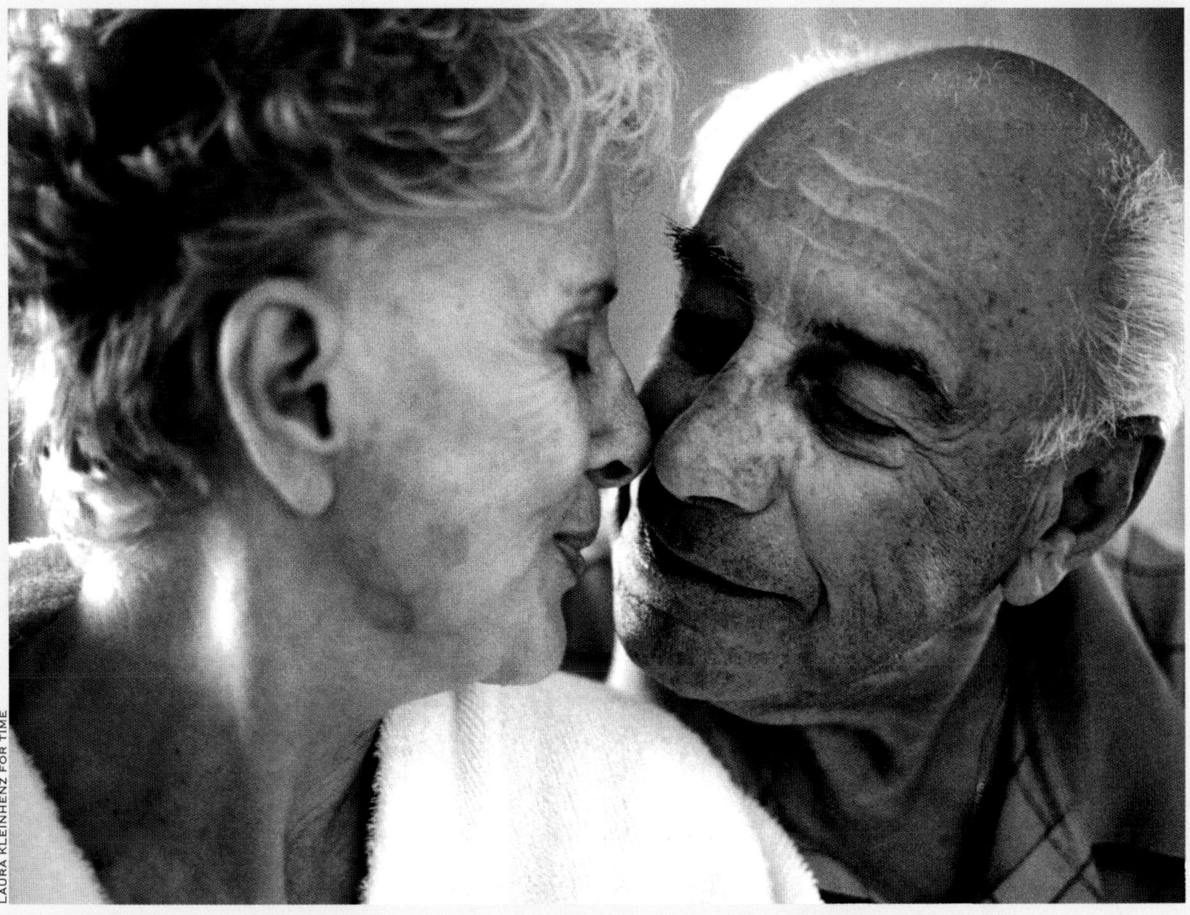
LAURA KLEINHENZ FOR TIME

As Baby Boomers Age, They Have a Question: Is There Sex After 60?

They are not yet eligible for Medicare, but you can tell from their sagging chins, receding hairlines and growing paunches that they are on the verge of major changes in mind and body. Yes, America's 77 million baby boomers are coming of age—old age. In 2006 the first offspring of the post–World War II generation (born from 1946 to 1964) will turn 60. What will that mean for the sons and daughters of the Age of Aquarius? Will passion diminish? Will performance decline or (gasp!) wither away?

Well, kids, check it out with any geezer you know who's receiving a Social Security check: the sexual impulse does not vanish with age, even if—how to say this delicately?—execution sometimes falters. There's plenty of evidence that healthy seniors, even residents of nursing homes, continue to have active sex lives. And why not? Without fear of an unwanted pregnancy—or worries about kids barging into the bedroom—older couples have much less reason to be uptight about sex. They are also much more likely to be adept at pleasing each other, knowing where and how to arouse.

So what's to fret about if you're only edging 60? Well, there are a few impediments. Erectile dysfunction, for example, is no joke; it afflicts about 1 of every 4 men over age 45 and half of all men over 75. Nowadays doctors can help many of them. Since Viagra's ballyhooed debut in 1998, the little blue pills and their progeny (Levitra and Cialis) have been doled out by the millions. They have been a boon for countless men (and, one hopes, their partners) while reducing demand for penile implants and other awkward mechanical aids.

Yet sexual dysfunction isn't just about male impotence. Both sexes experience failures as they age. And any number of health factors may be at fault, including poor circulation, diabetes, high blood pressure, heart disease, stress and alcoholism—to say nothing of the medications often prescribed for them. For women, the problem is often a decline in estrogen at menopause, usually around age 50. That may cause disconcerting hot flashes as well as dryness and a thinning of the vaginal wall that can make intercourse unpleasurable, if not painful. Production of the male sex hormone testosterone—which occurs in both sexes—also drops, and with that may come a diminished interest in sex.

Some doctors are prescribing testosterone as a libido booster for so-called low-T women, helping push testosterone sales to about $400 million annually. Variously given as a pill combined with estrogen or as a patch, cream or injection, testosterone remains unproven as a sex aid. Meanwhile, it can cause oily skin, unwanted facial hair, a lowered voice and an upsetting onslaught of sexual fantasies.

Most gerontologists recommend exercise and a healthy lifestyle as a far better route than hormones to prolonged sexual happiness. Says Dr. Jeffrey M. Drazen, editor in chief of the *New England Journal of Medicine:* "You're better off spending your money at a gym." ■

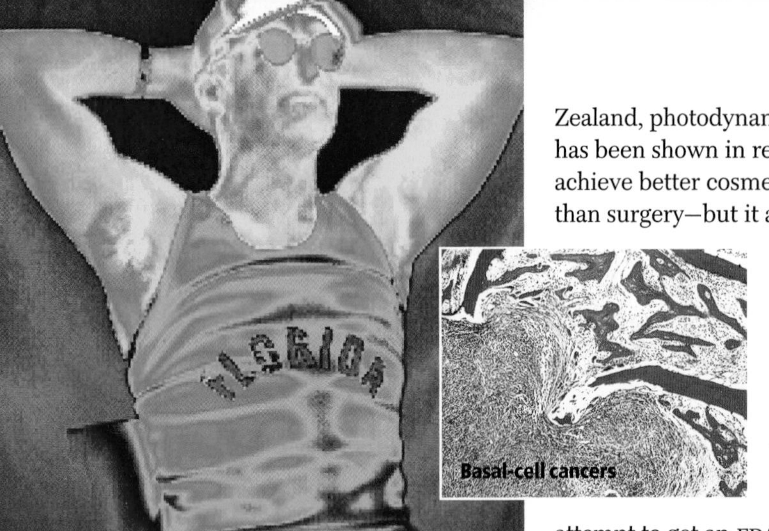

Basal-cell cancers

Skin Cancer

A new topical treatment helps clear up minor basal-cell cancers. Yet even minor skin lesions can lead to serious forms of cancer later on

On the Horizon The FDA is studying a new kind of treatment for skin cancers, in which medication within a skin cream is activated by exposure to laser light

Despite pleas from health experts to stay out of the sun, 1 million Americans are expected to develop skin cancer in 2004. The good news for die-hard sun worshippers is that treatments are improving. In July 2004, the FDA gave 3M Pharmaceuticals the go-ahead to market Aldara as a therapy for a common type of basal-cell carcinoma (BCC); it was the first topical treatment approved for BCC in 25 years. In trials, it cleared up cancerous lesions after three months for more than 80% of patients.

Though the new medication helps, it's no reason to throw common sun-sense to the wind. Aldara does not treat superficial BCC tumors larger in diameter than .8 in.; in those cases, surgery or other treatment will still be required.

Another new treatment for BCC may soon be available, but has not yet been approved by the FDA. Photodynamic therapy harnesses powerful cancer killers within a skin cream that are activated by exposure to a laser. Widely used in Europe, Australia and New Zealand, photodynamic therapy has been shown in recent tests to achieve better cosmetic results than surgery—but it also exposes patients to a greater risk of recurrence than more conventional approaches. Additional research is ongoing in an attempt to get an FDA green light for the photodynamic cream.

Why the concern over minor skin lesions? A 2003 study found that people who develop forms of skin cancer often considered harmless (such as BCC or squamous cell tumors) face a much higher risk of later developing more dangerous forms of skin cancer or deadly cancers in other parts of the body.

SUNNY-SIDE DOWN

Many skin cancers due to exposure to the sun may seem minor, but they can lead to more serious cancers later on

➤A New Gauge One tool for preventing skin cancer that already has been reformulated is the Federal Government's UV index, a measure of how much of the sun's skin-damaging rays reach the earth's surface on a given day. The new Global Ultraviolet Index was unveiled by the FDA and the National Weather Service in March 2004; it is a stricter standard intended to heighten our awareness of the need for caution when exposing ourselves to the sun.

For example, a Level 5 day, considered "moderate" on the old scale, is now rated "high." The index, which contains a new, "extreme category," brings U.S. reporting standards in line with similar yardsticks used around the world.

➤Instant George Hamilton At last, there's a safer alternative to reclining in the sun (or on a tanning bed) to achieve that golden-bronze look that Americans view as a badge of health and prosperity. The new tan comes in a can—an aerosol can. How does it work? A chemical solution that usually consists of aloe vera and dihydroxyacetone (DHA) —a sugar that reacts with the surface layer of skin cells, tinting them a light shade of brown—is applied either mechanically by sprayers inside a booth or by hand, via a device that resembles an airbrush.

The spray-on solution is completely harmless, and sessions cost as little as $15 for a real-looking tan that lasts about a week. Don't be fooled, though: spray-on tans do not offer any protection from the harmful rays of the sun, so a UV-resistant sunscreen is still strongly recommended for the can-tanned who venture outside on sunny days.

■ Resources

SKIN CANCER FOUNDATION SITE: *www.skincancer.org*

NIH WEBSITE: *www.nlm.nih.gov/medlineplus/sunexposure*

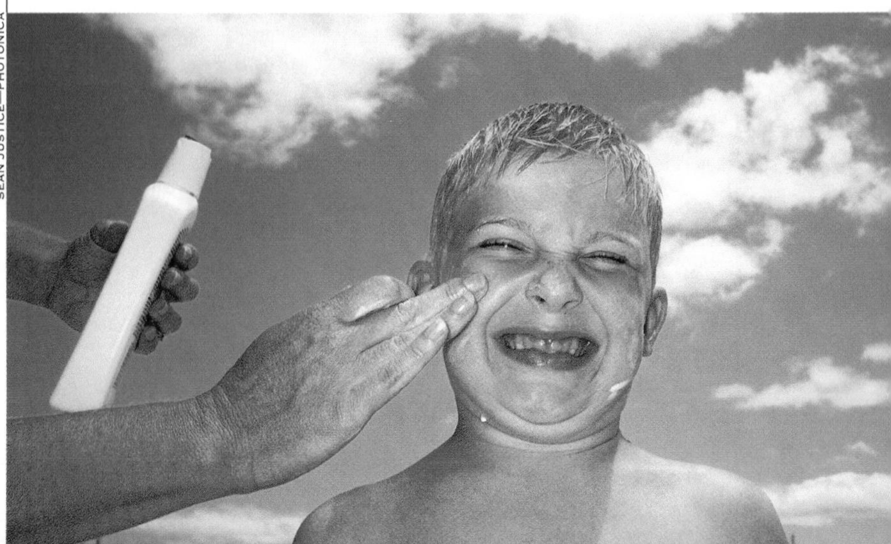
SEAN JUSTICE—PHOTONICA

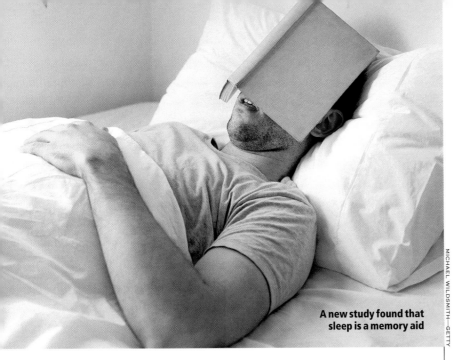
A new study found that sleep is a memory aid

MICHAEL WILDSMITH—GETTY

Sleep Disorders

The right mattress can improve your health, and a good night's sleep can improve your memory. But snoring isn't easy to stop

Goldilocks Was Right A study found that the best mattress for those with low-back pain was neither too firm nor too soft

Having trouble remembering your PIN? Try sleeping on it. Research has found that shut-eye improves recall. In a study, college students were asked to memorize a series of word sounds. Some were tested for their recall after being awake for 12 hours, others after 12 hours of slumber. The latter group was able to recall more sounds, leading the researchers to speculate that sleep may help etch things into our memory.

➤Mattress Matters Orthopedic physicians often recommend that patients sleep on firm mattresses to alleviate lower-back pain, but a recent study didn't concur. Subjects with chronic lower-back pain were assigned to either a firm or a medium-firm mattress to sleep on for three months. The result was good news for those of us who like a little give in our cribs: patients who slept on the medium-firm mattresses were twice as likely as those sleeping on firm ones to report reduced pain while lying in bed or getting up in the morning. They also had less disability associated with back pain and were less reliant on pain-killing drugs.

➤Too Much Sleep? Is there a quick fix for snoring? To find out, 40 volunteers tested three over-the-counter remedies: Snorenz (a lubricating spray), Breathe Right Strips (to enlarge nostrils) and the Snore-No-More (an ergonomic pillow). Sadly, none of the aids worked.

If a partner's snoring keeps you up, however, maybe you should be grateful. A 2004 study suggested that getting too much sleep may be harmful: test subjects who said they slept eight or more hours a night had a higher mortality rate than those who slept seven hours. As little as five or six hours of shut-eye didn't increase the risk of death from all causes, but death rates did rise in people getting less than 4.5 hours. Seven hours of sleep a night may be just about right.

■ Resources

NATIONAL CENTER ON SLEEP DISORDERS: *www.nhlbi.nih.gov/about/ncsdr*

Smallpox

Once wiped out, smallpox has returned as a potential terrorist tool. But some of those vaccinated for protection in 2003 were harmed

Payback The U.S. government has begun a program to compensate those harmed by the vaccine, used before the war with Iraq

When the possibility that Saddam Hussein might release smallpox against coalition troops during the Iraq war seemed troublingly real, the U.S. military undertook a major inoculation campaign. By June 2003, some 627,000 military employees and nearly 40,000 civilian first responders and health-care workers had been vaccinated. Although it now appears that Iraq did not have any stockpiles of smallpox, the news came too late for some. The civilian program reported close to 900 "adverse events" occurred within days of inoculation, including one confirmed death from the vaccine. The military has reported one death and 75 cases of heart inflammation caused by the vaccine.

In the summer of 2003, the Institute of Medicine, an independent agency that advises the Federal Government on health policy, concluded that widespread use of the smallpox vaccine would be both dangerous and unethical. In December, the U.S. Department of Health and Human Services launched a $42 million compensation program for those who were harmed by the vaccine.

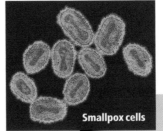

Smallpox cells

■ Resources

HHS COMPENSATION SITE: *www.os.hhs.gov/news/press/2003pres/20031212a.*

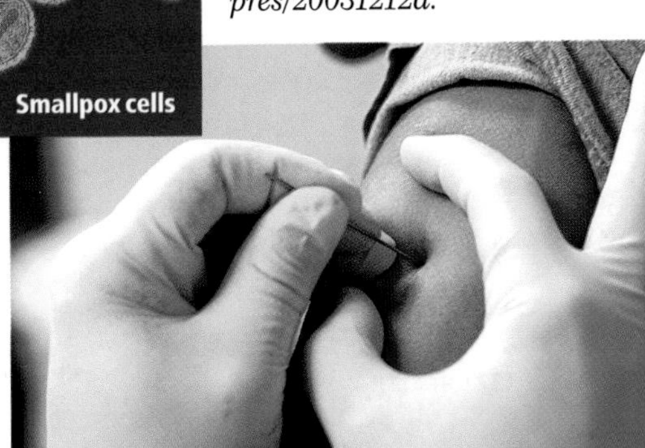

S

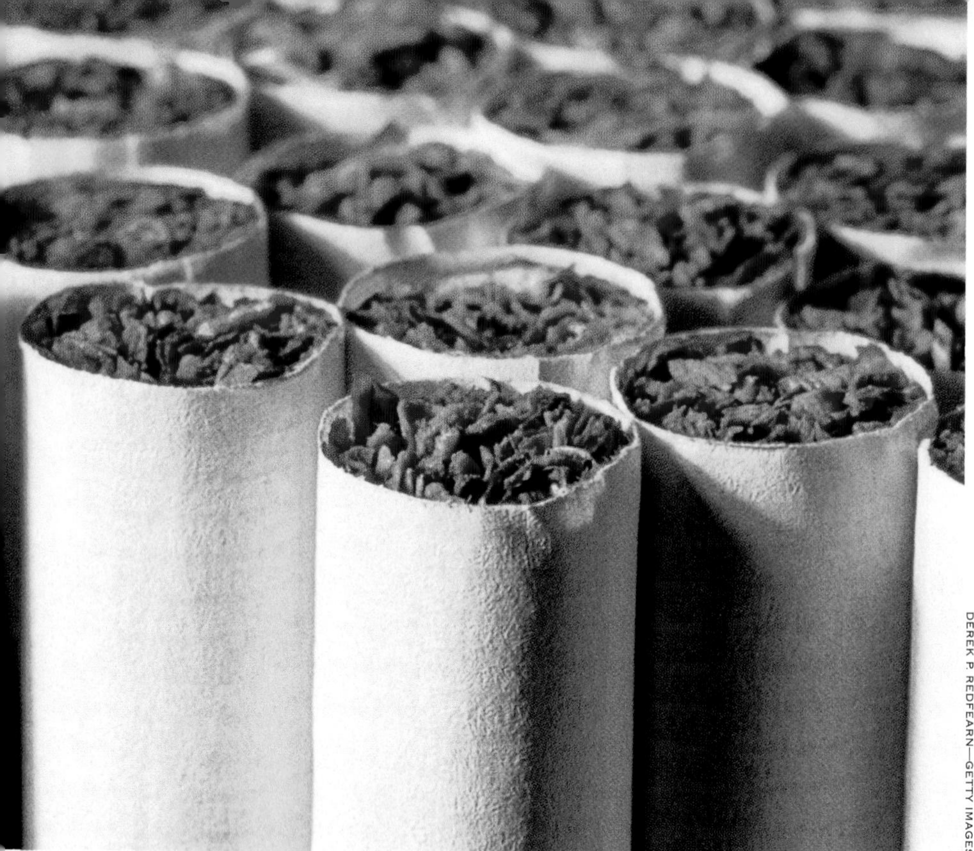

DEREK P. REDFEARN—GETTY IMAGES

Smoking

Fifty years ago in Britain, and 40 years ago in the U.S., doctors first warned us of tobacco's dangers. Some of us are slow learners ...

Second Hand News If you've ever complained about secondhand smoke and been accused of being overly sensitive—new research is on your side

A report issued by U.S. Surgeon General Richard H. Carmona in 2004 added several new maladies to the list of diseases believed to be caused by cigarette smoking: acute myeloid leukemia and cancers of the cervix, kidney, pancreas and stomach; abdominal aortic aneurysm; cataracts; periodontitis; and pneumonia. The report also suggested that smoking may be related to colorectal cancer, liver cancer, prostate cancer and erectile dysfunction.

This litany of ills only added to the existing list of diseases linked to smoking, which includes cancers of the bladder, esophagus, larynx, lung, mouth and throat, as well as chronic lung disease, chronic heart and cardiovascular disease, and reproductive problems. It adds up to more than 440,000 U.S. deaths each year—and more than 12 million since the first *Report on Smoking and Health* was issued in 1964.

➤**Grim Anniversaries** It's been 50 and 40 years, respectively, since British and U.S. medical experts first weighed in on the dangers of smoking. In July 2004, the *British Medical Journal* published a 50-year update of the massive research project on which its original paper was based. The longest smoking study ever, the British research calculated that cigarettes took an average 10 years off the lives of smokers who never quit. The study, which began in 1951 and ended in 2001, followed 35,000 male doctors and found that kicking the habit reduced mortality rates on a sliding scale. Quit at 60, and you gain three years of life; quit at 30, and it is almost as if you'd never smoked.

> **IT'S NEVER TOO LATE**
>
> Quit smoking at 60, and you may live three extra years; quit at 30, and it's almost as if you'd never smoked

Since the U.S. Surgeon General's office issued its 1964 report, the incidence of smoking among adult Americans has dropped, from 42% to 23%. That's good news, but it could be better—a lot better. The drop-off in smoking stalled in 1990 and has hardly budged since then. Surveys show that 70% of tobacco users want to quit yet struggle with this powerful addiction.

➤**Firsthand News About Secondhand Smoke** A small study conducted in Helena, Mont., yielded surprising results and provoked a new warning from the CDC about secondhand smoke. When the town passed an ordinance banning indoor smoking in 2002, Helena's only heart hospital recorded a 40% drop in the number of heart attacks (from an average of 40 every six months to just 24 in that city of 26,000). What's more, when a court order lifted the ban half a year later, the heart-attack rate bounced right back.

Dr. Robert Shepard, author of the Helena study, theorizes that the spike in heart-attack rates stems from the fact that secondhand smoke can make blood platelets stickier, causing clots and spasms within arteries, both of which can lead to heart attacks. Although the health risks posed by secondhand smoke had been documented previously, this new research showed that the damage may be both faster acting and more serious than previous studies suggested.

As a result, the CDC issued a new advisory in 2004, cautioning anyone at risk of heart disease to avoid entirely indoor public spaces where smoking is allowed. According to the new CDC warning, exposure to secondhand smoke for as little as 30 minutes can significantly increase the risk of heart attack.

Among the ramifications: some experts are convinced that the CDC will now have to revise upward its appraisal of the damage caused by secondhand smoke. Currently, the agency estimates that secondhand smoke leads to 35,000 deaths a year from heart disease in the U.S. But since 60% of Americans (smokers and nonsmokers) show biological effects from exposure to tobacco smoke, the effects of secondhand smoke may be more widespread than previously believed.

JUST SAY NO SMOKING

A new report found that the dangers posed by secondhand smoke are more serious than we had understood

About the only encouraging news from Helena was that city dwellers who have to pass through nicotine clouds every time they enter and leave an office building shouldn't worry too much: experts believe that exposure for a few seconds probably isn't harmful, because the toxins in cigarette smoke are quickly diluted in outside air.

➤Unsafe at Any Age Youth offers no protection against the health risks of cigarettes. Smokers under 40 are five times as likely to have a heart attack as their nonsmoking peers, according to a new study that analyzed WHO data from 21 countries. The study noted that about 80% of all heart-attack victims ages 35 to 39 were smokers and concluded that smoking in this age group causes 65% of nonfatal heart attacks in men and 55% of those in women.

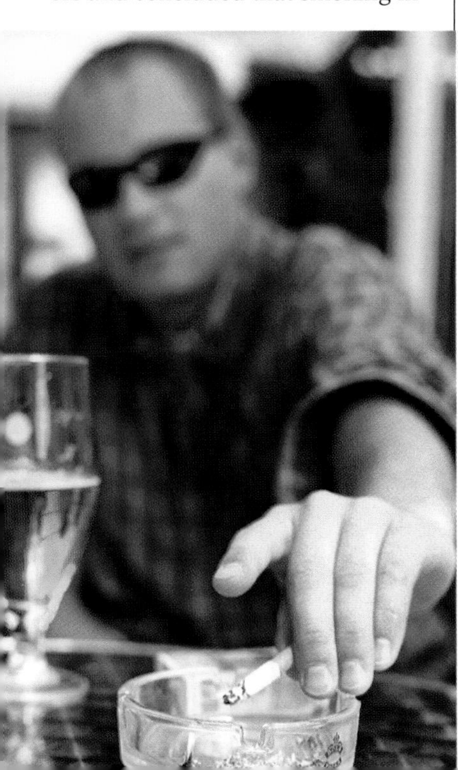

PROFIMEDIA—ALAMY

➤A Link to Drink Cigarettes and alcohol often share a barstool, and scientists believe they have found a physiological reason why: even a small amount of alcohol seems to significantly boost the pleasurable effects of nicotine. Researchers are testing drugs that can break this link, hoping to find a treatment that can help people kick both habits. That's good news, considering that 80% to 90% of alcoholics smoke, and alcoholism is 10 times as prevalent among smokers as among nonsmokers.

➤How to Beat the Habit What a lot of smokers don't realize is that the most popular method of quitting—simply stopping, a.k.a. going cold turkey—is the least effective. Studies show that getting intensive short-term counseling, taking drugs like Zyban (an antidepressant) or using one of the many nicotine aids (gum, patch, inhaler, nasal spray, lozenge) all double one's chance of success. Preliminary results suggest that combining these methods will increase success rates even more.

The good news: it's never too late to light up that last cigarette. As the years go by, an ex-smoker's risk of heart disease and stroke diminishes until it's close to that of a person who has never smoked. Unfortunately, an ex-smoker's risk of getting lung cancer never quite gets down to what it would have been without smoking. But even here, there is a subtle, if chilling, benefit: former smokers respond better to chemotherapy than patients who are still lighting up as they fight cancer.

■ Resources

NATIONAL CANCER INSTITUTE SITE: *cis.nci.nih.gov/fact/3_14.htm*

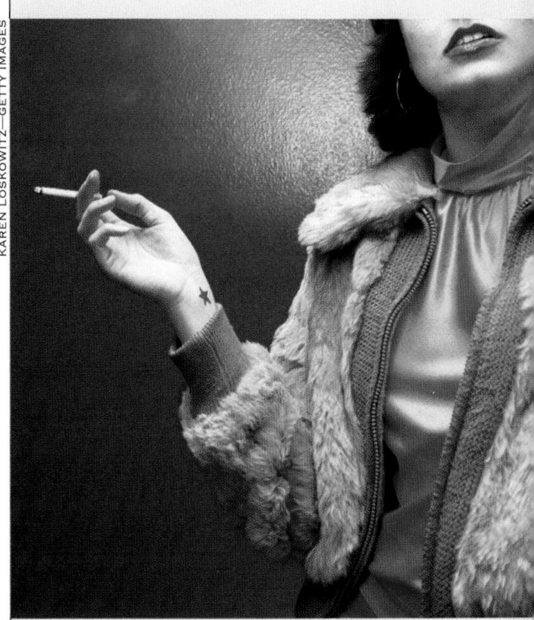

KAREN LOSKOWITZ—GETTY IMAGES

Damsels in Distress

Here's news for women who may need just one more reason to quit smoking: a new study suggested that women who smoke are twice as likely as male smokers to develop lung cancer. Using computed tomography (C.T.) scanning, researchers studied nearly 3,000 male and female smokers 40 and older. Not surprisingly, they found that the risk of developing lung cancer increased with the amount smoked as well as with age. Yet even independent of those two variables, the study found, women smokers still had double the cancer risk of men.

Breast cancer may be another smoking-related risk unique to women. The Surgeon General's 2004 report on smoking noted that while there is not enough evidence to establish a definite causal link between smoking and breast cancer, there does appear to be a relationship, especially in women with a genetic predisposition to breast cancer. The reasons for both of these elevated levels of risk remain unclear, but the prescription—quitting now—is not.

American women are not alone in facing graver risks from smoking. A separate report warned that the increase in lung-cancer deaths among U.S. women may soon be repeated in Asia and Africa, where taboos against women's smoking are weakening. The report called for further studies of the emerging links between smoking and gender. ■

S

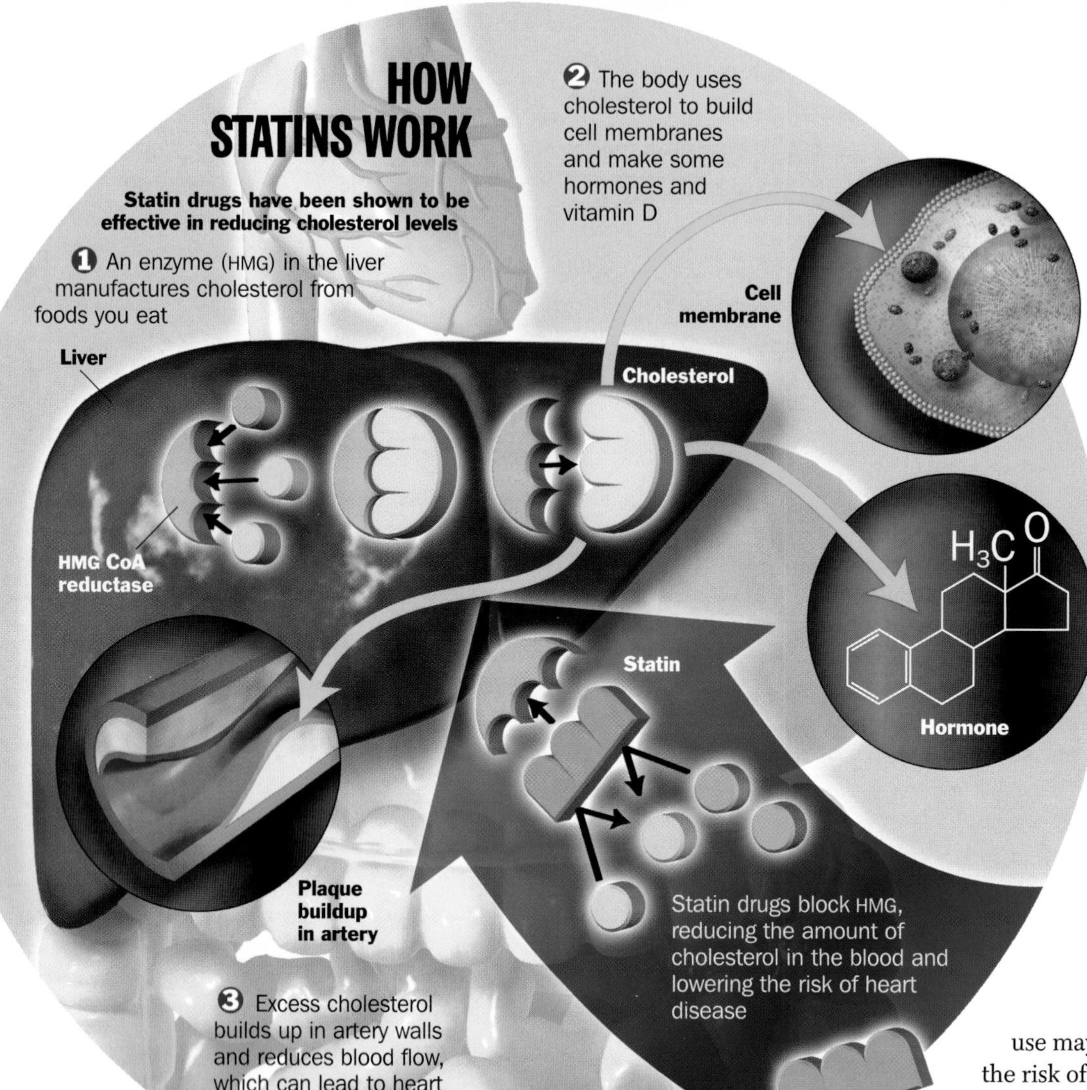
HOW STATINS WORK
Statin drugs have been shown to be effective in reducing cholesterol levels
1 An enzyme (HMG) in the liver manufactures cholesterol from foods you eat
Liver
HMG CoA reductase
2 The body uses cholesterol to build cell membranes and make some hormones and vitamin D
Cell membrane
Cholesterol
H_3C
O
Hormone
Statin
Statin drugs block HMG, reducing the amount of cholesterol in the blood and lowering the risk of heart disease
Plaque buildup in artery
3 Excess cholesterol builds up in artery walls and reduces blood flow, which can lead to heart disease
TIME Diagram by Joe Lertola

Statins

Move over, aspirin: statins are the wonder drugs of the new century. Their ability to lower cholesterol is only the beginning of their benefits

Full-Body Workout Statins may help treat ailments ranging from those of the eyes to the joints. They lower the risk of glaucoma; offer relief from arthritis; and help fight adult macular degeneration

Imagine a drug that effectively treats one of the leading killers confronting medical science, causes few side effects and shows promise as a therapy for more than a dozen other serious diseases. Some cardiologists joke that statins should be added to the water supply. Others aren't kidding when they suggest that everyone over age 55 could benefit by taking these drugs, which work by limiting the production of cholesterol in the liver.

What aspirin was for generations—an all-purpose miracle drug used to treat dozens of ailments—statins are arguably poised to become. Although statins have helped millions of heart patients lower their cholesterol level, evidence is piling up that they can help in numerous other ways as well. New studies show that in addition to lowering cholesterol levels, statins may also fight heart disease by reducing potentially dangerous inflammatory reactions in heart arteries. One 2004 study found that long-term statin use may lower the risk of glaucoma; another suggested that the drugs may offer relief from rheumatoid arthritis; a third found that statins may also help treat adult macular degeneration (AMD), the most common cause of irreversible blindness among older adults.

Other studies have indicated that statins may help prevent various types of cancer (including breast cancer) and that diabetes patients who take the drugs could cut their risk of stroke by half while reducing the likelihood of heart attacks by more than a third. (A separate study has found that the anti-stroke benefits extend to people without diabetes.) Ongoing research is exploring the potential of statins to treat or prevent such conditions as osteoporosis, multiple sclerosis and Alzheimer's.

WRITE YOUR OWN ...

In Britain statins are now classified as over-the-counter remedies; thus, no prescription is needed to buy them

➤**Who Benefits?** One piece of sobering news is that statins don't affect everyone the same way. A new study found the statin Pravachol was as much as 22% less effective in patients with two common variations in one of 10 genes involved in cholesterol metabolism. But even this small dark cloud held a silver lining: the findings suggested that doctors may someday be able to test patients' genes to determine in advance who will benefit most from the drugs.

➤**Untapped Potential** At least for now, the principal benefit that statins offer is their ability to lower cholesterol. Even this potential, though, seems barely to have been tapped—though statins now outsell all other classes of prescription drugs. In July 2004, U.S. health officials lowered the recommended cholesterol target levels, setting aggressive new goals that put almost 10 million more Americans into a category for whom statins are recommended *(see* Cholesterol). Officials estimate that less than half of all Americans who could benefit from statins take them.

➤**A New Leader** In July 2004, the FDA approved a new cholesterol medicine, Vytorin, which is a combination of two existing drugs, Zocor and Zetia. Zocor is a statin that suppresses the liver's production of cholesterol. Zetia is the first in a new class of drugs that work by preventing the absorption of cholesterol in the intestines. Together, they form a one-two punch that limits the amount of cholesterol made within a patient's body while blocking dietary cholesterol. The combined drug has been shown in clinical trials to lower cholesterol even more than the market leader, Lipitor, which accounts for almost half of all statin sales in the U.S.

➤**Safe for Kids ...** A two-year study published in the summer of 2003 suggested that children born with a genetic predisposition toward dangerously high cholesterol levels can lower their cholesterol safely by using statins. Researchers noted a one-fourth drop in cholesterol levels among young test subjects—and a reversal of the artery-narrowing effects of the disease, which occurs in one out of every 500 births—with no serious side effects.

Longer-term studies are needed to demonstrate conclusively that statins don't pose health risks for children, but this one is a relief to parents who have grappled with the difficulties of the only other anticholesterol therapy available for children: resin pills. These are less effective than statins, require up to six doses each day and can lead to side effects like constipation.

Gugul-plex

Gugul (short for gugulipid and no relation to Google.com) is a natural extract of the sap of an Indian myrrh tree that has been valued throughout Asia for 2,500 years for use in medicine. A folk remedy for obesity and arthritis, it is also used to make perfume and incense. In 2002, the list of maladies that gugul might help treat appeared poised to grow longer by one significant item: research in mice suggested that it could lower cholesterol as much as 12%.

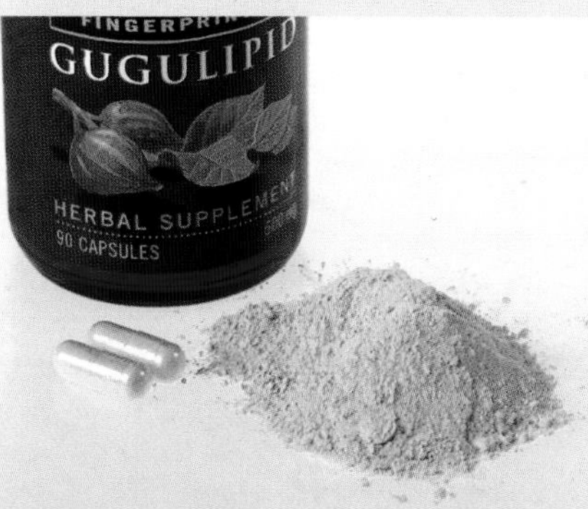

But a separate study, published in 2003, found that the herb not only failed to reduce cholesterol readings in human test subjects but also raised the amount of LDL, the bad cholesterol, as much as 5 points in some patients.

That wasn't the only bad news. Nine of the 67 people who participated in the trial also developed an itchy red skin rash over much of their bodies, though differences in genetics or diet may have been a factor in these cases. For now, don't drop statins for tree resin. ■

➤**... But Less Effective for Women** Research published in August 2004 suggested that women derive less benefit from statins than do male heart patients with a similar risk profile (e.g., age, weight, blood pressure and cholesterol level). The culprit, however, may not be the medication, but the fact the women generally face a slightly lower overall risk of heart attack than men.

➤**Over-the-Counter Statins** In May 2004, the U.K. became a statin island when British regulators approved Zocor as an over-the-counter (rather than prescription) medication. With statins draining more than $1.2 billion each year from Britain's National Health Service (which covers prescriptions but not OTC purchases), the move may have had as much to do with the bottom line as medical merits. Further such approvals are in the pipeline in Britain, and manufacturers (delighted because sales jump when drugs are easier to purchase) plan to apply for similar approvals in the U.S. before the end of the year 2004.

TAKA

■ Resources

NIH WEBSITE: *www.nhlbi.nih.gov/chd/meds1.html*

S

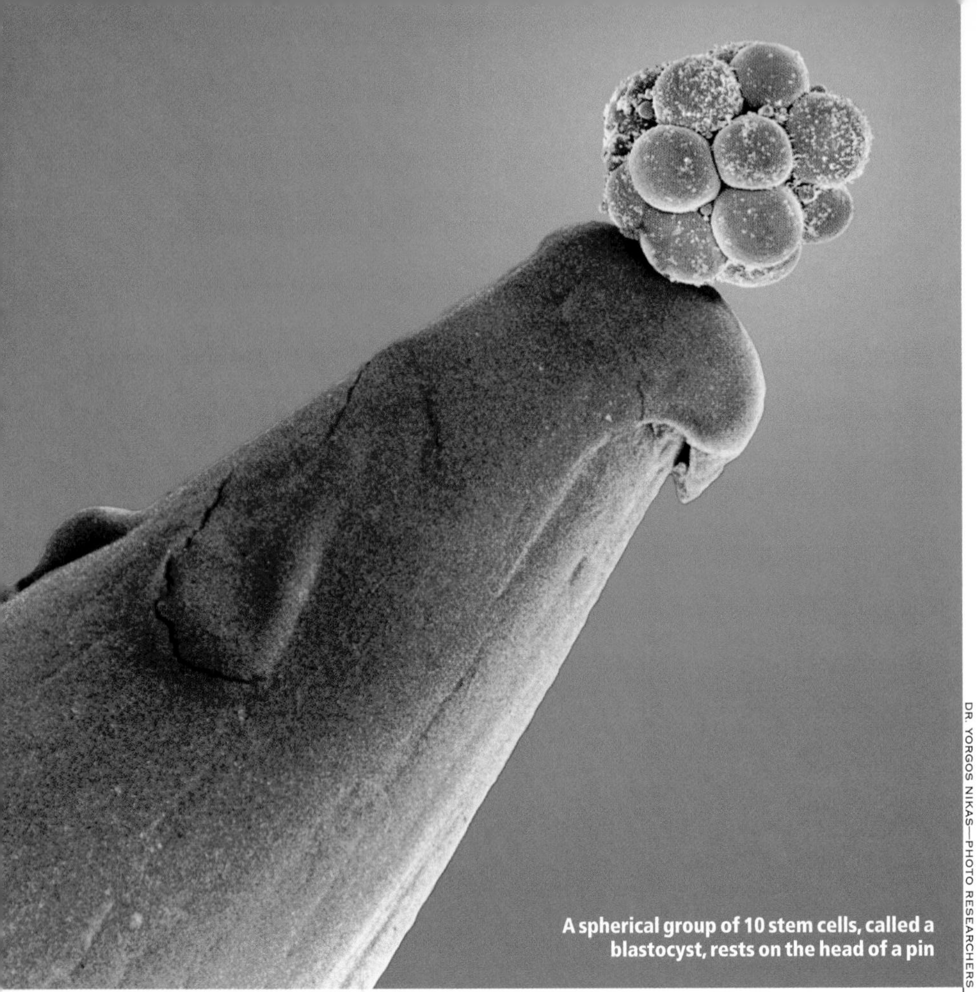

A spherical group of 10 stem cells, called a blastocyst, rests on the head of a pin

DR. YORGOS NIKAS—PHOTO RESEARCHERS

Stem Cells

Debate rages over the medical use of this raw material from which cells in human embryos develop hearts, eyes, teeth and other organs

Ethical? Stem cells for research come from various sources, including therapeutic cloning, but since each source involves intervening with a form of potential human life, many people oppose such research

Election-year politics and fresh news from the lab put the battle over the ethics of using human stem cells in medical research back on the front pages in 2004.

On the scientific front, advances ranged from the cosmetic but-potentially lucrative to the truly significant. In the first category, separate research teams figured out how to use stem cells to grow hair and teeth in laboratory animals. In more important developments, discoveries may lead to new treatments for some of the most serious human illnesses—as when two teams of scientists published research showing that stem cells can repair damaged tissues in the heart and brain.

Even advances that fell somewhere between these extremes managed to startle, if only because they broadened the frontiers of medicine in unexpected ways. In August 2004, a team of German doctors announced they had used stem cells to grow a replacement jaw bone in the shoulder of a man whose mandible (lower jaw) had been surgically removed because of mouth cancer.

But while the science of stem cells moved ahead with breathtaking dispatch, the ethics of using such cells crawled and plodded with agonizing hesitation. The Bush Administration's 2001 ban on federally funded research using any human stem-cell lines, other than those existing at the time of the policy's announcement, remained in force. (Only 19 of the supposed 78 lines turned out to be available, thus choking off most federal research funds to the field.)

In 2004, despite appeals by 58 Senators, 206 members of Congress and Nancy Reagan—who was convinced that the Alzheimer's disease that took her husband's life might have been beaten back by stem-cell research—the policy remained unchanged, even though a poll released in June showed that 3 out of 5 Americans favor stem-cell research.

Although the federal guidelines

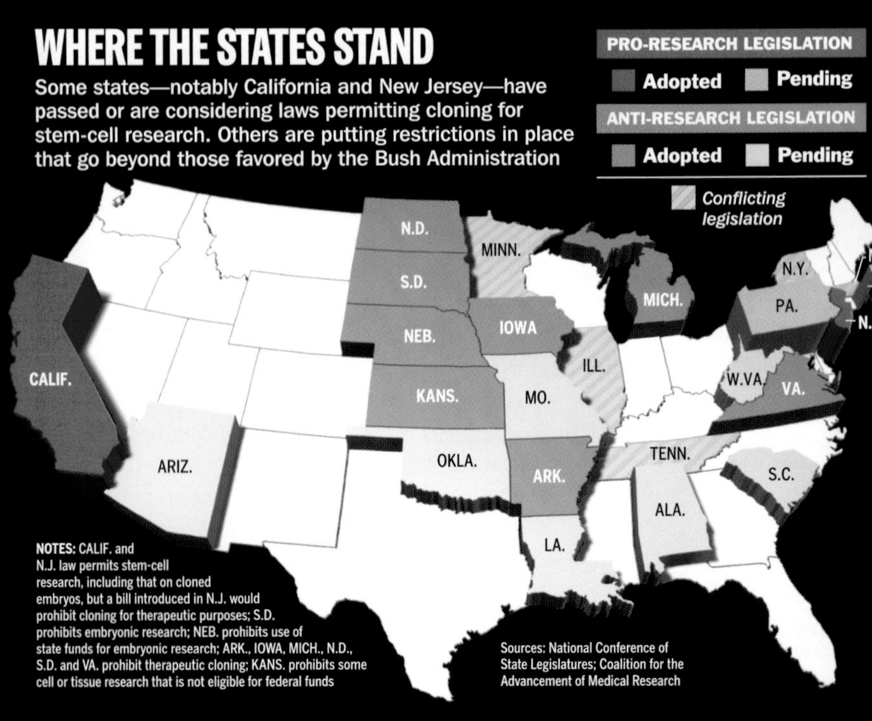

WHERE THE STATES STAND
Some states—notably California and New Jersey—have passed or are considering laws permitting cloning for stem-cell research. Others are putting restrictions in place that go beyond those favored by the Bush Administration
PRO-RESEARCH LEGISLATION
Adopted
Pending
ANTI-RESEARCH LEGISLATION
Adopted
Pending
Conflicting legislation
N.D.
MINN.
S.D.
N.Y.
MICH.
PA.
NEB.
IOWA
N.J.
CALIF.
ILL.
W.VA.
VA.
KANS.
MO.
TENN.
OKLA.
ARIZ.
ARK.
S.C.
ALA.
LA.
NOTES: CALIF. and N.J. law permits stem-cell research, including that on cloned embryos, but a bill introduced in N.J. would prohibit cloning for therapeutic purposes; S.D. prohibits embryonic research; NEB. prohibits use of state funds for embryonic research; ARK., IOWA, MICH., N.D., S.D. and VA. prohibit therapeutic cloning; KANS. prohibits some cell or tissue research that is not eligible for federal funds
Sources: National Conference of State Legislatures; Coalition for the Advancement of Medical Research

remain in place, new initiatives at the state level (and abroad) may make them irrelevant. By mid-2004, California and New Jersey had passed laws specifically authorizing the cloning of human eggs to create stem cells (so-called therapeutic cloning), and the legislatures of seven other states, including Illinois and New York, were considering similar bills. California was preparing a ballot measure authorizing up to $3 billion in state funding for stem-cell research over 10 years, which would dwarf federal outlays, which currently hover around $17 million annually.

Harvard and Stanford universities also announced that they were launching stem-cell research centers, for which they hoped to raise $100 million each.

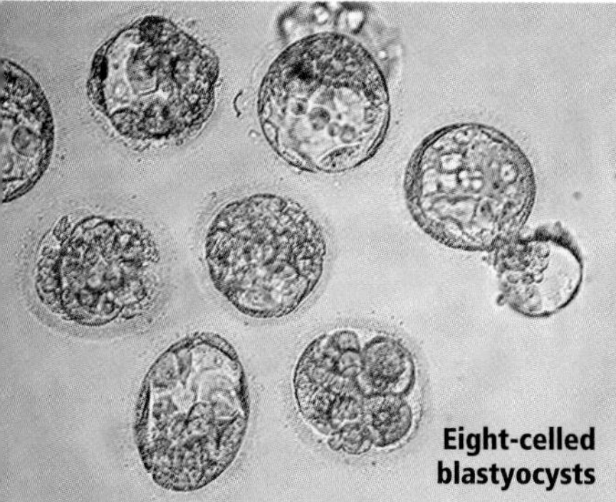
Eight-celled blastyocysts

AFP—GETTY IMAGES

All of which may (or may not) come just in time to prevent America's lead in stem-cell research from migrating overseas. One prominent U.S. researcher moved to Britain in 2004, where stem-cell research is encouraged—and where, in May 2004, medical authorities opened the world's first stem-cell "bank," which will cultivate, store and supply stem-cell lines for research. This initiative, coming just a few months after the stunning news that a South Korean research team had succeeded in creating a new stem-cell line from a cloned human embryo, left many American scientists feeling they were at a competitive disadvantage but determined to catch up.

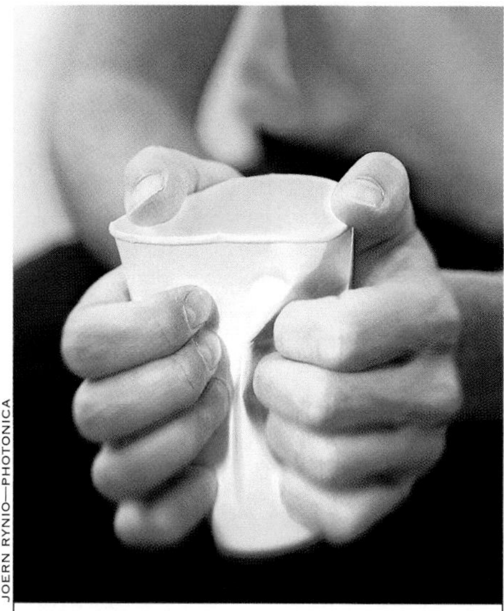

JOERN RYNIO—PHOTONICA

Stress

Anxiety can make us mentally tense and unhappy, but new research shows that stress actually causes changes in our immune systems

Take Charge To beat stress, experts say, you should confront it head on rather than seeking ways to compensate for it. Smoking or eating too much only builds more stress

Researchers conducting a new analysis of more than 300 previous studies involving some 19,000 subjects of stress arrived at some surprising conclusions. They found that modern stresses prompt complex reactions beyond the simple fight-or-flight response, the primordial motivator that sends your heart racing and pumps up your blood pressure. In particular, they found that stress triggers a variety of changes in the immune system—some beneficial, some decidedly less so—depending on how long the stress lasts and whether an end to it is in sight.

> **INVASION STRATEGIES**
>
> **The immune systems of patients switched on under high stress, as if their bodies had been invaded by infection**

When test subjects were asked to speak in public or do mental math in the lab, the tasks tended to mobilize their fast-acting immune response, the body's all-purpose defense system for fending off infection and healing wounds. Compared with controls, people subjected to such short-term stresses had up to twice as many natural killer cells in their blood, ready to fight the early stages of infection.

Short-term stressors faced with high stakes, like the SATs or the bar exam, appeared to hinder the immune response by suppressing Th1 cells, which normally activate killer cells and wound-healing chemicals called cytokines. This suppression can also boost the concentration of Th2 cells, which produce antibodies and can make allergies worse.

Chronic stress agents that alter a person's role in society or sense of self and show no sign of ending, such as unemployment, permanent disability or the need to care for a parent with dementia, are bad news. They have significantly negative effects on almost all immune functions.

Do people subjected to such stresses actually get sick? There have been surprisingly few studies to test that theory, but research on long-term hardship at work finds that stress is associated with an increase in heart disease. Other studies found that people suffering chronic stress on the job or in relationships are at least twice as likely to get sick from a cold or flu.

Experts suggest that those subject to stress apply management strategies that anyone can adopt. For example, avoid situations that you know cause stress. Discuss problems with friends, family or a mental-health professional before they become overwhelming. Face stress head on, and don't resort to coping mechanisms like smoking, eating more or exercising less; that only adds to the strain. And remember: you can't avoid stress altogether, but you can learn to keep it at bay.

■ **Resources**

NIMH WEBSITE: *www.nlm.nih.gov/medlineplus/stress.html*

S

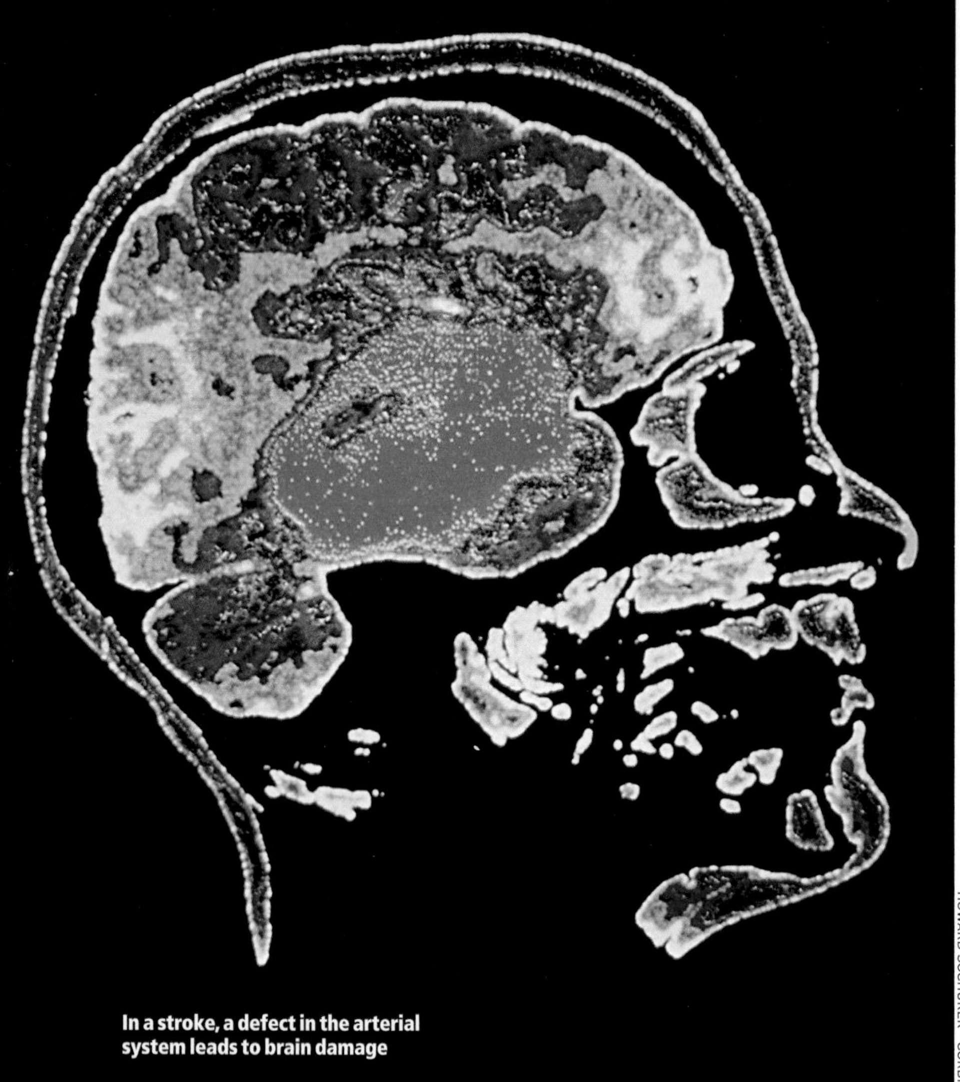
In a stroke, a defect in the arterial system leads to brain damage

HOWARD SOCHUREK—CORBIS

Stroke

Research reveals new ways to predict and prevent stroke, while doctors are finding better ways to help victims cope with life after one of these crippling brain seizures

What Is It? In a stroke, the arteries that supply blood to the brain either burst or are blocked, killing brain tissue and leading to subsequent loss of nerve and muscle control, often on one side of the body

Every 45 seconds, someone in America has a stroke; every three minutes, someone dies of one. That translates into 700,000 strokes and 165,000 deaths each year, making ischemia (the technical term for the most common type of stroke) the nation's No. 3 killer. (It's also the No. 1 reason America's elderly check into nursing homes.) Even among survivors, strokes can exact a terrible toll: after-effects range from difficulty walking, speaking and carrying out the everyday activities of life to depression and paralysis. Happily, new diagnostic tools are helping doctors better sort out the two major types of stroke, which require diametrically opposing treatments. Strokes caused by blood clots require clot-busting, or blood-thinning approaches, while strokes originating from burst vessels necessitate blood thickening agents.

A COMMON KILLER

Stroke is the No. 3 cause of death in the U.S. and the No. 1 reason senior citizens enter nursing homes

➤Prevention The best medicine, of course, is to prevent strokes from happening in the first place, and the prescription is clear. If you have high blood pressure, reduce it. If your cholesterol level is high, lower it. If you smoke, stop. If you drink, do so moderately. If you're overweight, try to drop a few pounds. If you are sedentary, exercise. These steps may sound difficult but consider the payoff: while reducing your risk of stroke, each of these measures will also reduce your risk of a heart attack.

➤Hidden Signs Strokes seem to come on with a frightening suddenness, but research published in the journal *Stroke* in January 2004 suggested that subtle signs may be measurable as much as 10 years before a stroke occurs. The finding arose from a study of 2,175 men and women ages 33 to 88 with no history of stroke or dementia. Researchers found that the risk of stroke increased—as indicated by variables like age, blood pressure, diabetes, smoking status and history of heart disease—in tandem with a decline in the subjects' cognitive functions, perhaps owing to minuscule changes in the brain.

➤Early Surgery A study published in May 2004 indicated that patients at risk of a stroke may benefit from having a carotid endarterectomy (traditional surgery to clear obstructions from the carotid artery, the vessel in the neck that carries blood to the brain) before the problem becomes urgent. More than 3,100 test subjects with partially blocked carotid arteries—a major risk factor for stroke—were divided into groups: those who elected to have the surgery early and those who waited until it was imperative. At the end of the study, 12% of the group who had deferred their surgery suffered strokes (about half of them fatal or resulting in serious disability), while only 6% of the patients who had opted for early surgery suffered strokes.

➤Poststroke Therapy Alexia, or a

loss of the ability to read, can be among the most heartbreaking after-effects of a stroke, amping up a patient's feelings of loss, isolation and dependence on others. Studies have shown that as many as 1 in 5 patients suffers from at least some loss of written or verbal communication skills within six months of suffering a stroke.

An experimental new technique, still being tested, may offer hope to stroke victims who suffer from alexia. The new therapy, "tactile-kinesthetic reading," teaches patients to recognize written words anew by tracing the shapes of letters on the palms of their hands. This practice seems to have the effect of rerouting the sensory input to the cerebral pattern-recognition centers of the brain while avoiding areas of the brain damaged by stroke. It's much too early to draw final conclusions from these initial experiments, but early results are promising, and research into this "touchy-feely" therapy for alexia is ongoing.

STARTING OVER

By tracing the shapes of letters on the palms of their hands, stroke victims rewire their brains to read again

■ Resources

AMERICAN STROKE ASSOCIATION
SITE: *www.strokeorganization.org*

To the Rescue: Vampire Bats, Corkscrews and Other Stroke Busters

The key to treating stroke is speed, as evidenced by the American Stroke Association's slogan: "Time lost is brain lost." The goal of treatment is to stop the death of brain tissue that results as its vital oxygen supply is shut off, whether by a blood clot or a burst artery, as soon as possible. The clot-busting drug TPA (tissue plasminogen activator), for example, has to be delivered within a critical treatment window that closes about three hours after the symptoms of stroke first appear.

The most exciting research presented at the 29th International Stroke Conference, held in San Diego in February 2004, consisted of advances aimed at opening that critical window a little wider. Among the new developments:

Cooler Heads

Researchers know lower temperatures protect the brain from injury, but cooling the brain usually cools the rest of the body as well, including the heart and immune system—and that's not favorable to victims fighting the first stages of a stroke.

In San Diego, a Japanese team reported that a helmet using a liquid-cooling technology developed by NASA and designed to cool only the head, not the rest of the body, shows great promise as a way to reduce the severity of neural damage in stroke.

The researchers hope such a helmet may someday be used by emergency medical personnel to slow the progression of a stroke and lengthen the time a patient is eligible for clot-busting therapy.

Vampire Bats

Paging Count Dracula! As the wily Transylvanian surely knows, nature has provided blood-sucking bats with a nifty little mechanism to keep their food supply fresh: a chemical in their saliva resists the process of blood clotting, keeping a victim's blood flowing. The chemical, desmoteplase, can also be used to dissolve clots; now researchers have developed a synthetic version of the compound that is so effective it can extend the time window for stroke treatment in some patients from three hours to as many as nine.

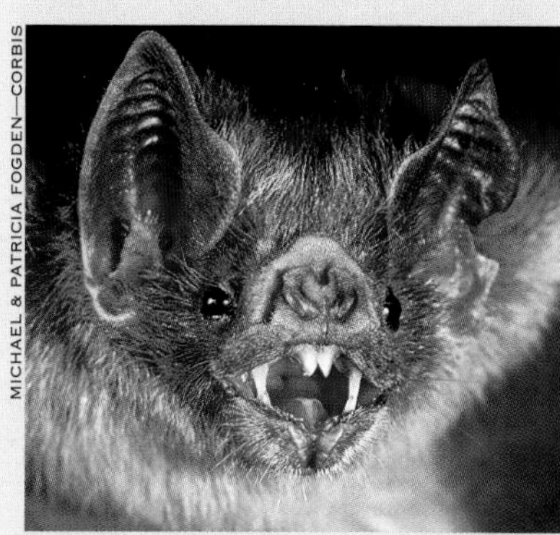
MICHAEL & PATRICIA FOGDEN—CORBIS

The Corkscrew

The most direct approach to fighting a clot-based stroke is to break up the offending clot, but doing so involves a risk: the clot may break into smaller particles that then lodge deeper in the brain. In August 2004 the FDA approved a new device, the Merci Retriever (Merci is an acronym for "mechanical embolus removal in cerebral ischemia"). This tiny corkscrew device, housed in a thin catheter, can snag blood clots and pull them out of an artery without disrupting them—stopping stroke damage almost immediately.

In tests at 25 medical centers around the U.S. (performed on more than 140 subjects who were not eligible for anticlotting drugs like TPA, which must be used within three hours of suffering a stroke), the Merci Retriever system restored blood flow in 54% of patients as long as eight hours after initial stroke symptoms appeared. In some of these cases, the corkscrew treatment resulted in an instant restoration of the ability to speak or move while the patient was still in the emergency room.

It may be some time, however, before this treatment is available at your local hospital. In the complex procedure, a catheter is inserted through the groin and snaked up into the brain, where a dye is released, outlining the obstruction and guiding doctors as they then insert the corkscrew. The operation requires extensive training and highly skilled specialists.

Prevention: Clearing Arteries

In August 2004 the FDA approved a new stent-and-filter system that is designed to prevent strokes before they occur by clearing blocked arteries leading to the brain. The stents open obstructed arteries in much the same way that similar devices clear blocked blood vessels close to the heart for cardiac patients. A mesh filter catches any debris as the obstructions in the artery break apart, preventing clot fragments from traveling to the brain and triggering a stroke. ■

Suicide

America's young people are taking their own lives far less frequently these days. The question is why

In Decline Between 1992 and 2001, the number of deaths from suicide in the U.S. among those aged 10 to 19 dropped, from 6.2 per 100,000 people to 4.6 per 100,000

If there's such a thing as good news about suicide, here it is: the CDC announced in April 2004 that the suicide rate among young Americans has dropped more than one-quarter since the early 1990s. Some of that reduction may be attributable to increased vigilance about risk factors, two of which made headlines in 2004: the popular class of antidepressants known as SSRIs, and the antimalaria drug Lariam, used by the U.S. military.

The FDA issued an advisory in 2004 cautioning that anyone taking SSRIs should be monitored for signs of emotional agitation, which can be a symptom of suicidal thoughts. Meanwhile, a string of suicides and murders among U.S. soldiers who had served in Iraq and had taken Lariam prompted the Federal Government to investigate a possible link to the medication.

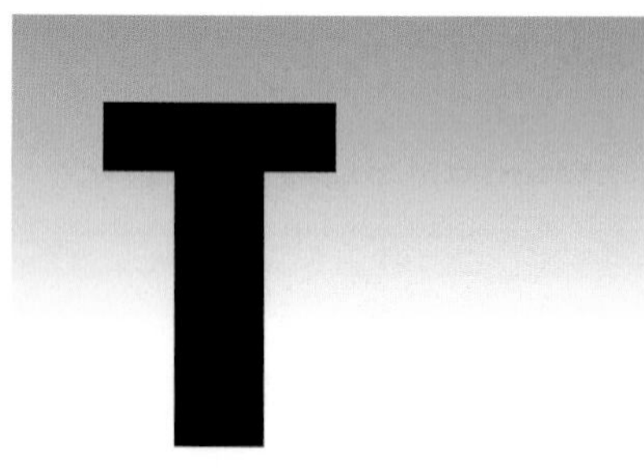

Testosterone

The male sex hormone has recently been described as a poison, a panacea and a potentially valuable therapeutic tool. Which is it?

Alzheimer's Link Men with low levels of testosterone appear to be at increased risk for Alzheimer's disease, a study found

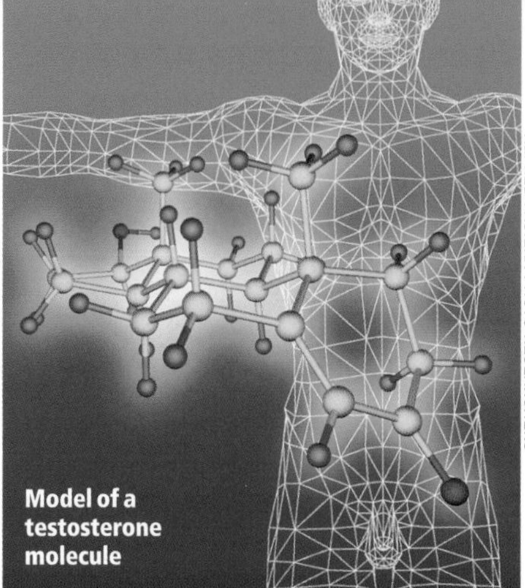
ALFRED PASIEKA–PHOTO RESEARCHERS

Model of a testosterone molecule

About the only point on which medical experts have reached a consensus concerning testosterone is that they don't know enough about it. In November 2003, a federal report warned that although dozens of studies have examined testosterone in recent years, most of them were small scale and short lived. In recent findings, one 2004 study reported that low levels of testosterone can put older men at greater risk of Alzheimer's, while another suggested that excessively high levels can increase the risk of prostate cancer. A third research team found that testosterone gel, applied to the skin in conjunction with Viagra, can help with erectile dysfunction in patients for whom Viagra alone is not effective.

■ Resources

NIH WEBSITE: *www.nih.gov/news/pr/jan2004/nia-26.htm*

Tonsillitis

Say ahhh ... Research shows that new, nonsurgical ways of treating tender tonsils are highly effective

Night Moves? If your child doesn't sleep well, it can lead to poor grades and other woes. The reason could be tonsil trouble

Tonsillectomies are not performed as often as they were decades ago, but some 400,000 of them take place every year. And they still hurt, even though the standard surgical technique, electrocautery, is a big improvement over the scalpel. A December 2003 study argued for an even kinder and gentler tool: the microdissection needle. Because it uses less energy and causes less pain, the needle moves kids swiftly to the ice-cream recovery stage.

Research published in July 2004 indicated that a newer surgical technique for tonsillectomies known as coblation (short for "controlled ablation," in which radiofrequency energy and a saline solution are used to dissolve tissue) may be just as effective as surgery while offering shorter recovery times and less postsurgical pain, as well as fewer side effects. Although approved by the FDA in 2001, coblation has been slow to catch on among physicians.

Research supplied further proof that sleep apnea, a childhood disorder characterized by troubled breathing during sleep, may be treated effectively by removal of the tonsils and adenoids. Sleep apnea has been linked to academic woes, short attention spans and impaired physical growth.

■ Resources

NIH WEBSITE: *www.nlm.nih.gov/medlineplus/tonsilstonsillectomy*

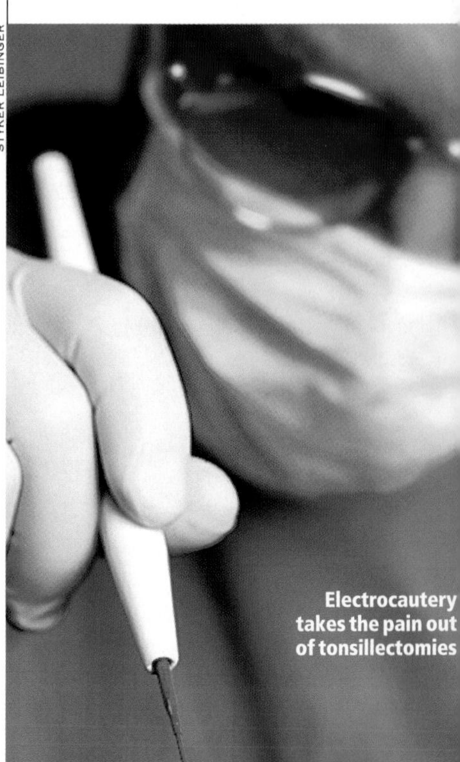
STYKER LEIBINGER

Electrocautery takes the pain out of tonsillectomies

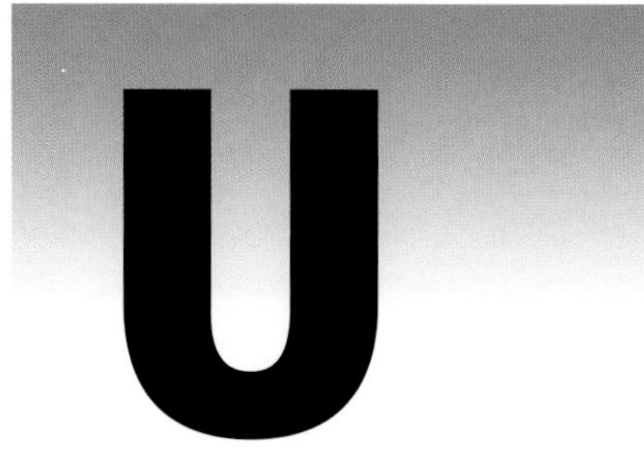

Ulcers

From orange juice to antibiotics, researchers are finding new ways to treat this irritating stomach ailment that's triggered by bacteria

Magic Wand In one new treatment, a wand inserted into the stomach sets off a reaction that kills the bug behind ulcers

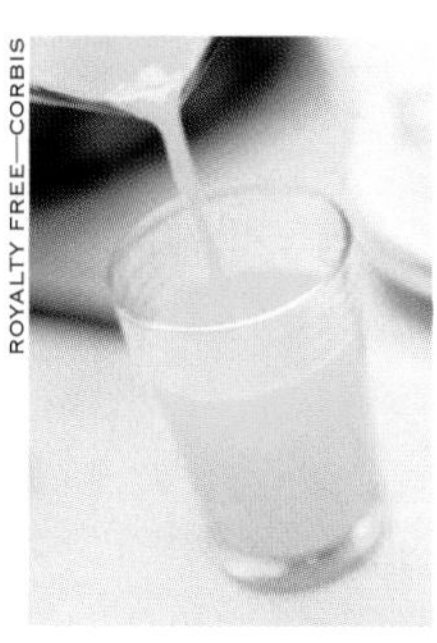

ROYALTY FREE—CORBIS

Can orange juice prevent ulcers? In a study of 7,000 Americans, researchers found that the lower the level of vitamin C in a person's blood, the more likely that he or she will be infected by the bacteria *Helicobacter pylori,* which is linked to ulcers and stomach cancer. Researchers do not yet know whether a low vitamin level is the cause or the effect of these infections. But even the latter is the case, the study's authors believe it prudent for people who test positive for the bug to increase their vitamin C intake.

Treating stomach ulcers caused by *H. pylori* with antibiotics may also help reduce the risk of stomach cancer, a new study determined. But the standard drug treatment for *H. pylori*—two different antibiotics, taken via as many as 20 pills each day, for weeks at a time—can be hard on patients. An experimental new procedure has raised hopes for a friendlier form of ulcer therapy. In this procedure, a light-emitting wand, inserted into the stomach by a flexible tube, emits pulses of blue light that trigger a chemical reaction that destroys *H. pylori.*

■ Resources

CDC WEBSITE: *www.cdc.gov/ulcer*

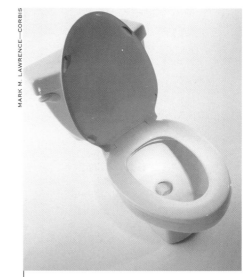

MARK M. LAWRENCE—CORBIS

Urinary Incontinence

Many women are troubled by this ailment, which can often be cured through simple lifestyle changes

Exercise Is Wise Simple precautions like doing Kegel exercises can help restore firmness to muscles key to bladder control

According to the American Urological Association, about 1 in 5 U.S. women over age 50 suffers from stress urinary incontinence (SUI), the tendency to leak urine when the bladder is stressed by running, jumping, sneezing, coughing or other activities. Whereas urge incontinence, the sudden unbearable need to urinate, is rare, SUI is remarkably common but also woefully underdiscussed.

Shame is a common side effect of SUI, and it often stops women from seeking treatment. This is especially unfortunate because 90% of women who seek help find relief, and new treatments are on the way. Although there is no drug available in the U.S. for SUI, duloxetine (which works by strengthening the urethral sphincter's contractions) has done well in trials, and the FDA is expected to approve it by 2006.

Currently, patients are often advised to make simple changes in behavior—losing weight, reducing intake of liquids or cutting back on irritants like caffeine, alcohol and cigarettes.

Women looking for a lasting remedy often choose surgery. Approximately 135,000 SUI operations are performed a year in the U.S., with a success rate of 75% to 95%. The two most common are the Burch procedure, which uses permanent stitches to support the bladder neck, and the sling procedure, which tightens the sphincter knot.

■ Resources

NIA WEBSITE: *www.niapublications.org/engagepages/urinary.asp*

A Firm Floor

Childbirth often damages the **pelvic muscles,** leading—sometimes years later—to stress incontinence. Kegel exercises can firm up these muscles and restore control

Side view of a woman's lower abdomen

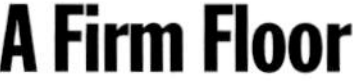

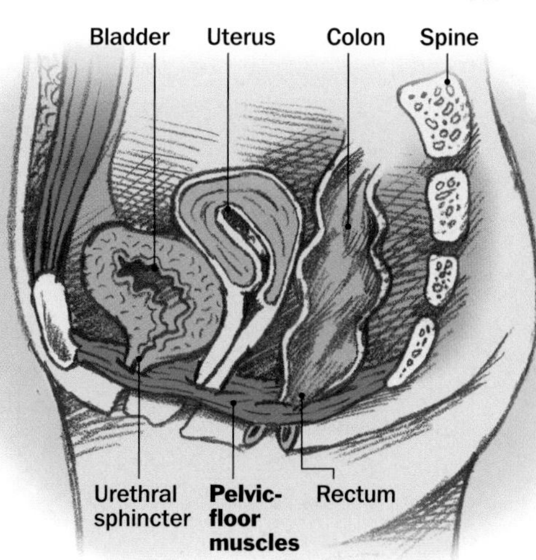

TIME Diagram Sources: *www.patient.co.uk; Atlas of Anatomy*

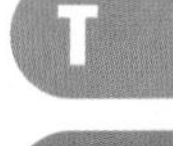

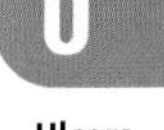

THE BATTLE WITHIN

A vaccine is nothing more than a cram course for the immune system, teaching it how to recognize and fight off potential invasions by hostile microbes. To create more effective vaccines, scientists have to understand the immune system's complex network of cellular sentries, which detect pathogens, and soldiers, which attack and destroy them

Pathogens

1 *B lymphocytes* seek specific pathogens

Pathogen is exposed

Identifie target pathoge

2 *Antigen presenting cell* uncovers pathogens

3 *Helper T cell* sounds alarm

SEARCHING FOR THE BAD BUGS . . .

1 Spotting the Enemy

Formed in bone marrow, **B lymphocytes** are the only immune cells that can make antibodies—the first line of immune defense. Antibodies are proteins that detect and bind themselves to invading pathogens in the blood. Once bound, the bugs can be neutralized

2 Exposing the Bad Guys

Often pathogens camouflage themselves against detection by antibodies with a cloak made of proteins called antigens. **Antigen presenting cells**—including macrophages and dendritic cells—strip away these cloaks by chopping up their proteins. Exposed, the pathogens become open to destruction

3 Sounding the Alarm

Helper T cells recognize and bind to bugs exposed by APCs. Once activated, helper T's secrete hormones called cytokines, which signal the immune systen to go into high gear and send more macrophages, B cells and T cells to destro the invaders, as well as more white blood cells containing enzymes that digest antigens

V

Vaccinations

Why vaccinate kids? Six Americans who had not been immunized in childhood came back from a trip abroad afflicted with measles, which can be deadly in adults

Say It Ain't So Two gigantic studies in Denmark refuted the widely suspected link between childhood vaccination and autism

The dangers of skipping childhood vaccinations were underlined in March 2004, when an Iowa college student whose family had chosen not to vaccinate him against measles as a child returned from a class trip to India infected with the disease. Although largely under control in the U.S., measles—which can cause high fevers, deafness, inflammation of the brain and even death—is endemic in India.

The young man wound up infecting at least one other person on the plane; a third person developed the disease on the ground. Altogether, six people in the student's group (which included several other people who had never been vaccinated) developed measles.

Thanks to an emergency program of vaccinations, examinations and quarantines mounted by Iowa health officials, the outbreak was contained. But it raised an important question: Why would anyone choose not to get vaccinated? For some it's a matter of religion. For others it's a concern about possible side effects. All vaccinations carry a small amount of risk. Some parents and even a few doctors suspect that recent increases in the rate of autism and earlier occurrences of Type 1 diabetes might have been caused by routine childhood vaccines.

The best and largest studies have proved that is not the case. In 2002, an enormous study of practically every child in Denmark found no causative link between autism and the so-called MMR shot—the triple vaccine against measles, mumps and rubella. Another large Danish study published in 2004 found no link between various childhood vaccines and Type 1 diabetes. As the Iowa incident demonstrated, when parents decide not to vaccinate their children, they are endangering not just their kids but everyone around them.

STATS NIX POX FIX

The protection offered by chickenpox vaccine weakens after a year and works poorly in tots under 15 months

TOM STEWART—CORBIS

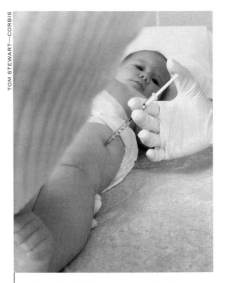

➤Better Than a Vaccine? As unpleasant as its itchy rash can be, enduring chickenpox may still be the best way to protect against catching it again, especially in the youngest tots. In a 2004 study, doctors from Yale and Columbia found that the chickenpox vaccine's ability to protect against the varicella virus weakens after the first year and that the vaccine is less effective in infants immunized before the age of 15 months.

■ Resources

NIH WEBSITE: *www.nlm.nih.gov/medlineplus/immunization.html*

Pathogen is exposed

4 B lymphocyte plasma cell releases ***antibody*** designed to kill specific pathogen

5 Killer T cell binds and destroys its target pathogen

6 Natural killer cell kills any invading bug in its path

... AND THEN DESTROYING THEM

4 Building the Bombs

After they encounter antigens in the blood, some B cells retreat to the lymph nodes, where they become **plasma cells** and churn out antibodies that can bind to these antigens

5 Going In for the Kill

Killer T cells must recognize antigens. Then they mature quickly to perform their second function—destroying pathogens. Killer T cells attach to a pathogen and douse it with a lethal toxin. Then they detach and go off to kill again, leaving the infected cell to die

6 Bringing In the Big Guns

Natural killer cells are the immune system's unspecialized fighters. They work like Killer T cells, flooding infected cells with toxins and destructive enzymes, but don't need to have the antigens presented by APCs first

Source: Dr. Gary Nabel, National Institutes of Health

TIME Graphic by Lon Tweeten, text by Michael D. Lemonick and Alice Park

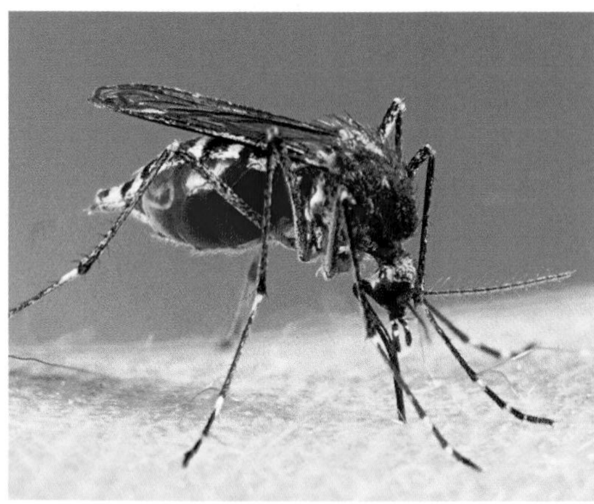

Viruses

An alarming uptick in the number of cases in which viruses native to animals are passed on to humans has virologists extremely concerned

Pet Peeve Scientists say one cause of the problem is the rising interest in keeping rare, undomesticated animals as pets

Virologists have been losing sleep over a number of emerging (or re-emerging) viruses—as well as new patterns in the way older viruses spread—that may soon pose serious hazards. One such threat is Eastern equine encephalitis (EEE), which usually strikes horses, rather than humans. When EEE does infect people, though, it is more than twice as deadly as West Nile virus (WNV). And EEE, which has been very rare for decades, may be on the rise. The number of cases in horses increased sevenfold in 2003, and the number of human cases was unusually high as well.

EEE is just one of a long list of diseases—including monkeypox, AIDS, SARS, West Nile virus and Lyme disease—that have lived in animal hosts for eons without affecting humans but that in the past 20 years have suddenly begun infecting people. Many experts say that animals are passing diseases to humans more rapidly, and in greater numbers, than ever before.

The change is probably driven in part by the conversion of former animal habitats, like rain forests and jungles, to human use. Human behavior is another engine of change: high-speed travel can spread a new virus around the world in 24 hours, while dietary choices like the civet cat, a delicacy in Asia, can carry infections and spread SARS. Human attempts to domesticate wild animals can also propagate disease: African prairie dogs imported as pets sparked the 2003 outbreak of monkeypox in the U.S. Midwest.

■ Resources

TULANE UNIVERSITY WEBSITE: *www.tulane.edu/~dmsander/garryfavweb.html*

Vitamins

We're still finding new ways these basic substances can help us stave off disease, including Alzheimer's

Miracle workers Both adult macular degeneration and depression may also be controlled with a regimen of vitamins

Health-care experts were stunned in January 2004 when research found that vitamins can play a role in preventing Alzheimer's disease. Some doctors had suspected that vitamins E and C (both antioxidants) can help stave off Alzheimer's disease. What they didn't know was how well. A recent study of 4,740 participants demonstrated that the two vitamins taken together in huge daily doses (at least 400 IU of E and more than 500 mg of C) could trim the risk of Alzheimer's by 78% in those who hadn't yet developed the disease.

➤Fighting Depression A 2003 Finnish study indicated that vitamin B_{12} might help clinically depressed patients beat their blues. Scientists monitored levels of the vitamin (found in meat, milk, eggs and fortified cereals) and determined that the patients who responded best to treatment were those who had high levels of B_{12} in their blood.

➤Saving Sight A November 2003 study confirmed earlier test results indicating that supplements of zinc combined with high doses of three antioxidants—vitamins C and E and beta-carotene—can help slow the progress of age-related macular degeneration (AMD), the leading cause of blindness in older adults. The new study also extrapolated these data to the general population and found that as many as 300,000 Americans at risk of losing their sight to AMD could improve their chances of keeping their sight with annual eye checkups and a diet rich in fruit and green vegetables, plus a daily multivitamin.

➤Preventing Birth Defects A May 2004 CDC report shows that the 1998 federally mandated program of adding folic acid to bread, pasta and other cereal grains has led to a 26% drop in two serious forms of birth defect: spina bifida (a crippling deformation of the spine) and anencephaly (a fatal disorder in which a child is born with much of the brain and spinal cord missing).

■ Resources

NIH SITE: *www.nlm.nih.gov/medlineplus/vitaminsandminerals.htm*

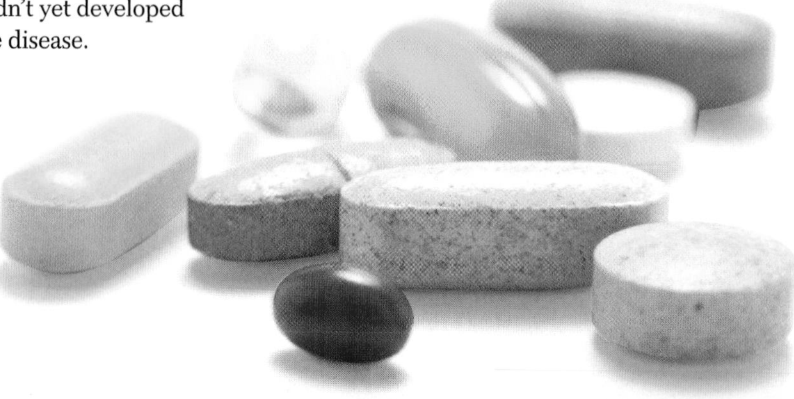

Update: The World of Vitamins

Vitamins are a group of chemical substances necessary for the body's normal metabolism, growth and development, as well as for the regulation of cell functions. Thirteen vitamins are essential for bodily functions, but we can only synthesize two of them, vitamins D and K. All vitamins can be obtained from food; an excessive amount of some of them can actually have toxic effects.

VITAMIN A
(retinol)

BENEFITS: Forms healthy teeth, skeletal and soft tissue, mucous membranes and skin. The name retinol comes from vitamin A's role in generating the pigments in the retina. It may also be required for reproduction and breastfeeding

SOURCES: Eggs, meat, milk, cheese, cream, liver, kidney, cod and halibut fish oils. Beta-carotene (a precursor) is found in plants like carrots, pumpkin, sweet potatoes, winter squashes, cantaloupes, pink grapefruit, apricots, broccoli, spinach and most dark-green leafy vegetables

THE LATEST: Beta-carotene may help slow the advance of macular degeneration in the eye

RDA: 3,000 mcg (women/men)

VITAMIN B_1
(thiamin)

BENEFITS: Helps cells convert carbohydrates into energy. Essential for the heart, muscles and nervous system

SOURCES: Fortified breads, cereals, pasta, whole grains (especially wheat germ), lean meats (especially pork), fish, peas and soybeans

RDA:
1.1 mg (women)
1.2 mg (men)

VITAMIN B_2
(riboflavin)

BENEFITS: Aids body growth and red blood cell production and helps in releasing energy from carbohydrates

SOURCES: Lean meats, eggs, legumes, nuts, green leafy vegetables, dairy products, milk. Breads and cereals are often fortified with riboflavin

RDA:
1.1 mg (women)
1.3 mg (men)

VITAMIN B_3
(niacin, nicotinic acid)

BENEFITS: Aids general health, growth and reproduction. Supports digestive system, skin and nerves. Helps convert food to energy

SOURCES: Dairy products, poultry, fish, lean meats, nuts and eggs

RDA:
14 mg (women)
16 mg (men)

VITAMIN B_6
(pyridoxine)

BENEFITS: Supports synthesis of antibodies by the immune system. Helps maintain normal nerve function and assists in the formation of red blood cells and in digestion of proteins

SOURCES: Vitamin B_6 is found in beans, nuts, legumes, eggs, meats, fish, whole grains and fortified breads and cereals

RDA:
1.5 mg (women)
1.6 mg (men)

VITAMIN B_9
(folate, folic acid, pteroylglutamic acid)

BENEFITS: Helps the body digest and utilize proteins and synthesize new proteins. Helps produce red blood cells and synthesize DNA. Assists tissue growth and cell function. Helps increase appetite and stimulates the formation of digestive acids

SOURCES: Beans and legumes, citrus fruits and juices, wheat bran and other whole grains, dark green leafy vegetables, poultry, pork, shellfish and liver

THE LATEST: Prevents neural tube defects. May decrease the reblockage of coronary arteries after angioplasty; may prevent spina bifida and other birth defects. Linked to lower risk of Alzheimer's disease

RDA: 400 mcg (women/men)

VITAMIN B_{12}

BENEFITS: Helps regulate metabolism and form red blood cells. Supports the central nervous system. Helps in synthesis of DNA. While most vitamins are not stored in the body, substantial amounts of this vitamin are maintained in the liver

SOURCES: Eggs, meat, poultry, shellfish, milk and milk products

RDA: 2.4 mcg (women/men)

VITAMIN B
(pantothenic acid)

BENEFITS: Supports metabolism of proteins and carbohydrates. Aids in the synthesis of hormones and cholesterol

SOURCES: Eggs, fish, milk and other dairy products, whole-grain cereals, legumes, yeast, broccoli (and other cabbages), white and sweet potatoes, lean beef

RDA: 5 mg (women/men), an estimate: no RDA established

VITAMIN B
(biotin)

BENEFITS: Helps us break down and utilize food. Supports metabolism of proteins and carbohydrates and synthesis of hormones and cholesterol

SOURCES: Eggs, fish, milk and dairy products, whole-grain cereals, legumes, yeast, broccoli (and other cabbages), white and sweet potatoes, lean beef

RDA: 30 mcg (women/men), an estimate: no RDA established

VITAMIN C
(ascorbic acid)

BENEFITS: Promotes healthy teeth and gums, helps absorb iron, helps maintain connective tissue, promotes wound healing, assists the body's immune system

SOURCES: Citrus fruits and juices, green peppers, strawberries, tomatoes, broccoli, turnip greens and other greens, sweet and white potatoes and cantaloupe

THE LATEST: May help slow the advance of adult macular degeneration. Some researchers claim a beneficial role for vitamin C in the prevention of heart disease, some kinds of cancer and the common cold. None of these claims have yet been verified

RDA:
75 mg (women)
90 mg (men)
+35 mg for smokers

VITAMIN D
(the "sunshine" vitamin)

BENEFITS: Promotes absorption of calcium (essential for healthy teeth and bones). Helps maintain adequate blood levels of calcium and phosphorus, essential minerals

SOURCES: Dairy products (especially cheese, butter, cream and fortified milk), fish, oysters and fortified cereals—and sunshine

RDA:
200 IU (under 50)
440 IU (51 to 70)
600 IU (over 70)

VITAMIN E
(tocopherol)

BENEFITS: This antioxidant protects body tissue from damage caused by unstable substances called free radicals. Helps form red blood cells and assists in metabolism of vitamin K

SOURCES: Wheat germ, corn, nuts, seeds, olives, spinach (and other green leafy vegetables), asparagus and vegetable oils (corn oil, sunflower oil, soybean oil, and cottonseed oil)

THE LATEST: May help slow the advance of macular degeneration in the eye, may reduce the risk of Alzheimer's disease and may prevent coronary heart disease

RDA: 15 mg (women/men)

VITAMIN K

BENEFITS: Essential to clotting of the blood. May help maintain strong bones in elderly

SOURCES: Cabbage, cauliflower, spinach (and other green leafy vegetables), cereals, soybeans. Vitamin K is also made by the bacteria that line the gastrointestinal tract

RDA:
65 mcg (women)
80 mcg (men)

KEY

RDA: recommended dietary allowance for adults, per day

mg = milligram

mcg = microgram

IU = international unit

Sources: The National Medical Library, National Institutes of Health; *Merck Manual of Medical Information*

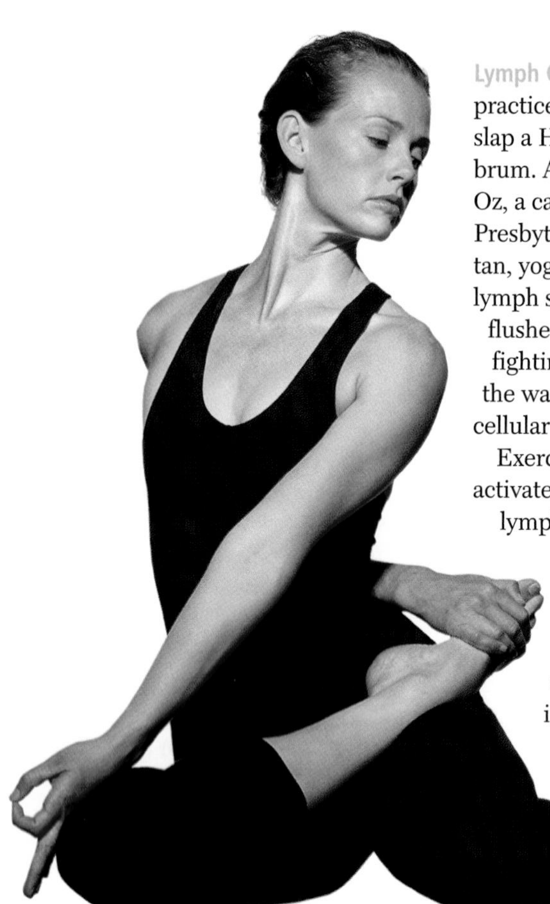

by adhering to a series of lifestyle changes, including yoga. In 2003 Ornish announced that he had achieved similar positive results in treating men with prostate cancer on a regimen consisting of diet, yoga and meditation.

Lymph Cleanser The sensible practice of yoga does more than slap a Happy Face on your cerebrum. According to Dr. Mehmet Oz, a cardiac surgeon at New York Presbyterian Hospital in Manhattan, yoga can also massage the lymph system—the network that flushes our body of infection-fighting white blood cells and the waste products of cellular activity.

Exercise in general activates the flow of lymph, but yoga in particular promotes the speed of the lymphatic system's draining process. Certain yoga poses stretch muscles that are known from animal studies to stimulate the lymph system. Researchers have documented the increased lymph flow that results when dogs' paws are stretched in a position similar to the yoga position called "downward-facing-dog."

➤Stress Fighter Yoga relaxesyou and, by relaxing, heals. At least that's the theory. "The autonomic nervous system," explains Richard Faulds, president of the Kripalu Center for Yoga and Health in Lenox, Mass., "is divided into the sympathetic system, which is often identified with the fight-or-flight response, and the parasympathetic, which is identified with what's been called the Relaxation Response. When you do yoga—the deep breathing, the stretching, the movements that release muscle tension, the relaxed focus on being present in your body—you initiate a process that turns the fight-or-flight system off and the Relaxation Response on. That has a dramatic effect on the body. The heartbeat slows, respiration decreases, blood pressure decreases."

Says Dr. Timothy McCall, an internist and yoga teacher: "We know that a high percentage of the maladies that people suffer from have at least some component of stress in them, if they're not overtly caused by stress. Stress causes a rise of blood pressure, the release of catecholamines [neurotransmitters and hormones that regulate

LAND OF LIMBER-TY

Today some 15 million Americans include some form of yoga in their fitness regimen; 75% of all U.S. health clubs offer yoga class. Seniors say it provides a low-impact workout

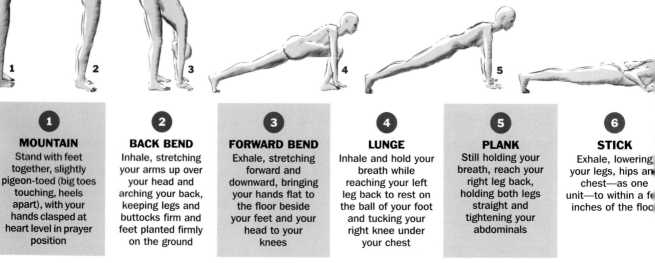

THE SUN SALUTATION

Often used as a warm-up, this series of poses-

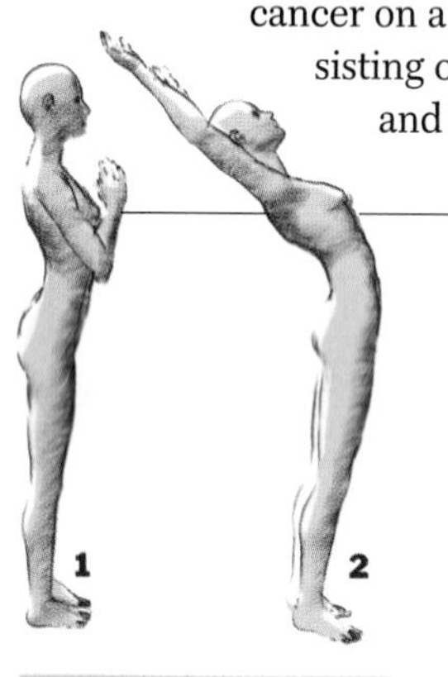

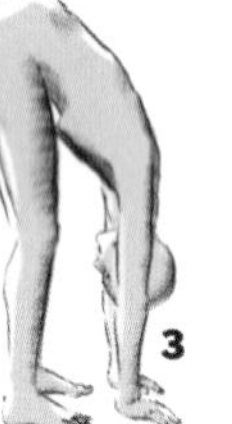

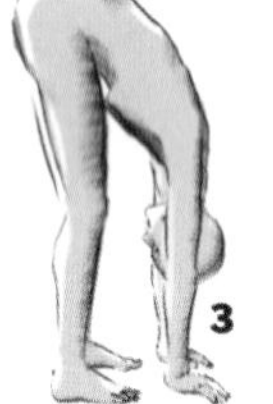

1 MOUNTAIN Stand with feet together, slightly pigeon-toed (big toes touching, heels apart), with your hands clasped at heart level in prayer position

2 BACK BEND Inhale, stretching your arms up over your head and arching your back, keeping legs and buttocks firm and feet planted firmly on the ground

3 FORWARD BEND Exhale, stretching forward and downward, bringing your hands flat to the floor beside your feet and your head to your knees

4 LUNGE Inhale and hold your breath while reaching your left leg back to rest on the ball of your foot and tucking your right knee under your chest

5 PLANK Still holding your breath, reach your right leg back, holding both legs straight and tightening your abdominals

6 STICK Exhale, lowering your legs, hips an chest—as one unit—to within a f inches of the floo

ILLUSTRATIONS BY LON TWEETEN

many of the body's metabolic processes]. We know when catecholamine levels are high, there tends to be more platelet aggregation, which makes a heart attack more likely."

So instead of a drug, say devotees, prescribe yoga. "All the drugs we give people have side effects," McCall says. "Well, yoga has side effects too: better strength, better balance, peace of mind, stronger bones, cardiovascular conditioning, lots of stuff."

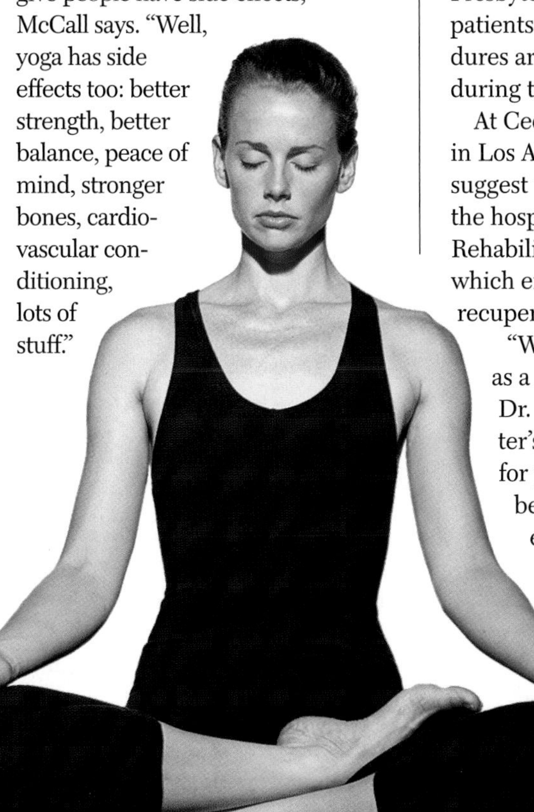

McCall, it should be said, is a true believer who teaches at the B.K.S. Iyengar Yoga Center in Boston. But more mainstream physicians seem ready to agree. At New York Presbyterian, all heart patients undergoing cardiac procedures are offered massage and yoga during the recovery period.

GETTING STARTED

You don't need special gear to take up yoga: just bring loose-fitting clothes. Since you work barefoot, no $125 sneakers are required

At Cedars-Sinai Medical Center in Los Angeles, cardiac doctors suggest that their patients enroll in the hospital's Preventive and Rehabilitative Cardiac Center, which employs yoga, among other recuperative therapies.

"While we haven't tested yoga as a stand-alone therapy," says Dr. Noel Bairey Merz, the center's director, patients opting for yoga do show "tremendous benefits." These include lower cholesterol levels and blood pressure, better cardiovascular circulation and, as the Ornish study showed, reversal of arterial blockage in some cases.

Yoga may also help women past menopause. Practitioners at Boston's Mind-Body Institute have incorporated forward-bending poses that massage the organs in the neuroendocrine axis (the line of glands that include the pituitary, hypothalamus, thyroid and adrenals) to bring into balance whatever hormones are askew, thus alleviating the insomnia and mood swings that often accompany menopause.

In our media-blitzed modern maelstrom, yoga's tendency to stasis and silence—to freeze-frame the frenzy—seems at first insane, then inspired. Modern science is only now catching up to what Eastern yoga practitioners seem to have known all along—that the notion of bodies at rest becoming souls at peace is reactionary, radical and liberating. Or, as Buddha is reputed to have said: "Don't just *do something*—stand there!"

■ Resources

THE YOGA JOURNAL
www.yogajournal.com

erformed in one flowing movement—is an easy way to build strength and flexibility

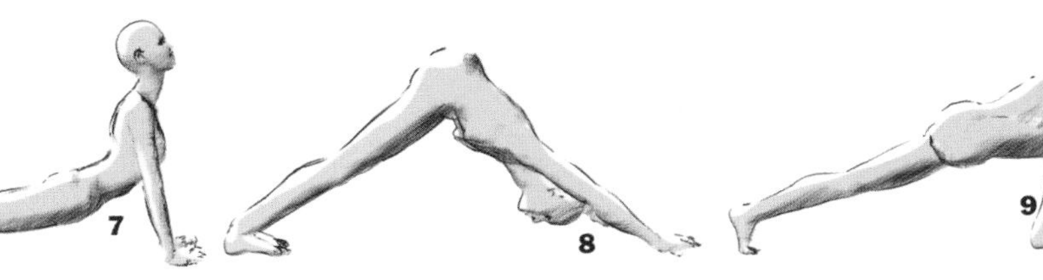

COBRA
Lower your hips, oint your feet and nhale, lifting your chest toward the sky, with elbows slightly bent and ressed into your ribs

DOWNWARD DOG
Tuck toes under and exhale, lifting buttocks and bringing your body into an inverted V. Press your heels down

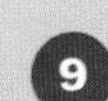

LUNGE
Lift your head and inhale, bringing your right foot forward between your hands

FORWARD BEND
Exhale and bend forward, bringing your left leg up to meet the right, and dropping your head to your knees

ARCHING BACK
Inhale and straighten your back, bringing your arms above your head. Look up and arch your back while remaining rooted to the ground

MOUNTAIN
Exhale, returning your hands to the prayer pose. Repeat the entire sequence, this time stepping back with the opposite leg

Index

Index